MOSBY'S
STERILE COMPOUNDING
for Pharmacy Technicians

MOSBY'S
STERILE COMPOUNDING
for Pharmacy Technicians

PRINCIPLES AND PRACTICE

Edition
2

Karen Davis, AAHCA, BHS, CPhT

Pharmacy Technician Program Director

Penn Foster Career School

Scranton, Pennsylvania;

Consultant and Trainer

Accreditation Alliance Consulting Services

Owner and Author

Society for the Education of Pharmacy Technicians (SEPhT)

Lyons, Georgia

ELSEVIER

Elsevier
3251 Riverport Lane
St. Louis, Missouri 63043

Notices

Knowledge and best practice in this field are constantly changing. As new research and experience broaden our understanding, changes in research methods, professional practices, or medical treatment may become necessary.

Practitioners and researchers must always rely on their own experience and knowledge in evaluating and using any information, methods, compounds, or experiments described herein. In using such information or methods they should be mindful of their own safety and the safety of others, including parties for whom they have a professional responsibility.

With respect to any drug or pharmaceutical products identified, readers are advised to check the most current information provided (i) on procedures featured or (ii) by the manufacturer of each product to be administered, to verify the recommended dose or formula, the method and duration of administration, and contraindications. It is the responsibility of practitioners, relying on their own experience and knowledge of their patients, to make diagnoses, to determine dosages and the best treatment for each individual patient, and to take all appropriate safety precautions.

To the fullest extent of the law, neither the Publisher nor the authors, contributors, or editors, assume any liability for any injury and/or damage to persons or property as a matter of products liability, negligence or otherwise, or from any use or operation of any methods, products, instructions, or ideas contained in the material herein.

Publishing Director: Kristin Wilhelm
Senior Content Development Manager: Luke Held
Senior Content Development Specialist: Kelly Skelton
Publishing Services Manager: Deepthi Unni
Project Manager: Radjan Lourde Selvanadin
Design Direction: Amy Buxton

Printed in India

Last digit is the print number: 9 8 7 6 5 4 3 2

Working together
to grow libraries in
developing countries

www.elsevier.com • www.bookaid.org

Reviewers

Sara Byars, BS, CPhT, PhTR
Clinical Liaison & Lead Faculty—Pharmacy Tech
  Program
San Jacinto College
Houston, Texas

Amanda Daniels, CPhT, BS
Clinical Coordinator/Instructor
Atlanta Technical College
Atlanta, Georgia

Lorraine Gaston, BS, CPhT
Adjunct Faculty and Laboratory Technician
Cuyahoga Community College
Highland Hills, Ohio

Carol Hasegawa, MEd
Corporate Director of Accreditation and Curricula
Delta College of Arts and Technology
Baton Rouge, Louisiana

Elena Bablenis Haveles, BS Pharmacy, PharmD, RPh
Adjunct Associate Professor of Pharmacology
Old Dominion University
Norfolk, Virginia

Marcia Janos, BS, CPhT
Faculty, Pharmacy Technician Program
Pikes Peak Community College
Colorado Springs, Colorado

Lorrenda Merritt, BA, CPhT, CSPT
Pharmacy Technology Program Coordinator
Somerset Community College
Somerset, Kentucky

Lourdes M. Rivera Alvarez, MS, BS
Pharmacy Technician Coordinator
Columbia Central University
Caguas, Puerto Rico

Preface

As health care continues to evolve and practices align more closely with patient safety and a demand for more patient-centered care, the importance of education and training for pharmacy technicians is even more important for practice. Recently, the standards for preparation of sterile products have been updated and more, with increased public awareness because of serious medication errors that have been publicized and arose from the inadequate training and environment for this area of practice. As an instructor and current manager of educators, I know how critical it is that compounding personnel and those instructing them understand the importance of their role and feel confident in practice. This book is dedicated to concepts and specifics of aseptic preparation with step-by-step instructions for a basic understanding of intravenous preparations.

Preparers will use this book to learn the history and principles of aseptic technique, as well as to learn the basic steps of sterile preparation. They will have guides for laboratory competencies and self-assessments to ensure a basic understanding before entering the field.

The more depth of understanding that pharmacy technicians have of aseptic practice, the safer all patients will be. It is imperative to maintain a sterile environment and provide a quality intravenous product. Technicians who go through this advanced practice will be validated and enter the pharmacy profession a step above their peers trained on these concepts through lecture and demonstrations. The students will perform each major step in aseptic technique and will be able to perform at externship with minimal supervision. The content is sufficient to prepare a certified pharmacy technician (CPhT) for the CSPT, the specialized certification in sterile preparation from PTCB, which will help advance their career.

ORGANIZATION

The book starts with the history of aseptic technique, details new USP standards, and then discusses the equipment, environment, training, documentation, quality control, and basic skills and techniques used. The progression allows students to understand how and when they will use these skills, and then allows them to perform each step through a series of hands-on laboratory exercises, self-assessments, and critical thinking activities.

DISTINCTIVE FEATURES

The book is aligned to the CSPT test domains, the advanced-level ASHP goals and objectives, and follows the most current version of the USP chapters <797>, <800>, and <825> guidelines. The students have detailed self-assessments, as well as critical thinking and real-world examples to ensure their understanding and performance of hands-on skills. These detailed checklists can be provided as documentation for ASHP-accredited programs, as well as for prospective employers.

LEARNING AIDS

A variety of pedagogic features are included in the book to aid in learning:

- **Learning Objectives** listed at the beginning of each chapter clearly outline what students are expected to learn from the chapter materials.

> ### Learning Objectives
> 1. Explain why certain medications must be sterile.
> 2. Discuss common terms used in sterile compounding.
> 3. Differentiate between asepsis and sterile.

- A list of **Key Terms** follows the Learning Objectives and identifies new terminology, the understanding of which is vital to success on the job. Key Terms are also highlighted in text discussions and combined into a glossary for reference.

> ### Terms & Definitions
> **Asepsis** Condition free from germs, infection, or any form of life
> **Centers for Disease Control and Prevention (CDC)** United States Federal Agency under the Department of Health and Human Services concerned with control and prevention of diseases

- **Tech Alerts** alert the student to drug look-alike and sound-alike issues.

> **Tech Alert!**
> According to the CDC website, in 1995 nosocomial infections caused one death every 6 minutes and cost an estimated $4.5 billion dollars.

- Helpful **Tech Notes** are dispersed throughout the chapters and provide critical, need-to-know information regarding dispensing concerns and interesting points about pharmacology.

 Tech Note!

Staphylococci is a naturally occurring bacteria or type of normal flora present on our hands all the time.

- **Lab Activities** allow students to perform basic aseptic manipulations in lab.

LAB ACTIVITY

For the following solutions or medications, use the resources provided to answer the questions:
1. What is the pH of premixed cimetidine HCL? How does it come (mg in solution)? If mixed with warfarin, describe what visual precipitate occurs.
2. Name two solutions that vancomycin can be mixed in. How long does the manufacturer state that it is good for when mixed with D5NS? If mixed with methotrexate, describe what precipitate occurs.
3. How is ceftriaxone (Rocephin) packaged? For IM injection, how much diluent would you use for a 500 mg vial? If using SWFI and the concentration is 250 mg/mL, how long is it stable at 4°C? How long is the frozen premixed solution stable?

- **Competency Checklists** provide measurable outcomes that reflect mastery of the task.

COMPETENCIES

EQUIPMENT AND FACILITIES (USP 797) GUIDELINES FOR ASEPTIC COMPOUNDING

Evaluation Key: S=Satisfactory   NI=Needs Improvement

Name: Quarter: Date:

COMPETENCIES	STUDENT			INSTRUCTOR		
Student will be able to:	S	NI	Comments	S	NI	Comments
Define *aseptic techniques*.						
Discuss USP 797 and its primary goal.						
Identify common equipment used in aseptic compounding.						
Discuss environment and quality control for the aseptic compounding area.						
Identify common personal protective equipment (PPE) and why USP 797 garbing procedures are used.						
Explain cleaning procedures for the laminar airflow workbench (LAFW).						
List the common duties that can be performed in the ante area.						
List common duties performed in the buffer area.						
List several USP 797 guidelines to follow when working in the buffer area.						
Discuss the daily and monthly cleaning procedures for the aseptic compounding area.						
Discuss garbing procedures according to the USP 797 guidelines.						

Review each concept to ensure that the learning objectives for the chapter have been met. Your instructor or supervisor will evaluate this as well.

- **Quiz and Critical Thinking Questions** further enhance student review and retention of chapter content by testing them on the key content within the chapter and helping them prepare for classroom and board exams.

REVIEW QUESTIONS

1. The first line of defense against the spread of microorganisms is:
   A. sterile environment
   B. good handwashing
   C. wearing gloves
   D. PPE
2. Personnel protective equipment include the following except:
   A. non-sterile gloves
   B. gown
   C. gloves
   D. mask

CRITICAL THINKING

1. You are a technician supervisor at a large hospital and recently have hired two new technicians for the intravenous room. How would you explain why using aseptic technique is imperative to the hospital patient's health?
2. You are a technician supervisor for the local hospital. Recently, a technician student asks you, "Why are most of the supplies used when preparing intravenous drugs disposable? Doesn't that cost a lot of money?" How would you explain the cost effectiveness of disposable supplies over reusable supplies like syringes and needles?

- The **Bibliography** provides a list of sources that students and instructors can use for additional information on the chapter's topic.

BIBLIOGRAPHY

1. General Chapter <797> Pharmaceutical Compounding-Sterile Preparations. Retrieved August 26, 2018. http://www.usp.org/compounding/general-chapter-797.
2. American Society of Health-System Pharmacists: ASHP Guidelines on Quality Assurance for Pharmacy-Prepared Sterile Products. Accessed August 26, 2018 at http://www.ashp.org/s_ashp/docs/files/BP07/Prep_Gdl_QualAssur Sterile.pdf.
3. Centers for Disease Control and Prevention: Guideline for hand hygiene in health-care settings: recommendations of the healthcare infection control practices advisory committee and the HICPAC/SHEA/APIC/IDSA hand hygiene task force, *MMWR* 51(RR-16:2, 29-33). October 2002: http://www.cdc.gov/mmwr/PDF/rr/rr5116.pdf. Accessed August 27, 2018.
4. *Dorland's illustrated medical dictionary*, ed 31, Philadelphia, 2007, Saunders.

EVOLVE RESOURCES

FOR THE INSTRUCTOR

We offer several assets on the Evolve Resources site to aid instructors:
- **Test Bank:** An ExamView test bank of 500 multiple-choice questions that feature rationales, cognitive

levels, mapping to learning objectives, mapping to CSPT examination blueprint, and page number references to the text. This can be used as review in class or for test development.

- **Image Collection**: The images from the book are available as JPGs and can be downloaded into PowerPoint presentations. These can be used during lectures to illustrate important concepts.
- **Correlation Guides**: The book content is mapped to the ASHP and ABHES accreditation standards and to the CSPT blueprint.
- **Short Answer Review Questions**: Critical thinking questions for each chapter will give students extra practice.
- **TEACH**: This includes lesson plans, answer keys, student handouts, and PowerPoint slides, all available via Evolve. TEACH provides instructors with customizable lesson plans and PowerPoints based on learning objectives. With these valuable resources, instructors will save valuable preparation time and create a learning environment that fully engages students in classroom preparation. The lesson plans are keyed chapter-by-chapter and are divided into logical lessons to aid in classroom planning. In addition to the lesson plans, instructors will have unique lecture outlines in PowerPoint with talking points, thought-provoking questions, and unique ideas for lectures. Student handouts provide a summary of the PowerPoint slides with room for note-taking, and answer keys address text Quiz and Critical Thinking questions as well as practice exercises.

FOR THE STUDENTS

Student assets on the Evolve Resources site will provide students extra practice and examination preparation:

- **Chapter Quizzes:** Approximately 300 multiple choice questions will help students master the book content.
- **Sample CSPT Exam:** A 75-question practice exam will give students extra preparation for the Certified Compounded Sterile Preparation Technician Exam.

NOTE TO STUDENTS

The pharmacy technician is such an incredible and important part of health care and the pharmacy industry. Never stop learning and progressing in your career. This book will allow you to complete a program with an advanced understanding of intravenous preparation, and employers will seek that out. The sky is the limit and I am living proof. You may want to write and teach one day, and there is no reason you can't. I encourage you to gain as much knowledge as you can, and institutional practice is a great field to work towards.

Karen Davis, AAHCA, BS, CPhT

Acknowledgment and Dedications

I would like to dedicate this book to the first pharmacist, Billy Kittrell, who taught me intravenous preparation over 30 years ago. I have had many great mentors along the way in my career, and to each of them I would like to say "Thank you." I would also like to say thank you to the Elsevier team which has been more supportive than I could ever imagine. Also, a special thank you to my family, especially my husband, who has always encouraged me and tells me every day that he is proud of me. I couldn't have done this without each of you.

Contents

Introduction to Sterile Compounding

Learning Objectives

1. Explain why certain medications must be sterile.
2. Discuss the history of aseptic preparations and the organizations that provide guidelines.
3. Describe aseptic technique, including handwashing, standard precautions, and personal protective equipment (PPE).
4. Discuss the training and responsibility of personnel when performing aseptic technique.
5. Identify common settings where aseptic technique is performed.

Terms & Definitions

Asepsis Condition free from germs, infection, or any form of life

Centers for Disease Control and Prevention (CDC) United States Federal Agency under the Department of Health and Human Services concerned with the control and prevention of diseases

Compounded sterile preparations (CSP) Medications prepared using sterile technique

Infection control Policies and procedures organizations put in place to prevent the spread of infection

The Joint Commission The shortened term for the Joint Commission on Accreditation of Healthcare Organizations; a nonprofit, private organization that evaluates medical facilities to ensure good patient care

Microorganism An organism (such as a bacterium, virus, or protozoan) of microscopic size

Normal flora Bacteria that resides on the skin's outer surface but does not cause disease

Parenteral Any medication route other than the alimentary canal (digestion system)

Pyrogen Fever producing substance

Standard precautions CDC guidelines that promote hand hygiene and the use of personal protective equipment (PPE)

Sterile Free of living organisms, especially microorganisms

United States Pharmacopoeia (USP) Nongovernmental, nonprofit public health organization that set standards for over-the-counter (OTC) and prescription medicines and other healthcare products in the United States; its main goal is to ensure public health

USP<797> Chapter in the USP concerning parenteral medications compounding and equipment endorsed by The Joint Commission and American Society of Health-System Pharmacists (ASHP)

INTRODUCTION

Preparing sterile medications is one of the most complicated tasks a pharmacy technician can perform in a pharmacy setting. It requires additional training and following strict guidelines with attention to detail. In this chapter, we will discuss the history and concept of asepsis, along with the terminology and responsibilities of personnel who prepare intravenous admixtures. Medication errors are now the third leading cause of death in the US, and contamination of sterile products is significant. As recent as 2012, more than 200 patients contracted fungal meningitis from a sterile preparation of methyl prednisolone prepared in a compounding pharmacy (ISMP, 2018).

Pharmacy technicians must have a good understanding of aseptic technique and the practices surrounding the preparation of sterile products to ensure safety, accuracy, and correctness of the medication. Following required proper procedures is the only way to ensure that contamination does not occur when performing aseptic technique.

The art of compounding aseptic or sterile preparations has been performed since the beginning of pharmacy. Pharmacy personnel must prepare intravenous medications when other routes, such as oral tablets or liquids, may not be appropriate because the patient cannot take them by mouth, or in emergency situations where rapid absorption is required. This route is known as parenteral, which is derived from two Greek words: *para*, meaning around, and *enteron*, meaning the intestines. These medications must be free from pyrogens or microbes that cause infection, since they are administered directly into the body via the bloodstream and bypass many of the body's natural defenses.

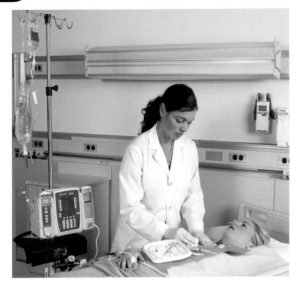

Fig. 1.1 A patient receiving intravenous therapy in a hospital. (Courtesy CareFusion, San Diego, CA.)

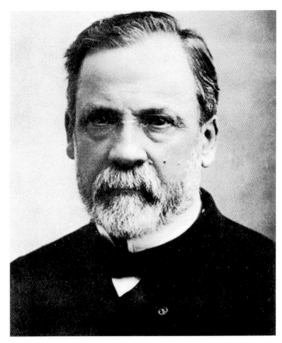

Fig. 1.2 Louis Pasteur, 1822–1895. (From US National Library of Medicine, Bethesda, MD.)

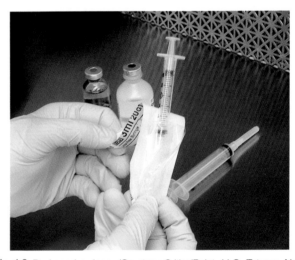

Fig. 1.3 Packaged syringe. (Courtesy CriticalPoint, LLC, Totowa, New Jersey.)

Patients receiving intravenous medications are often hospitalized and immune compromised, and they are more susceptible to infection (Fig. 1.1). Since sterile intravenous products can be prepared in many settings, such as hospitals, outpatient pharmacies and clinics, doctor's offices, and in a patient's home, the need for extremely clean or sterile preparation is imperative to ensure the wellbeing of these patients. Typically, the normal bacteria that we all have on the surfaces of our body do not affect us because we are healthy, but to a sick person, these can cause significant harm, and since patients receiving intravenous therapy are usually the most critical, every precaution must be taken to avoid contamination. The personnel responsible for their preparation must follow certain rules and guidelines, as well as use specialized equipment. Technicians perform most of the preparation duties today, under the direct supervision of a pharmacist.

HISTORY OF ASEPTIC PREPARATIONS

The practices of medicine advanced very quickly during the early 19th century and researchers discovered that germs and unknown organisms caused certain diseases. In the 1600s people believed that microorganisms spontaneously came from decaying nonliving matter.

Louis Pasteur's germ theory in the early 1800s specified that bacteria caused diseases (Fig. 1.2). Practices that are common today, such as handwashing, were not practiced routinely. As a result, many deaths were attributed to the unclean conditions of operating rooms and personnel practices. A person was more likely to die of postoperative gangrene than the surgery itself. In addition, transference of the germs went from patient to patient because of the improper sterilization of items or the person not performing proper hygiene precautions. As a result, many changes in the

practices were established. In 1865, Sir Joseph Lister, a well-known surgeon, read a paper by Louis Pasteur and learned about the germ theory of disease. He stated that if infections were caused by microbes, the best way to prevent infections would be to kill the microbes before they reached the open wound. Lister used carbolic acid to kill germs. He wrote about the use of this acid in his work, *Antiseptic Principle of the Surgery Practice* (essortment.com).

The use of sanitary dressings and instruments led to the development and use of disposable supplies, such as syringes, needles, and other intravenous supplies in the 1920s (Fig. 1.3). This allows the supplies sealed in packaging from the manufacturer to be opened in a controlled environment, used once, and discarded. Even though this may be most costly, the decrease of medication errors and better patient safety far outweighs the cost. Sterile solutions and equipment became accepted in health care in the 1930s. In the 1960s following a host of serious patient complications, the National Coordinating Committee on Large Volume Parenterals (NCCLVP) published the first set of recommendations for pharmacy and other healthcare professionals. In 1972 the Baxter Corporation produced a training manual, which was later revised in 1990. Following these guidelines, American Society of Health-System Pharmacists (ASHP) and United States Pharmacopoeia (USP) published updated guidelines that are considered standard practices for pharmacy personnel, when preparing sterile preparations or **compounded sterile preparations (CSPs)**.

Aseptic technique is required when preparing any medication that enters the body through a parenteral or ophthalmic route. According to the USP<797>, these preparations may include compounded biologics, diagnostics, drugs, nutrients, radiopharmaceuticals, eye preparations, and tissue implants.

 Did You Know?

Diagnosing a bacteria type is done by Gram staining. This process was discovered by Hans Gram in 1883, and the procedure is still used today.

Bacteria are stained with a substance called *crystal violet*. Those that retain the color are gram positive, and those that lose the color are gram negative. Antibiotic drugs are grouped together or classified based on their activity against gram-positive organisms, such as *staphylococci* or against gram-negative organisms, such as aminoglycosides activity against diplococci (Fig. 1.4). Once the bacteria is determined to be gram positive or gram negative, a physician can prescribe the medication that works most effectively for either a gram-positive or a gram-negative bacteria.

Today, industry standards for the preparation of intravenous products include the use of proper practices or aseptic technique, specific procedures, equipment, training of personnel, and storage recommendations (Fig. 1.5).

These guidelines are provided by the USP, which is an official standards-setting organization made up of a volunteer body of experts in the medical field.

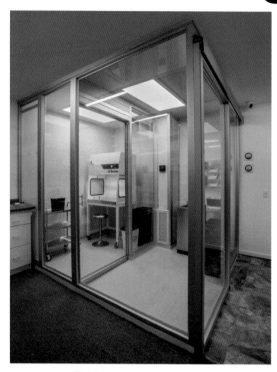

Fig. 1.5 Intravenous (IV) room.

Chapter 797, which was written in 2004, was the first enforceable document to outline the practices associated with sterile compounding. These guidelines were recently updated and continue to provide the best practices associated with sterile preparation of intravenous medications. In the 1980s a document known as *ASHP Guidelines on Quality Assurance for Pharmacy-Prepared Sterile Products by the American Society of Health-System Pharmacists* was published and supported the USP<797> guidelines for the pharmacy industry. Both of these organizations address quality assurance and medication error prevention activities for CSPs and are endorsed by The Joint Commission on Accreditation of Hospitals. The Joint Commission is a nonprofit organization that accredits more than 16,000 healthcare organizations and programs in the United States. Their main focus is on patient rights, treatment, and infection control, while using the standards of USP for compounding. The purpose of the USP<797> and ASHP guidelines is to describe practices and environmental conditions that prevent harm or even death to patients. To achieve these standards, facilities must provide minimum practices and quality standards that include:

- Establishment of Policy and procedures for compounding
- Staff training and evaluation of competencies requirements per USP<797>
- Environmental facilities and air quality controls to ensure that sterile conditions are available for aseptic compounding
- Establishment of storage and beyond use dates for sterile products
- Hygiene procedures to include garb and handwashing.

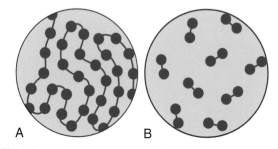

Fig. 1.4 (A) Gram-positive bacteria. (B) Gram-negative bacteria.

ASEPTIC TECHNIQUE

Aseptic technique refers to manipulation of medications or fluids from one container to another, and its primary goal is to maintain asepsis or keep all products free from contamination from microbes. This requires special training, special procedures, and special equipment. The personnel preparing aseptic products must always remember to keep any potential harm from befalling the patient.

According to the **Centers for Disease Control and Prevention (CDC)**, the first line of defense against the spread of microorganisms is good handwashing. There are always bacteria present on our bodies and hands known as normal flora. These bacteria are a basic defense mechanism for our bodies and are found on the skin, in the vagina, and intestines. Some, such as *Escherichia coli*, are necessary in the digestive process in the colon. However, to a patient who has an immune compromised system, they can cause harm, infection, and even death, because the person is susceptible to infection as a result of their alteration in normal immune function.

 Tech Note!

Staphylococci is a naturally occurring bacteria or type of normal flora present on our hands all the time.

HANDWASHING AND STANDARD PRECAUTIONS

One of the most important aspects of proper aseptic technique is proper handwashing. The most common type of contamination is touch, and since we have bacteria on our body surfaces at all times, it is important to avoid the transfer of these to any product going directly into a person's bloodstream. Organizations, such as the CDC, have standards known as standard precautions for the healthcare industry to prevent the transfer of microorganisms. This organization is a government agency that is part of the Department of Health and Human Services. Their main task is to formulate safety guidelines concerning the spread of infection, which is a significant part of aseptic technique guidelines.

 Tech Note!

The route of administration for parenteral medications is directly into the bloodstream; therefore injectable medications must be prepared aseptically, always remembering the increased risk of infection.

The observance of handwashing precautions and performing aseptic technique is imperative to ensure patient safety and the sterility of the intravenous admixture. The result of a compromised admixture can result in a nosocomial infection, which is an infection the patient receives during healthcare treatment. Patients receiving sterile compounds often have compromised immune systems, and even the slightest exposure to bacteria can cause extreme harm or even death. This can also eventually lead to significant costs to the healthcare system.

 Tech Alert!

According to the CDC website, in 1995 nosocomial infections caused one death every 6 minutes and cost an estimated $4.5 billion dollars.

PERSONAL PROTECTIVE EQUIPMENT

Along with proper handwashing and aseptic technique, wearing appropriate personal protective equipment (PPE) is also required. Personnel compounding or performing aseptic technique must wear sterile gloves, gown, protective eyewear, mask, beard covers, and shoe covers. We will discuss the procedures for their use in Chapter 4.

TRAINING AND RESPONSIBILITY OF PERSONNEL

When performing aseptic technique, there are basic duties for which intravenous or compounding technicians will be responsible. These are determined by the facility's policies and procedures, as well by as industry standards and USP<797> guidelines for personnel training. This will usually include periodic observation of technique, validation of completed products, and documentation of common tasks required, such as cleaning logs. In addition, technicians will perform calculations, data entry, labeling, and delivery. Even though the pharmacist must provide the end check, that does not mean that the technician is not responsible for being as accurate and correct in the procedure, as they can possibly be. This takes a conscientious and detailed approach to technique and proper preparation.

 Tech Alert!

If you know a preparation has been contaminated, consult the pharmacist, and it should be thrown away and redone immediately. Even though the pharmacist may not see this action, it is still an error.

It is extremely important that the finished product is free of contaminates and correctly prepared and labeled. As part of the USP<797> guidelines, there should be a quality control (QC) or quality assurance (QA) program in place to include validation of performance, preparations, and environmental controls. Each step of the process should be recorded and evaluated regularly for improvement. Once this is in place, it will provide a mechanism to monitor, evaluate, and improve the activities and processes used.

ENVIRONMENT

Another important aspect of aseptic manipulations is the environment in which it must be performed.

USP<797> designates the space or areas that compounding must take place, along with guidelines for temperature and air quality, cleaning, and proper equipment placement to prevent contamination of prepared sterile products. The designated area or room should be away from the flow of regular traffic and only authorized, trained personnel should be allowed. This space is separated into two areas, the ante room and the buffer room where the actual compounding takes place. These areas must be temperature and humidity controlled and only trained and properly garbed personnel are allowed. This will be discussed in detail in Chapter 9.

SETTINGS FOR INTRAVENOUS THERAPY ADMINISTRATION AND PREPARATION

The administration and preparation of sterile products most often occur in an institutional setting, such as the hospital, but can also take place in a long-term care facility, retail pharmacy, and even physicians' offices. Since the population of older people is increasing because of extended life expectancy, there is often a need for home health intravenous therapy, and these medications are prepared in a facility and delivered to the patient's home. It is imperative that the preparer have a good understanding of the medications, their storage, proper techniques when preparing, and delivery systems being used, such as pumps. Patient education should also be stressed, especially in a home healthcare setting.

REVIEW QUESTIONS

1. The first line of defense against the spread of microorganisms is:
   A. sterile environment
   B. good handwashing
   C. wearing gloves
   D. PPE
2. Personnel protective equipment include the following except:
   A. non-sterile gloves
   B. gown
   C. gloves
   D. mask
3. _____ is a naturally occurring bacteria or type of normal flora present on our hands all the time.
   A. Staphylococci
   B. E. coli
   C. Streptococcal
   D. Clostridium difficile
4. When bacteria are stained with crystal violet, those that retain the color are gram _____, and those that lose color are gram _____.
   A. positive, neutral
   B. neutral, positive
   C. negative, positive
   D. positive, negative

5. Which of the following is not one of the different settings where compounding sterile products takes place:
   A. long-term facilities
   B. nurses' residence
   C. physicians' offices
   D. retail pharmacy
6. Parental medications are given by which route?
   A. PO (by mouth)
   B. IM (intramuscular)
   C. IV (intravenous)
   D. PR (rectal)
7. Aseptic technique is required when preparing any medication that enters the body through a _____ or _____ route.
   A. parental, rectal
   B. parental, ophthalmic
   C. ophthalmic, intramuscular
   D. ophthalmic, rectal
8. The (high-efficiency particulate air [HEPA] filter can remove particles that are _____ microns or larger.
   A. 0.1 microns
   B. 0.5 microns
   C. 0.4 microns
   D. 0.2 microns
9. Biological safety cabinets (BSCs) are used when compounding _____ drugs.
   A. ophthalmic
   B. intramuscular
   C. hazardous
   D. parental
10. The minimum practices and quality standards of the USP<797> and ASHP guidelines include all of the following except:
    A. Staff training and evaluation of competencies requirement per USP<797>
    B. Establishment of storage and beyond use date for sterile products
    C. Establishment of policy and procedures for creating packages
    D. Hygiene procedures to include garb and handwashing

CRITICAL THINKING

1. You are a technician supervisor at a large hospital and have recently hired two new technicians for the intravenous room. How would you explain why using aseptic technique is imperative to the hospital patient's health?
2. You are a technician supervisor for the local hospital. Recently, a technician student asked you, "Why are most of the supplies used when preparing intravenous drugs disposable? Doesn't that cost a lot of money?" How would you explain the cost effectiveness of disposable supplies over reusable supplies like syringes and needles?

COMPETENCIES THE BASICS OF ASEPTIC PREPARATIONS

Evaluation Key: S = Satisfactory   NI = Needs Improvement

Name: _____   Quarter: _____   Date: _____

COMPETENCIES	STUDENT			INSTRUCTOR		
Student will be able to:	S	NI	Comments	S	NI	Comments
Define aseptic technique.						
Discuss USP<797> guidelines and the importance of these standards.						
List preparations included in USP<797> that are considered compounded sterile preparations (CSPs).						
Discuss the basis for using parenteral medications.						
Discuss the importance of normal bacteria and why it does not cause infection in healthy persons.						
Discuss the responsibilities of a compounding technician.						
Discuss settings where parenteral medications may be administered.						

Review each concept to ensure that the learning objectives for the chapter have been met. Your instructor or supervisor will evaluate this as well.

BIBLIOGRAPHY

1. General Chapter <797> Pharmaceutical Compounding-Sterile Preparations. Retrieved August 26, 2018. http://www.usp.org/compounding/general-chapter-797.
2. American Society of Health-System Pharmacists: ASHP Guidelines on Quality Assurance for Pharmacy-Prepared Sterile Products. http://www.ashp.org/s_ashp/docs/files/BP07/Prep_Gdl_QualAssurSterile.pdf. Accessed August 26, 2018.
3. Centers for Disease Control and Prevention: Guideline for hand hygiene in health-care settings: recommendations of the healthcare infection control practices advisory committee and the HICPAC/SHEA/APIC/IDSA hand hygiene task force, *MMWR* 51(RR-16:2, 29-33). October 2002: http://www.cdc.gov/mmwr/PDF/rr/rr5116.pdf. Accessed August 27, 2018.
4. *Dorland's illustrated medical dictionary*, ed 31, Philadelphia, 2007, Saunders.
5. ISMP: Sterile Compounding Tragedy is a Symptom of a Broken System on Many Levels. Retrieved September 28, 2018. https://www.ismp.org/resources/sterile-compounding-tragedy-symptom-broken-system-many-levels.
6. Sir Joseph Lister. Developer of Antiseptic Surgery. *essortment* (website): http://www.essortment.com/sir-joseph-lister-developer-antiseptic-surgery-37935.html. Accessed September 2, 2018.
7. MD. Medical Errors-Third Leading Cause of Death (website): https://www.mdmag.com/conference-coverage/aapa-2017/medical-errors-the-third-leading-cause-of-death-in-the-united-states. Accessed September 17, 2018.
8. Mitchell J, Haroun L: *Introduction to health care*, ed 2, Clifton Park, NY, 2007, Thomson Delmar Learning.
9. The Joint Commission: Medication—Sterile Compounding—Compounding Staff Competency Requirements: https://www.jointcommission.org/standards_information/jcfaqdetails.aspx?StandardsFaqId=1624&ProgramId=46. Accessed September 2, 2018.

Medications and Disease Management

Learning Objectives

1. Discuss the four steps of pharmacokinetics.
2. Discuss special dosing considerations to consider when determining the correct dosages for parenteral medications.
3. Name at least two references that can be used to find the storage requirements for a parenteral medication.
4. Discuss the characteristics of different solutions used in intravenous therapy.
5. List several factors that affect the compatibility of intravenous fluids.

Terms & Definitions

Absorption Movement of a drug into the circulatory system

Admixture The preparation of an intravenous (IV) medication that requires a mixture of medications

Adverse effects Drug effects that are unexpected and unwanted and are usually reported in only a few patients

Antagonistic effect The action of one drug preventing the action of another drug or preventing the action of a messenger on a receptor site in the body

Clarity Clear and free of visible particulate matter

Compatibility Ability to combine drugs or substances without interfering with their action

Coring Breaking off small pieces of the rubber stopper on vials and allowing them to enter the solution or IV fluid

Distribution Movement of a drug through the body into tissues, membranes, and then organs

Excretion Removal of a drug from the body

Hypertonic Any solution containing a higher concentration of dissolved substances than red blood cells

Hypotonic Any solution containing a concentration of dissolved substances less than red blood cells

Incompatibility Drugs, or drugs and fluids, that cannot be put together because of the incident of unwanted or unexpected effects

Isotonic Any solution containing a concentration of dissolved substances, such as salts, that are the same as the concentration found in human red blood cells

Metabolism Changing of the chemical structure of a drug by the body

Osmolarity Number of dissolved particles in a solution per liter of solution

Osmosis Movement of a solvent (water) across a cell membrane from a lower osmolality to a higher osmolality

pH Degree of alkalinity or acidity of a solution. Acidity is usually between 0 and 6, while alkalinity is between 8 and 14. Neutral pH is around 7.

Precipitation Solid material or deposits that are separated from a solution often caused by reactions between drugs or drugs and certain fluids

Reconstitution Process of adding a diluent to a powder form of a medication

Side effects Drug effects that are predictable, widely reported, and can be found in literature

Synergistic effect The action of two drugs working together to produce effects

Therapeutic effect The intended effect of a drug

Tonicity The osmolarity of a solution or the effect of the concentration of dissolved particles in the solution.

INTRODUCTION

Technicians are required to prepare intravenous (IV) admixtures using aseptic technique with the correct fluids and knowledge of what they are for and how they react in the body. Medications often have special considerations because of the processes they go through in the body. A technician must be aware of the medication's properties, its interactions and side effects, and any special considerations that need to be followed when preparing the drug to ensure patient safety and medication accuracy. In this chapter, we will discuss concepts of pharmacokinetics, dosing information, and the references that are available (Fig. 2.1).

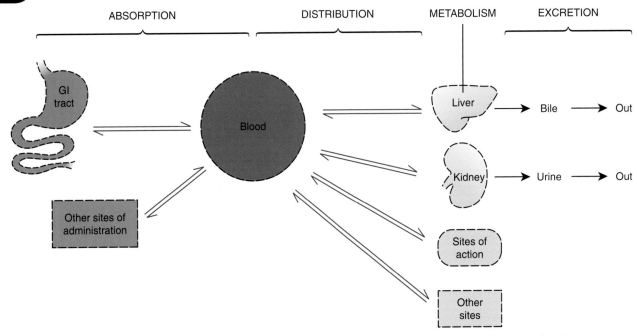

Fig. 2.1 The four basic pharmacokinetic processes. Dotted lines represent membranes that must be crossed as drugs move throughout the body. *GI,* Gastrointestinal. (From Burchum JR, Rosenthal LD: *Lehne's pharmacology for nursing care,* ed 10, St Louis, 2019, Elsevier.)

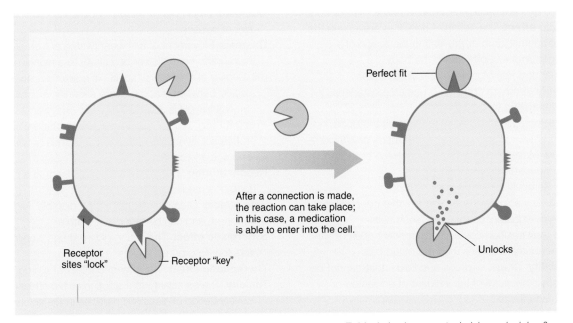

Fig. 2.2 The "lock and key" mechanism of receptor sites. (From Hopper T: *Mosby's pharmacy technician: principles & practice,* ed 3, St Louis, 2012, Elsevier Saunders.)

PHARMACOKINETICS FOR PARENTERAL MEDICATIONS

Manufacturers create medications with the ability to release and be distributed over a certain period of time. The process that drugs go through in the body is known as *pharmacokinetics* and includes four different steps. The first step is known as **absorption**. This process is the movement of the drug through barriers, such as the digestive tract, into the bloodstream where it can be distributed to the target organs or tissues.

With parenteral medications, there are no barriers to slow the movement of drugs into the bloodstream because they bypass these digestive processes. This allows the second step or **distribution** of drugs to occur. This distribution process is what allows the drug to reach its target cells and exert its action. Target cells have special places where drugs go to allow a specific action to take place. These places are known as *receptor sites*. This is sometimes referred to as a *"lock and key"* mechanism, which describes the interactions of the drug at the receptor sites on the target cell (Fig. 2.2).

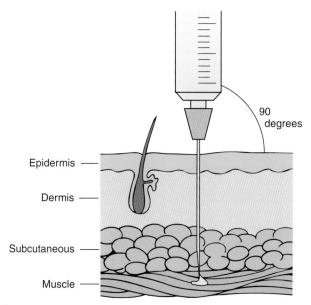

90 degrees

Epidermis

Dermis

Subcutaneous

Muscle

Fig. 2.3 An intramuscular (IM) injection. (From Clayton BD, Stock YN, Cooper SE: *Basic pharmacology for nurses*, ed 15, St Louis, 2010, Mosby Elsevier.)

Everything happens at a cellular level, and since parenteral forms of medications are injected into the bloodstream and are allowed to bypass natural defenses, such as the gastrointestinal (GI) tract, they reach the target cell quickly. Drugs have to reach the blood and be distributed before they act on the body. The third step in the drug's life is to be metabolized in the liver, and this is an actual chemical alteration of the original drug. The primary enzyme system responsible for **metabolism** is the cytochrome P450. **Excretion** is the fourth and last phase of a drug's life, and often occurs in the kidneys. Drugs are eliminated from the body a number of ways but most commonly through urine, feces, breast milk, and sometimes sweat.

If a drug is given intravenously, it bypasses the GI system and goes directly to the bloodstream, where it is distributed throughout the body. When a drug is given via an intramuscular (IM) injection, it is absorbed through tissue membranes and then enters the bloodstream (Fig. 2.3).

Drugs administered orally must be absorbed in the stomach before reaching the blood for circulation. This is why IV medications have the most rapid onset of action or begin to work the fastest.

SPECIAL DOSING CONSIDERATIONS FOR PARENTERAL MEDICATIONS

The dose of a drug is the amount of drug given at one time, and this varies with each patient. The recommended dose of a drug to produce the desired effect is known as the **therapeutic effect**. This means the dose given will be the most effective. If too little of a dose is administered, it can be subtherapeutic, which means it is not enough to be effective. If too much of a dose is administered, it can cause toxic or adverse effects, or in extreme cases be fatal.

All drugs produce certain effects, wanted and unwanted, including therapeutic effects, side effects, and adverse effects. Therapeutic effects are the desired effects of the drug. The dose required to achieve the desired therapeutic effect is somewhere between the smallest effective dose that can be given and the largest dose that is safe. **Side effects** can be found in the manufacturer's literature for a medication and are usually widely reported. Side effects are what patients experience from using the medication or during clinical trials. Common side effects include nausea, dizziness, and dry mouth. **Adverse effects** are usually unexpected and often require a dose change or possibly stopping the drug altogether. These effects may cause harm to the patient and with parenteral medications are even more dangerous because these drugs enter the bloodstream directly.

Tech Note!

When drugs are given to a patient, all three types of effects may occur. Adverse drug reactions (ADRs) should be reported to the US Food and Drug Administration (FDA) through their system known as *MedWatch* (http://www.fda.gov/medwatch/). A special FDA program to report ADRs for vaccines is called the *Vaccine Adverse Event Reporting System (VAERS)*.

DISEASE STATES OR EXISTING CONDITIONS

Certain types of patients are considered contraindicated and should not take certain forms of medications. When dosing a patient, individual factors must be taken into consideration.

A patient may have other diseases that may affect the processes of pharmacokinetics, such as liver, kidney, or cardiovascular disease. If the liver does not function properly because of impairment caused by a disease or a decrease in function because of deteriorating body functions (the aging process), drugs may not be metabolized properly. If there are cardiovascular problems, the blood supply may be less than normal for the distribution process. If the kidneys have failed, drugs will not be excreted or removed from the body at the correct rate. This could mean a smaller dose would be required because of the impairment of vital organs.

AGE

Low weight in neonates and infants usually causes a reduction in the dosage of medication, but there are many other factors to consider when dosing medication for these patients (Box 2.1).

Neonates and infants have smaller skeletal structures, and this can affect the absorption of medication just as much (Fig. 2.4). Since there is limited physical activity in these patients, there is a decrease in blood flow to the muscles. This causes slower absorption of

Box **2.1**   Age Variables

Neonates—up to 1 month after birth
Infant—between 1 month and 2 years
Child—between age 2 and 12 years
Adolescent—between 13 and 19 years
Adult—between 20 and 70 years
Elderly—older than 70 years

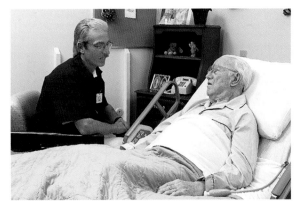

Fig. 2.5 A geriatric patient. (From Sorrentino SA: *Mosby textbook for nursing assistants*, ed 6, p. 92, Fig. 6-8, St. Louis, 2004, Mosby.)

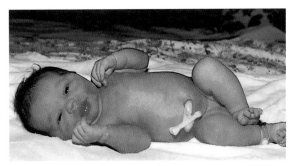

Fig. 2.4 A neonate. (From Thibodeau GA, Patton KT: *The human body in health & disease*, ed 5, St Louis, 2010, Mosby Elsevier.)

Tech Alert!

According to the FDA, benzyl alcohol, a preservative in bacteriostatic water for injection, which is used regularly to dilute some powder forms of IV medication, has been associated with toxicity in neonates.

the medication and increases the risk of muscle and nerve damage with any IM injection, since the medication is not absorbed into the bloodstream as quickly as with an adult. Several factors, such as blood flow and metabolism, influence how much of a drug reaches its organ or area of the body. Various organs, such as the liver and kidneys, have the largest blood supply.

In addition, the adult brain has a protective barrier called the *blood brain barrier*, which protects it from water-soluble substances. Drugs must have a certain degree of lipid- or fat-solubility to penetrate this barrier and get to the brain. Liver function and the blood brain barrier are still immature in pediatric patients, and they have a higher percentage of body water and a lower percentage of body fat than adults. If a lipid-soluble drug is administered to a pediatric patient, there is decreased distribution of the drug to the organs and body tissues because of the lower percentage of fat in the body. This causes more of the medication to stay in the blood longer, causing higher drug blood levels. In comparison, a water-soluble drug can cause lower drug blood levels when administered because the percentage of water is higher in the body, and there is more peripheral drug distribution as a result.

Plasma protein in pediatric patients is lower than in adults, and this allows more of a drug to remain unbound or "free" in the body. Since only unbound medications exert a drug effect, the pediatric patient may have a greater intensity of a drug effect. The liver and the kidneys are not fully developed in pediatric patients. This causes metabolism and excretion to occur more slowly than in adults and allows the drug to stay in their body longer. Since the drug stays in the child's body longer, this can lead to a build-up of the drug, causing toxicity.

Elderly patients experience many differences in the pharmacokinetic processes as aging occurs (Fig. 2.5). Cardiac output decreases significantly with age, which affects the amount of blood that the kidneys and liver receive. Since these organs should have the most blood flow, along with the brain, the metabolism and excretion processes are slower in this population, which allows the drug to stay in the body longer, potentially leading to drug accumulation and toxicity. Drug distribution is greatly affected in the aging adult because the percentage of lean body mass or muscle and the total percentage of body water are lower than in the younger adult. Drug concentration levels in the body are less because there is less water for a drug to be distributed in. Since the amount of body fat increases with age, lipid- (fat-) soluble drugs are widely distributed in those organs that contain the most adipose tissue. This causes the drug to be diverted from the kidneys and liver, where the metabolism and excretion processes should take place. This slows the elimination of the drug from the body and causes it to have a longer half-life and toxicity because of the increased levels of medication in the bloodstream. Elderly patients are generally more sensitive to medications than younger people. This sensitivity often requires a reduction in the usual adult dosage. In an elderly person, the same dosage amount may produce a greater pharmacologic effect.

Did You Know?

Foods like broccoli act as a natural blood thinner and patients taking anticoagulants, such as warfarin (Coumadin), must avoid large amounts of these foods and other leafy green vegetables.

DRUG INTERACTIONS

Drug-drug and drug-food interactions are also a concern. Often drug interactions will occur, and this can be a significant problem with parenteral medications. Since the medication enters the bloodstream and distribution occurs almost immediately, the effects can be magnified. Once the medications are administered, stopping their effects is almost impossible. Some drugs will potentiate the effects of another. In other words, the drug prolongs or magnifies the effect of another being given at the same time. An example would be a sleep aid that acts on the central nervous system combined with drinking alcohol. Some drugs, when given together, can increase each other's effects, such as naprosyn and aspirin, and may require a decreased dosage of both drugs to get the desired therapeutic effects. There are also some drugs that negate the action of another. These drugs may not be taken together, such as azithromycin (Zithromax) and antacids like Rolaids and Maalox.

Chart of Common Drug-Drug Interactions

Antagonist—When one medication stops the action of another

Agonist—When one medication increases the action of another

Synergist—When two medications work together

There are also drug-food interactions. This occurs when a food affects the effectiveness or safety of a drug. For example, heparin is an IV anticoagulant and should not be taken with broccoli because they both thin the blood, and together they may cause internal bleeding.

! Tech Alert!

Medications, such as heparin and insulin, are considered high alert drugs because of the dosing and the significant chance of causing harm to a patient. For a list of the most common high alert medications, see the Institute for Safe Medication Practices website, http://www.ismp.org/Tools/highalertmedications.pdf.

BODY WEIGHT

The amount of drug required is related to weight because it determines the concentration of drug in the body. Pediatric patients, for instance, do not weigh what an average adult weighs, and dosages need to be adjusted. Formulas using body weight are often used to calculate a pediatric dose.

ROUTES OF ADMINISTRATION

There are some drugs that cannot be given orally because of the breakdown that occurs in the GI system. For example, heparin is destroyed by stomach acid and is therefore only available in injectable form.

Injectable medications have to be in an aqueous solution form to allow them to be injected into the body. They may be packaged as a solution and require preparation using a syringe to withdraw the desired amount; or, they may be packaged as a powder, which requires dilution with a specific fluid called a *diluent*.

The injectable medications will either be transferred to an IV solution container of fluid, usually in a plastic bag, drawn up in a syringe for IV push, or be manufactured as a ready-to-use premixed product. Examples of products available today are prefilled syringes, vials, or heat-sealed glass containers known as *ampules*. All of these products are considered sterile, and all manipulations require aseptic technique (Fig. 2.6).

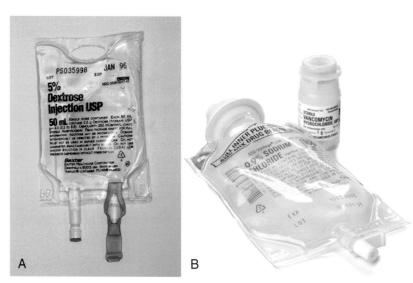

Fig. 2.6 (A and B) Intravenous (IV) products. (A, Brown M, Mulholland JL: *Drug calculations: process and problems for clinical practice*, St. Louis, 2007, Mosby Elsevier. B, Courtesy Hospira Inc., Lake Forest, IL.)

REFERENCES AND STORAGE INFORMATION

All drug products have a National Drug Code (NDC) for identification (Fig. 2.7). This enables the technician to verify the exact product, because it identifies the specific drug, the manufacturer, and the package size.

The packaging information is the best source of information regarding the medications. The label of every drug package must include the following information:
- Brand and generic name
- Liquid forms of medications include the total volume of the container and the concentration, such as 25 mg/mL
- Powder forms provide the information required to dilute the powder, including the concentration and directions for reconstituting the drug
- If it is a prescription medication, the label reads "Federal Law Prohibits Dispensing Without a Prescription" or "RX ONLY"
- Name and address of manufacturer
- Precautions associated with the drug
- Possible side effects and adverse effects
- Storage requirements, including refrigeration information, if needed.

Other common reference sources to use for IV medications include *Drug Facts and Comparisons 2014*, the *Physicians' Desk Reference*, and the *Handbook on Injectable Drugs* by Lawrence A. Trissell. *Drug Facts and Comparisons* and the *Handbook on Injectable Drugs* contain the most current drug information. The *Handbook for Injectable Drugs* is used mostly in the hospital setting because it provides comprehensive compatibility information in chart form, such as to which fluids a medication can be added, storage requirements, stability, and preparation directions. In addition to these references, there are some quick-reference compatibility charts that some hospitals or facilities may use based on the literature made available from the manufacturers.

SOURCES OF INFORMATION AND REFERENCES AVAILABLE

Once the order for an IV admixture is written, the next step for the technician is to verify that the components can be safely mixed, and if so, what concentrations they should be and in what order if any. Certain medications come in powder form and are to be diluted with certain fluids according to the manufacturer (Table 2.1).

Once the medication is diluted if necessary, the next step is choosing a proper IV solution to which the medication can be added. This can be found in literature, such as the package insert, Trissel's *Handbook on Injectable Drugs*, electronic databases, and incompatibility charts. Storage information can be found in these resources as well.

It is very important to label the final product with any storage information that is necessary, such as the expiration date, refrigeration if required, and any other special manufacturer's considerations. Whenever possible, avoid incompatibilities to ensure safe and effective patient care. For example:
- Always take the time to consult reference sources for information about the proper preparation required
- Always be aware of special storage requirements
- Always dilute with proper fluids according to the manufacturer's guidelines or literature
- Always double-check calculations
- Always note any interactions with certain types of containers, such as plastic or aluminum
- If the final product is not to be used immediately, it is best to refrigerate if appropriate.

A technician must always be aware of the medications and any special considerations concerning storage, mixing, and proper handling when performing aseptic technique. The patient's safety depends on it.

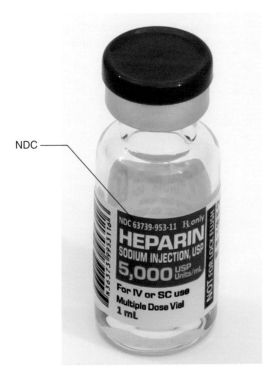

NDC

Fig. 2.7 The National Drug Code (NDC) appears on this vial.

Table 2.1	Example: Ceftriaxone Sodium (Rocephin).
Vial Size	**Volume of Diluent**
For Intramuscular Use	
250 mg	0.9 mL
500 mg	1.8 mL
1 g	3.6 mL
2 g	7.2 mL
For Intermittent Intravenous Infusion	
250 mg	2.4 mL
500 mg	4.8 mL
1 g	9.6 mL
2 g	19.2 mL

Technicians must be familiar with the content for various references to verify information about medications. These references are provided at the facility and should be updated continuously to ensure the most recent information. There are also continuing education lessons offered in magazines, such as "Drug Topics," "Pharmacy Times," and other publications, that are designed for technicians to stay current with the latest marketed drugs.

Errors can occur at any time, but when technicians prepare admixtures, chances are significantly increased because of the complexity of special procedures, equipment, and fluids that must be used. Often there is minimal supervision during the actual process, and this requires technicians to be even more conscientious about their technique and understanding of the medications that they are preparing. In this chapter, we will discuss common IV fluids, their industry abbreviations and their characteristics, compatibilities, and reference sources that are available for the technician to use.

CHARACTERISTICS OF DIFFERENT SOLUTIONS USED IN INTRAVENOUS THERAPY

IV solutions used in parenteral administration must be prepared using aseptic technique and have certain characteristics. They must be sterile (i.e., free from bacteria). They must also have **clarity**, which means clear and free of visible particulate matter. In addition to the clarity and being bacteria free, the solutions also have certain characteristics that determine how they will act once they are in the blood stream. The **tonicity** of the fluid determines which direction the fluid will pass between the extracellular and intracellular compartments. **Osmosis** is the passage of water particles from an area of lower concentration to an area of higher concentration across a barrier, such as a cell membrane. The number of these dissolved particles per liter of solution is known as **osmolarity**. The **pH** of the solution is also very important because the body's fluid is slightly alkaline or about 7.4 (Fig. 2.8).

Fluid entering the bloodstream that is too acidic or too alkaline can cause pain or discomfort, and damage to the red blood cells should be avoided if possible. The fluid inside the cell contains dissolved substances, such as sugars and salts. The cell membrane is designed to allow fluid to pass freely from one membrane to another but not the substances. **Isotonic** fluids have the same osmolarity as normal body fluid. These solutions

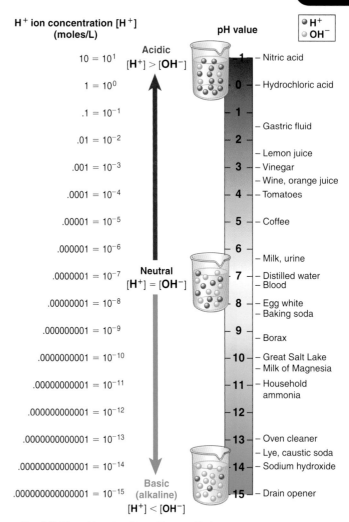

Fig. 2.8 The pH scale. (From Patton KT, Thibodeau GA: *Anatomy & physiology*, ed 8, St Louis, 2012, Mosby Elsevier.)

are the closest to the red blood cells because the concentration of the salt and other substances are the same as those found in red blood cells. Both 5% dextrose and 0.9% sodium chloride are examples of isotonic fluids. If the solution contains a concentration of dissolved substances less than red blood cells, it is known as **hypotonic**. This means fluid will move into the cells and cause swelling. If the solution contains a higher concentration than the red blood cells, it is **hypertonic** and cells can shrink because of the movement of fluids out of the cells. Both of these types of fluids can cause stinging because the cells are trying to either swell or shrink, to handle the fluids introduced (Fig. 2.9).

There are several common IV fluids available today. Medications that are added to the fluid are known as *additives*, whereas the final product is known as the **admixture**. Common IV fluids include sodium chloride injection, dextrose injection, and lactated Ringer's solution for injection (Fig. 2.10). Dextrose injection (glucose) is primarily used as a carbohydrate for nutrition and as a source of fluid. It is usually given in 5% concentration. Sodium chloride is used as a source of

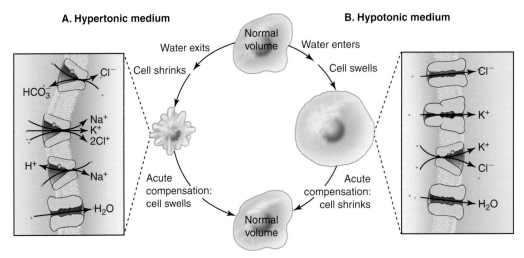

Fig. 2.9 Cell behavior in hypotonic and hypertonic solutions. Cl^-, Chloride; H^+, hydrogen; H_2O, water; HCO_3^-, bicarbonate; K^+, potassium; Na^+, sodium. (From Pollard TD, Earnshaw WC: *Cell biology*, ed 2, Philadelphia, 2008, Saunders Elsevier.)

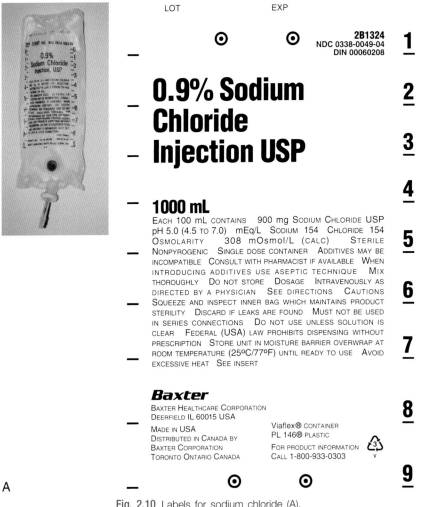

Fig. 2.10 Labels for sodium chloride (A),

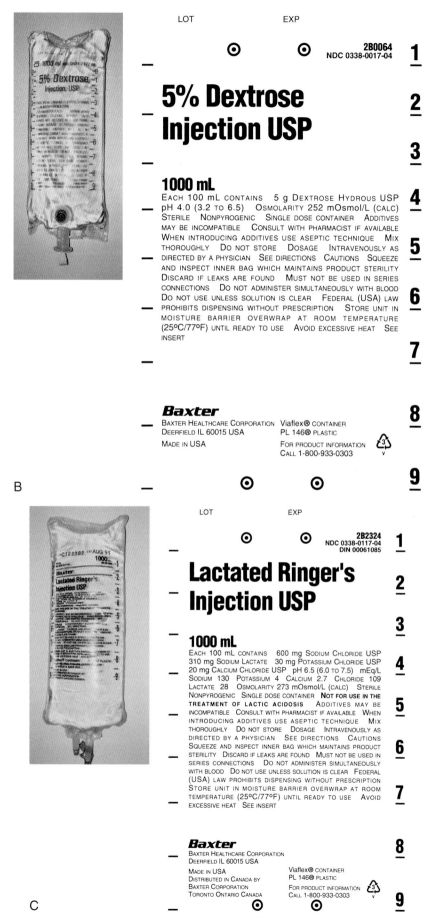

LOT   EXP

NDC 0338-0017-04   **2B0064**

1

5% Dextrose Injection USP

2

3

1000 mL

EACH 100 mL CONTAINS   5 g DEXTROSE HYDROUS USP
pH 4.0 (3.2 TO 6.5)   OSMOLARITY 252 mOsmol/L (CALC)
STERILE   NONPYROGENIC   SINGLE DOSE CONTAINER   ADDITIVES
MAY BE INCOMPATIBLE   CONSULT WITH PHARMACIST IF AVAILABLE
WHEN INTRODUCING ADDITIVES USE ASEPTIC TECHNIQUE   MIX
THOROUGHLY   DO NOT STORE   DOSAGE   INTRAVENOUSLY AS
DIRECTED BY A PHYSICIAN   SEE DIRECTIONS   CAUTIONS   SQUEEZE
AND INSPECT INNER BAG WHICH MAINTAINS PRODUCT STERILITY
DISCARD IF LEAKS ARE FOUND   MUST NOT BE USED IN SERIES
CONNECTIONS   DO NOT ADMINISTER SIMULTANEOUSLY WITH BLOOD
DO NOT USE UNLESS SOLUTION IS CLEAR   FEDERAL (USA) LAW
PROHIBITS DISPENSING WITHOUT PRESCRIPTION   STORE UNIT IN
MOISTURE BARRIER OVERWRAP AT ROOM TEMPERATURE
(25°C/77°F) UNTIL READY TO USE   AVOID EXCESSIVE HEAT   SEE
INSERT

4

5

6

7

Baxter
BAXTER HEALTHCARE CORPORATION   Viaflex® CONTAINER
DEERFIELD IL 60015 USA   PL 146® PLASTIC
MADE IN USA   FOR PRODUCT INFORMATION
          CALL 1-800-933-0303

8

B

9

LOT   EXP

NDC 0338-0117-04   **2B2324**
DIN 00061085

1

Lactated Ringer's Injection USP

2

3

1000 mL

EACH 100 mL CONTAINS   600 mg SODIUM CHLORIDE USP
310 mg SODIUM LACTATE   30 mg POTASSIUM CHLORIDE USP
20 mg CALCIUM CHLORIDE USP   pH 6.5 (6.0 TO 7.5)   mEq/L
SODIUM 130   POTASSIUM 4   CALCIUM 2.7   CHLORIDE 109
LACTATE 28   OSMOLARITY 273 mOsmol/L (CALC)   STERILE
NONPYROGENIC   SINGLE DOSE CONTAINER   **NOT FOR USE IN THE
TREATMENT OF LACTIC ACIDOSIS**   ADDITIVES MAY BE
INCOMPATIBLE   CONSULT WITH PHARMACIST IF AVAILABLE   WHEN
INTRODUCING ADDITIVES USE ASEPTIC TECHNIQUE   MIX
THOROUGHLY   DO NOT STORE   DOSAGE   INTRAVENOUSLY AS
DIRECTED BY A PHYSICIAN   SEE DIRECTIONS   CAUTIONS
SQUEEZE AND INSPECT INNER BAG WHICH MAINTAINS PRODUCT
STERILITY   DISCARD IF LEAKS ARE FOUND   MUST NOT BE USED IN
SERIES CONNECTIONS   DO NOT ADMINISTER SIMULTANEOUSLY
WITH BLOOD   DO NOT USE UNLESS SOLUTION IS CLEAR   FEDERAL
(USA) LAW PROHIBITS DISPENSING WITHOUT PRESCRIPTION
STORE UNIT IN MOISTURE BARRIER OVERWRAP AT ROOM
TEMPERATURE (25°C/77°F) UNTIL READY TO USE   AVOID
EXCESSIVE HEAT   SEE INSERT

4

5

6

7

Baxter
BAXTER HEALTHCARE CORPORATION
DEERFIELD IL 60015 USA
MADE IN USA   Viaflex® CONTAINER
DISTRIBUTED IN CANADA BY   PL 146® PLASTIC
BAXTER CORPORATION
TORONTO ONTARIO CANADA   FOR PRODUCT INFORMATION
          CALL 1-800-933-0303

8

C

9

Fig. 2.10, cont'd dextrose (B), and lactated Ringer's solution (C). (From Brown M, Mulholland JL: *Drug calculations: process and problems for clinical practice,* ed 8, St Louis, 2007, Mosby Elsevier.)

Table 2.2	Standard Abbreviations and Tonicity of Intravenous Solutions.		
Intravenous Solution	**Abbreviation**	**Tonicity**	
5% Dextrose	D5W	Isotonic	
0.9% Sodium chloride	NS (normal saline)	Isotonic	
Lactated Ringer's solution	LR	Isotonic	
10% Dextrose	D10W	Hypertonic	
0.45% Sodium chloride (normal saline)	1/2NS	Hypotonic	
5% Dextrose and 0.9% sodium chloride	D5NS	Hypertonic	
5% Dextrose and 0.45% sodium chloride	D51/2NS	Hypertonic	
5% Dextrose and 0.2% sodium chloride	D51/4NS	Isotonic	
Lactated Ringer's solution and 5% dextrose	D5LR	Hypertonic	

fluid and electrolytes. It is usually given in 0.9%. Lactated Ringer's solution for injection contains primary electrolytes found in plasma and is used for fluid replacement or as a source of electrolytes.

 Tech Note!

If any of the fluids listed in Table 2.2 are manufactured with additives already added, the bag would have the additive written in red, such as dextrose 5% and 0.9% normal saline, with 20 mEq of potassium chloride (D5NS20KCL).

All of these fluids can be found in various combinations and can also be manufactured with certain additives already in them. There are also standard abbreviations that are used when writing orders or prescriptions with which technicians should be familiar (see Table 2.2).

COMPATIBILITY AND INCOMPATIBILITY OF INTRAVENOUS FLUIDS

When combining medications in IV fluids, the **compatibility** of the admixture must be considered. Often there are drugs that cannot be combined safely with a particular IV fluid for various reasons. There may be a physical change (such as color or clarity) or a formation of particles called *particulate matter*. These IV admixtures are known as **incompatible** and must not be given to the patient. When preparing IV admixtures, carefully inspect the completed product visually and look for any obvious changes. Any leaks, tears, or changes in the bag of fluid should be observed while still in the hood.

Look for the following characteristics:
- Particles floating, such as rubber from the stopper of the vial (known as **coring**)

- Any color changes
- Haze or turbidity
- Solid particles or filaments formed (particulate matter).

Some incompatibilities cannot be seen with visual inspection but are just as important. These factors can affect the compatibility and/or stability of the drugs in an IV admixture, and reference materials, such as package inserts or Trissel's *Handbook on Injectable Drugs*, will provide storage and compatibility information about each drug specifically.

Some of these factors are discussed in the following sections.

 Tech Note!

Always refer to medication information concerning compatibility. Color changes or particulate matter does not always form immediately. It may take hours for this to happen, and in that amount of time the IV may be delivered to the patient for administration.

TEMPERATURE

Drugs often degrade because of storage in improper temperatures. Some drugs must be refrigerated, some kept at room temperature, and some may even be frozen for storage. For example, metronidazole (Flagyl) should be kept at room temperature because refrigeration causes precipitate to form.

LIGHT

Some drugs must not be exposed to light and should be protected by a light-blocking protective bag or cover because the medication will be destroyed or degraded. Often, vials of medication are packaged in colored or tinted containers to protect them. During administration, the admixture is protected from light by using special brown bags that block the light.

TIME

Once medications are added to an IV fluid, the amount of time that they are stable may vary from the manufacturer's information provided in the packaging. This is because the drug has been taken from its original packaging and added to a sterile solution, which changes how it reacts with that fluid.

For instance, once a vial of cefazolin is reconstituted and added to a bag of 0.9% sodium chloride, the admixture is only good for 7 days; at 4°C in its original vial, it will be good for years.

DILUTION

Medications can often be added to an IV fluid in certain concentrations and be compatible, but they will produce participates if they are added in higher concentrations. For example, when mixing calcium and phosphates, only 15 mEq of calcium can be added to a liter of fluid containing 30 mEq of phosphate without precipitating.

COMPATIBILITY

Some drugs will interact with certain metals, such as cisplatin (a chemotherapy drug) and aluminum. There are also medications that interact with polyvinyl chloride plastic, and contact between them should be avoided.

pH

If the fluid and medication to be added have conflicting pH values, this may cause the drug to either degrade or form a precipitate. An example is ampicillin, which is an antibiotic that has a pH of 8 to 10 as packaged in a vial from the manufacturer. As an admixture, the fluid of choice is sodium chloride 0.9%. Sodium chloride is preferred over dextrose because of the decomposition of the drug when mixed in dextrose during clinical studies.

 Did You Know?

Some medications (such as intravenous immunoglobulin [IVIG], a plasma replacement therapy, and insulin, used for diabetes) cannot be shaken after **reconstitution** because of the excess foam that will develop.

INTRAVENOUS SOLUTION

Some drugs are only compatible with certain IV fluids, and the reference materials will indicate this. For example, ampicillin cannot be mixed in lactated Ringer's solution because the ampicillin will degrade within about 24 hours. However, when ampicillin powder is reconstituted or diluted and then added to a bag of sodium chloride (as recommended by the manufacturer's instructions), it is stable for 8 hours at room temperature. Other drugs cannot be added to the same IV fluid at the same time, such as furosemide and chlorpromazine, because **precipitation** will occur immediately.

ORDER OF MIXING

Some drugs can be mixed together only if they are mixed well in the fluid before the next additive is mixed. If they are given the opportunity to be diluted individually before immediately adding the next drug, then the chance of them coming into direct contact with each other will be decreased and will allow them to be added to the same fluid.

 Tech Alert!

When in doubt about compatibility with drug-drug or drug-fluid, always refer to reference sources. Some incompatibilities do not always show up visually.

Common Parenteral Medications Types

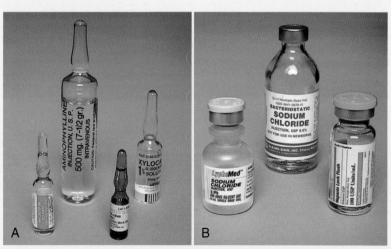

Perry AG, Potter PA, Ostendorf WR: *Nursing interventions & clinical skills*, ed 7, St Louis, 2020, Elsevier.

Antibiotic therapy—IV antibiotic medications are often administered to patients with infections in order to reach the blood stream quicker and start to work. This may be a one-time injection, such as a Rocephin intramuscular shot followed by an oral drug, or a regimen of 7 to 10 days via an IV preparation.

Fluid replacement—Often IV medications are used in cases of dehydration, such as with Lactated Ringers, which is very close to the body's normal fluid.

Antineoplastic (Chemotherapy)—Many cancer treating medications are supplied for intravenous use and can be given as weekly treatments in outpatient facilities.

Nutrition—Provision of nutrition for patients who cannot digest or process food because of trauma or some GI conditions are given intravenously.

Pain management—Some patients receive IV pain medications through a pump, which can be programmed for dosing.

Biologics—Some newer medications that are derived from deoxyribonucleic acid of living organisms and used to treat many diseases, such as Crohn diseases or rheumatoid arthritis, are available as injections that can be given monthly.

Trauma (emergency)—In cases of emergency, many medications must be given to save or prolong life, and the quickest method is injectable.

REVIEW QUESTIONS

1. The number of dissolved particles in a solution per liter of solution is:
   A. precipitation
   B. osmolarity
   C. tonicity
   D. hypertonic

2. The factors that can affect the compatability and/or stability of the drugs in IV admixtures are listed subsequently, except:
   A. temperature
   B. dilution
   C. light
   D. excessive plastic

3. When preparing IV admixtures, carefully inspect the completed product. Look for the following characteristics, except:
   A. any color changes
   B. excessive foam
   C. particles floating
   D. haze of turbidity

4. Which process is not a process of pharmokinetics?
   A. Distribution
   B. Digestion
   C. Absorption
   D. Metabolism

5. All drug products have a National Drug Code (NDC) for identification. The NDC contains all of the following, except:
   A. specific drug
   B. the package size
   C. quality of the drug
   D. manufacturer

6. The recommended dose of a drug to produce the desired effect is known as _____.
   A. side effect
   B. therapeutic effect
   C. adverse effect
   D. administered effect

7. The process of adding a diluent to a powder form of a medication is:
   A. reconstitution
   B. admixture
   C. isotonic
   D. tonicity

8. Osmosis is the passage of water particles from an area of _____ concentration to an area of _____ concentration across a barrier.
   A. neutral, higher
   B. higher, neutral
   C. neutral, lower
   D. lower, higher

9. The changing of the chemical structure of a drug by the body is called:
   A. Osmolarity
   B. Distribution
   C. Excretion
   D. Metabolism

10. The movement of a drug into the circulatory system is called:
    A. Metabolism
    B. Excretion
    C. Absorption
    D. Incompatibility

CRITICAL THINKING

For the following scenarios, use the most appropriate resource and answer the questions:

1. A nurse calls the pharmacy and asks if she can add some morphine sulfate to a bag of heparin that is already hanging in the patient's room. Where can she find this information? Are these two drugs compatible with each other?

2. As a technician in an IV room, there is an order for ampicillin 1 g stat to be given. Is it compatible with lactated Ringer's solution?

3. A nurse calls to ask if ceftazidime and ciprofloxacin are compatible.

4. The same nurse calls later and asks if heparin can be given with ciprofloxacin.

5. A nurse calls and states that she found a bag of ready-to-use metronidazole IV fluid on the counter in the nurse's office for a patient who has gone home. It was there when she left last night, and she wants to know if it can be credited and reused for another patient.

6. A technician is preparing an order for vancomycin on December 15, 2019, and finds one that has been credited in the refrigerator. It was made and dated December 10, 2019. Is this appropriate to reuse for this patient?

7. Your patient is a 67-year-old woman who weighs 97 pounds. She has been diagnosed in the past with kidney problems. She presents to the emergency room complaining of extreme nausea and vomiting. She is dehydrated and needs fluids immediately. Your choice for medication is promethazine (Phenergan) IV or orally (PO). Which route would you use and why? Would the average adult dosage be appropriate? Why or why not?

8. Your patient is a 6-year-old child weighing 45 pounds. She presents to the emergency room with a rash, and the mother states that she had received a phenobarbital injection for seizures approximately 2 weeks ago, but has recently started being irritable and unable to sleep through the night. Just last night, the mother noticed her slurring her words and became concerned. What type of effects do these reactions indicate? What should be done, if anything, for this patient?

9. The use of digoxin, a heart medication, has been associated with an increase in risk of falls in the elderly patient, as well as an increase of toxic effects. Explain why this may occur. (Use a drug reference for your drug information.)

10. Using a drug reference of your choice, answer the following questions:
    - What is the generic name for Synercid?
    - What is it used to treat?
    - Explain how it is packaged and prepared for injection.
    - Name one contraindication for using Synercid.
    - Can this medication be used in pediatric patients?
    - How should this medication be stored?

COMPETENCIES

INCOMPATIBILITIES, COMPATIBILITIES, AND STORAGE REQUIREMENTS FOR INTRAVENOUS MEDICATIONS

Evaluation Key: S = Satisfactory   NI = Needs Improvement

Name: _____   Quarter: _____   Date: _____

COMPETENCIES	STUDENT			INSTRUCTOR		
Student will be able to:	S	NI	Comments	S	NI	Comments
Describe visual incompatibilities, concentration effects, and pH.						
Discuss isotonic, hypotonic, and hypertonic fluids.						
Discuss common IV fluids and the abbreviations used.						
Describe particulate matter inspection.						
Explain how to perform visual inspection of a parenteral solution.						
List various reference materials and the type of information they include pertaining to IV preparations.						
List several ways to avoid IV preparation incompatibilities.						

Review each concept to ensure that the learning objectives for the chapter have been met. Your instructor or supervisor will evaluate this as well.

PATIENT CONSIDERATIONS FOR INTRAVENOUS MEDICATIONS

Evaluation Key: S = Satisfactory   NI = Needs Improvement

Name: _____   Quarter: _____   Date: _____

COMPETENCIES	STUDENT			INSTRUCTOR		
Student will be able to:	S	NI	Comments	S	NI	Comments
Discuss the processes of pharmacokinetics for parenteral medications.						
Discuss the differences in pediatric patients and the need for dose adjustment.						
Discuss the differences in elderly patients and the need for dose adjustment.						
Discuss factors that must be considered when using IV medications.						
Identify at least two reference sources for IV medication information.						
Discuss side effects, adverse effects, and therapeutic effects and the differences between them.						
Using provided reference materials, identify drug information, such as storage, indications, contraindications, how supplied, NDC number, and interactions.						

Review each concept to ensure that the learning objectives for the chapter have been met. Your instructor or supervisor will evaluate this as well.

LAB ACTIVITY

For the following solutions or medications, use the resources provided to answer the questions:

1. What is the pH of premixed cimetidine HCL? In what form does it come (mg in solution)? If mixed with warfarin, describe what visual precipitate occurs.
2. Name two solutions that vancomycin can be mixed in. How long does the manufacturer state that it is good for when mixed with D5NS? If mixed with methotrexate, describe what precipitate occurs.
3. How is ceftriaxone (Rocephin) packaged? For IM injection, how much diluent would you use for a 500 mg vial? If using sterile water for injection (SWFI) with a concentration of 250 mg/mL, how long is it stable at 4°C? How long is the frozen premixed solution stable?
4. How is amphotericin B administered normally? Name any special considerations used when preparing an infusion. Name two solutions that are incompatible and describe what occurs.
5. Using the online resource, GLOBALRPh, at www.globalrph.com, search for "New Drug Approvals," and list the brand and generic names of two drugs under the cardiology category. Then discuss the mechanism of action, therapeutic use, usual adult dosage, and classification.
6. Using the online resource www.pdr.net (*Physicians' Desk Reference*), answer the following questions about Phenergan: What is the generic name? What is the indication? What is the therapeutic class? Is this drug available in an injectable form? Name an adverse effect. Name a drug interaction.
7. Using the online resource GLOBALRPh, at www.globalrph.com, and under the *Dilutions* category at the top, look up FORTAZ and enter the following information found: With what fluids can this powdered drug be diluted? If diluted with sterile water for an IM injection, how many days will the drug maintain potency if refrigerated? Name two indications for using this drug.

BIBLIOGRAPHY

1. Blanchard, Loeb: *Nurse's handbook of I.V. drugs*, ed 3, Burlington, MA, 2009, Jones & Bartlett.
2. Delgin JH, Vallerand AH: *Davis' drug guide for nurses*, ed 11, Philadelphia, 2009, F.A. Davis Company.
3. Gahart BL, Nazareno AR: *2008 Intravenous medications*, ed 24, St Louis, 2007, Mosby Elsevier.
4. Phillips L: *Manual of I.V. therapeutics: evidence-based practice for infusion therapy*, ed 5, Philadelphia, 2010, F.A. Davis Company.
5. Trissel LA: *Handbook on injectable drugs*, ed 15, Bethesda, MD, 2008, American Society of Health-System Pharmacists.
6. U.S. National Library of Medicine: *MedlinePlus: Drugs, Supplements, and Herbal Information* (website): http://www.nlm.nih.gov/medlineplus/druginformation.html. Accessed March 1, 2013.
7. *Drug facts and comparisons 2013*, ed 68, Philadelphia, 2013, Lippincott Williams & Wilkins.
8. *Global RPH*: http://www,globalrph.com.
9. *Physicians' desk reference*, ed 2013, Montvale, NJ, 2012, PDR Network.
10. *Taber's cylopedic medical dictionary*, ed 22, Philadelphia, 2013, F.A. Davis Company.
11. Trissel LA: *Handbook on injectable drugs*, ed 15, Bethesda, MD, 2008, American Society of Health-System Pharmacists.

Communication Within and Beyond the Pharmacy

3

INTRODUCTION

Communication within the pharmacy, as well as with the patient and other caregivers, requires a focused approach. Delivery of an intravenous (IV) medication is often time consuming because of preparation and order complications, and the additional requirements of working in the environment itself. Preparing an IV is not like pulling an oral medication from the shelf or automated system and administering it to the patient within just a few minutes. "Time is money," as they say, and an unorganized process can produce additional costs and waste. Good communication skills can eliminate mistakes, emergency situations, and enhance patient safety (Fig. 3.1).

SITUATIONS FOR IV MEDICATION THERAPY

IV medication therapy may often involve several healthcare providers. The order may be initiated by a physician in a variety of ways. The administration may occur in a variety of settings as well, which can offer challenges to costs, product integrity, and time required in the process. Some of the most common include:

- Inpatient setting—Hospital-based patient on IV therapy and medication is prepared each shift for a 24-hour supply. The medications, such as antibiotics, coagulation therapy, and fluid replacement can be prepared in batches and are routinely delivered to the floor. If there are STAT orders or on-demand IV orders, this can lead to rushed work and possibly compromise safe guards, such as proper technique, in the compounding process (Fig. 3.2).

- Home infusion—Patient may be discharged from a facility or be deemed appropriate for receiving an IV regimen at home. They may be assisted by caregivers within the home, a visiting nurse, or themselves. Challenges can include teaching difficulties for lay persons, unsanitary conditions, and delivery or storage issues for medications, such as those sent in weekly deliveries (Fig. 3.3).

- Hospice in-patient—This may require an order to be sent to a local pharmacy where delivery is required to the facility. In this environment, it may be short notice and require an emergency type preparation. Often, this may involve pain management medications, which adhere to special requirements for dispensing, which can cause delays in the process.

- Chemotherapy or Infusion centers—The facility may have its own IN-HOUSE compounding pharmacy that prepares IV medications ahead, for patients who come on site for regular scheduled times. These medications may require additional shipping time and special storage (Fig. 3.4).

BUILDING A COLLABORATIVE TEAM

The healthcare environment today looks much different than in the past. The approach is patient-centered care, or is centered on creating a relationship where the patient is aware of their disease state and has input into the therapy. For patients receiving IV medication therapy, there are additional complications that they should understand, which will ultimately increase compliance. Rather than just receiving an order for antibiotic therapy at home and sending the medication,

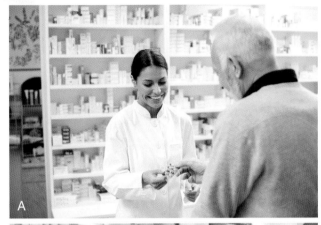

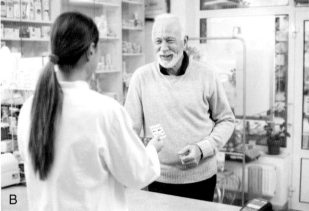

Fig. 3.1 Good communication skills can eliminate mistakes, emergency situations, and enhance patient safety. (A and B, Copyright © Gligatron/iStock/Thinkstock.com.)

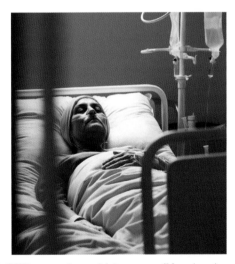

Fig. 3.2 STAT or on-demand intravenous (IV) orders in a hospital setting can be a challenge. (Copyright © KatarzynaBialasiewicz/iStock/Thinkstock.com.)

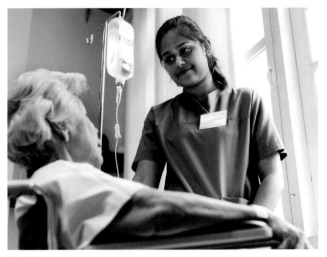

Fig. 3.3 Home infusion can present challenges, such as teaching difficulties for lay persons, unsanitary conditions, and delivery or storage issues. (Copyright © Rawpixel/iStock/Thinkstock.com.)

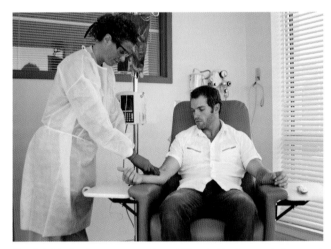

Fig. 3.4 Medications may require additional ship time and storage at infusion centers. (Copyright © Trish233/iStock/Thinkstock.com.)

the pharmacy compounding personnel should be aware that the patient may or may not have an outside healthcare professional coming to administer and that they may be doing this themselves.

The 21st century will push the boundaries for collaborations between health professionals to provide comprehensive and quality care for patients. Each person on the team should use their personal skill set to align with others to share resources, information, and problem-solving talents.

For instance: if you receive an order for a new IV therapy medication and find out that it will have to be drop shipped and take 3 days to arrive, you should immediately notify the Pharmacist, so they can communicate options with the ordering physician and other team members involved. Being alert and working together starts with individuals and should continue to grow throughout your career (Fig. 3.5).

ELEMENTS OF AN EFFECTIVE COLLABORATIVE TEAM MEMBER

As the compounding technician, the need to be prepared and properly trained in your tasks is key to fulfilling your part of the team's responsibilities. It should not stop there, however. Knowing the roles for the other team members allows you to see further than just your compounding responsibilities. Knowing the

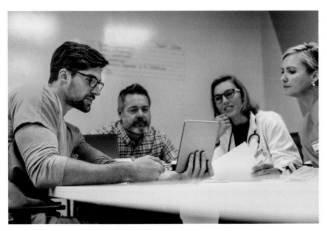

Fig. 3.5 Being alert and working together starts with individuals and should continue to grow throughout your career. (Copyright © jacoblund/iStock/Thinkstock.com.)

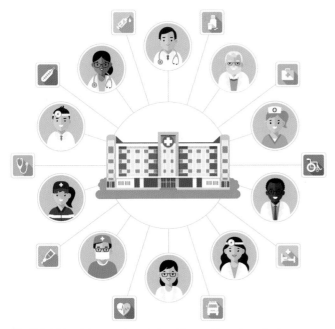

Fig. 3.6 Maintaining trusting relationships and knowing who is responsible for each element of care is the best way to assure the patient gets quality care. (Copyright © bluebearry/iStock/Thinkstock.com.)

inventory process, such as turnarounds, periodic automatic replenishment (PAR) levels, and accessibility to common IV medications, assist with cost containment and quicker response times on orders.

Maintaining trusting relationships and knowing who is responsible for each element of the process is the best way to assure the patient gets quality care (Fig. 3.6). There are some key elements which you should strive for:

Assertiveness—ask questions, challenge yourself to learn daily and stay current in your field. Go to the source instead of a third-party. If you see a potential problem, address it as early as possible.

Awareness—be aware of other's roles/responsibilities on the team, such as who to contact, and how your actions affects the entire process. Do not think of your role as isolated. If you see a potential problem, try to work to help it get solved, even if it is not your specific role.

Active—be an active listener. If you are communicating with a health team member, ask direct questions and listen to answers. Repeat back if you are unsure.

Case Study

As the compounding technician in a busy infusion center, you are to prepare the next day's dose for Ms. Smith's chemotherapy treatment. She is a regular patient and you usually order one kit ahead for her each month. Looking in the refrigerator, you cannot seem to find her medication. After asking the Infusion Manager, he states that a new patient came in yesterday and they used it on them. You ask the inventory manager to order another one for Ms. Smith and go back to work.

Which Key element would apply best here to avoid coming to the center tomorrow and not getting her dose? Explain why, and what you would do.

Assertiveness—Look on her profile and contact her nurse at the clinic. Explain that you will not have her medication for her appointment tomorrow and request she let the patient know to change her appointment until the next day. This will keep the patient from coming twice in the same week.

Case Study

A nurse comes to the window with a STAT order for a drug that you just found out yesterday was recalled. The technician working at the front tells the nurse she will get that to the IV room and deliver it to her as soon as it is made. You are really busy, so you go back to work and assume the Pharmacist will discover this once they begin to enter the order in the system.

Which key element would apply best here and what should they have done?

Awareness—you should inform the Pharmacist immediately what you know, which will allow them to inform the nurse and ultimately the physician who may make a change.

Case Study

The technician working with you today comes to the IV room and informs you there is a new order coming for an antibiotic IV therapy that needs to be delivered today. When you turn around to ask her who the patient is so that you can look for it, she is gone. You ask the other technician in the room with you to repeat what she said, and she tells you there was Vancomycin order coming. You know this is usually 1g/D250 mL and 7 to 14 bags. Since the mediation is in a powder vial, you start to dilute the vials, so you can be ahead of the order. When the order finally comes, it is not for Vancomycin, but another antibiotic and now the diluted vials will have to be wasted.

What key element could have helped avoid this and how?

Active listening is an important skill, and instead of asking a third person what was said, they should have asked the initial person or waited to know exactly what was needed. Assuming what they thought they heard cost the pharmacy the price of the medication as well as the time involved its preparation.

HOW TO BUILD A COLLABORATIVE TEAM

Each member of the healthcare team has strengths and weaknesses. As a compounding technician, it is important to be aware of these for yourself. Here are some elements a manager may look for to ensure the team's productivity and communication within and outside.

- Does the individual have personal goals and align them with the team's goals?
- Does the individual have mutual respect for their colleagues?
- Does the individual share their skills and knowledge as well as appreciate knowledge from others?
- Does the individual appreciate input from others and have a willingness to learn from their mistakes?
- Does the individual strive to stay current in their field and changes in practice?
- Does the individual use effective listening skills with others?

As a compounding technician, you will be faced with challenges in a strict and fast paced environment. The USP<797> guidelines cannot be neglected or bypassed, regardless of how immediate the need for the IV medication therapy is needed. The handwashing, garbing, and environmental practices must be followed in every instance. This is why it is so important to be aware of the practices surrounding your particular role and how what you do affects the entire process (Fig. 3.7).

COMPOUNDING TECHNICIANS ROLE IN IV MEDICATION THERAPY PROCESS

With the current revisions to USP<797>, most facilities use a centralized compounding space because of costs and environmental restrictions. This approach requires a workflow system to be in place to maintain efficiency and best practices. The compounding technicians are an integral part of the delivery process of services and medications. Managing wastes and awareness of supply are ways to keep costs low and provide timely services. Every member should be aware of providing the most efficient and quality IV medication therapy and what types of technology can be used. In some settings the use of automated compounders can help manage costs and save preparation time. This may require additional training and workflow processes that include different team members. Regardless of each team member's role, the ultimate goal is timelier and safer patient care. Working alongside nursing and other departments, the use of IV smart pump technology and other advances in administration can also be integral for **patient-centered care** and services, which may also reduce costs and provide better efficiency (Fig. 3.8).

ELECTRONIC COMMUNICATION AND RESOURCES

With the changes in technology and patients being more involved in their own disease management and wellness decisions, IV medication therapy can be complicated and may involve virtual patient care as well as telepharmacy. There is also social media, internet-based physician video sharing, applications via phone, and email. Today's approach to patent care is often fast paced and required to be available 24/7. It may include a virtual visit, followed by an emailed prescription. Communication through these electronic sources can be tricky and sometimes lead to miscommunication with spelling and incorrect punctuation. Maintaining

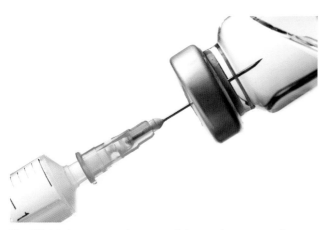

Fig. 3.7 It is important to be aware of the practices surrounding your specific role and to know how what you do affects the entire process. (Copyright © Esben_H/iStock/Thinkstock.com.)

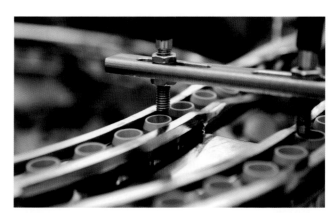

Fig. 3.8 The use of intravenous (IV) smart pump technology and other advances in administration can also be integral for patient-centered care and may also reduce costs and provide better efficiency. (Copyright © Neznam/iStock/Thinkstock.com.)

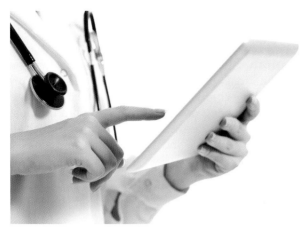

Fig. 3.9 Communication between internal and external members is key to a productive team. (Copyright © Neznam/iStock/Thinkstock.com.)

patient confidentiality is also required, and without any nonverbal cues, sometimes an email or text message can come across as something entirely unintended.

 Tech Note!

When in doubt; ask for a repeat or clarification. DON'T ASSUME!

USING TRUSTED SOURCES AND SHARING OF INFORMATION

Compounding sterile products will require the use of reference sources, many of which are on the internet now. Always use a trusted source, and if you have questions, be ASSERTIVE and ask. Team members should collaborate to share information and learn from each other. Communication between internal and external members is key to a productive team (Fig. 3.9).

Some of the most common resources include:
• Handbook of Injectable Drugs
• Drug Facts and Comparisons
• Physician Desk Reference
• Global RPh at https://globalrph.com/

 Tech Note!

Remember: Once it is on the web, it is out there. Always maintain patient confidentiality.

REVIEW QUESTIONS

1. The practice model of taking care of patients and their families is called:
   A. healthcare
   B. patient-centered care
   C. home infusion
   D. hospice in-patient

2. Some key elements which an effective collaborative team member should strive for include the following, except:
   A. awareness
   B. active
   C. assertiveness
   D. aggression

3. The model in which patients may be discharged from a facility or be deemed appropriate for receiving an IV regimen at home is called:
   A. hospice in-patient
   B. infusion center
   C. inpatient setting
   D. home infusion

4. Good communication skills can eliminate the following, except:
   A. mistakes
   B. enhance patient safety
   C. on-time deliveries
   D. emergency situations

5. Each person on the collaborative team should use their personal skill set to align with others to share the following, except:
   A. information
   B. resources
   C. personal issues
   D. problem-solving talents

6. Delivery of an IV medication is often time consuming because of the following:
   A. preparation
   B. additional requirements of working in the environment itself
   C. order complications
   D. automated system

7. An order sent to a local pharmacy where delivery is required to the facility is called:
   A. hospice in-patient
   B. infusion center
   C. home infusion
   D. inpatient setting

8. The USP<797> guidelines cannot be neglected or bypassed, regardless of how immediate the need for the IV medication therapy is. The following must be adhered to in every instance except:
   A. garbing
   B. noncompliance
   C. handwashing
   D. environmental practices

9. Hospital-based patients on IV therapy and medication is prepared each shift for a 24-hour supply is called:
   A. home infusion
   B. hospice in-patient
   C. inpatient setting
   D. infusion centers

10. The facility may have its own IN-HOUSE compounding pharmacy that prepares IV medications ahead for patients who come on site, for regular scheduled times. This is called:
    A. home infusion
    B. chemotherapy infusion centers
    C. hospice in-patient
    D. inpatient setting

CRITICAL THINKING

1. You are a technician supervisor at a large hospital and have recently hired two new technicians for the intravenous room. How would you go about evaluating their strengths and place on the team? (Use at least two questions a manager would use to decide).

2. You answer the phone and the nurse states that she is calling in an injection for a home patient. The order is a little confusing, but before you can ask for a repeat, they hang up. Should you go with the closest spelling you know, ask the Pharmacist, or call them back? Which is most appropriate and why?

BIBLIOGRAPHY

1. Pharmacy's Critical Role in the IV Medication Therapy Process—Cerner. Retrieved February 22, 2019 from https://www.cerner.com/blog/pharmacy-role-in-the-iv-medication-therapy-process.

Infection Control and Waste Management

4

Learning Objectives

1. Discuss the links in the chain of infection.
2. Discuss the importance of proper handwashing, as well as demonstrate proper handwashing and garbing procedures required for preparing sterile medications.
3. Identify environmental controls and waste management as part of infection control measures.

Terms & Definitions

Garbing Donning (putting on) protective personal equipment in a specific method

Parenteral route Puncture, injection, or some method to enter the bloodstream directly

Pathogen Any disease-causing agent or microorganism

PPE Personal protective equipment to include gown, gloves, hair, foot covers, masks, and eye protection

Standard of care Precautions, such as hand washing, use of PPE, proper disposal of waste, and respiratory hygiene

Transmission Interaction between infectious agents and a susceptible host

Universal precautions Methods to prevent contamination or transference of infection, such as protective barriers

INTRODUCTION

Since the use of intravenous medications requires a direct entry into the blood stream, it is important to have a basic understanding of the immune system, the ways an infection travels, and common infections associated with intravenous (IV) infusions. When preparing sterile medications, the most common way contamination occurs is by touch. Each preparer must be trained properly and adhere to strict guidelines for hand hygiene, proper dress, and disposal of hazardous waste.

CHAIN OF INFECTION

Any patient receiving an invasive procedure, such as a parenteral medication therapy, is susceptible to risk of infection because there is nonintact skin, which is a direct portal of entry for pathogens. This may be caused by the insertion of a catheter line, which remains open to the outside for an extended period of time, or a needle puncture for an injection. These patients are often hospitalized and compromised for many reasons and can require medication immediately because of trauma, infections, hydration, or nutrition. If the medication was not prepared aseptically, or free from contamination of a pathogen, the preparer can transfer an infection causing agent to the patient.

The transmission of diseases or infections follows a path known as the *"six chains of infection."*

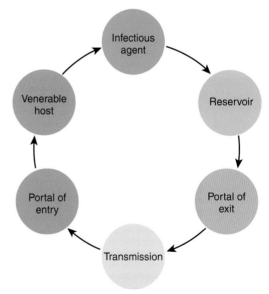

- **Infectious agent**—a pathogen or disease-causing agent. This can be found on the hands or clothing of the preparer if proper hand washing or garbing has not occurred.
- **Reservoir**—source of the infectious agent. This can be the preparer who may or may not know they are carrying the agent.

- **Portal of exit**—site through which the microorganisms enters the host. In parenteral therapy, this is through the opening into the skin made with either a catheter or needle
- **Mode of transmission**—how the organism is transferred from one host to the next. In aseptic technique, this can be the transfer from the preparer to the product and then to the patient.
- **Portal of entry**—how the organism enters the body, which in parenteral therapy is through the opening into the skin made with a needle or catheter for an IV line.
- **Susceptible host**—a person is at risk for infection. Since parenteral therapy requires an opening into the skin, the patient is vulnerable because they have a ready portal of entry directly into the blood stream. If the preparer has not followed proper universal precautions, contamination of the product will allow a pathogen a direct method of entry into a vulnerable patient.

 Tech Note!

ANY break in the chain will stop the process of transferring the infection. By understanding the proper techniques for hand hygiene, garbing, and aseptic technique, the preparer can stop the transfer of microorganisms.

UNIVERSAL PRECAUTIONS

United States Pharmacopoeia (USP<797>) requires that "compounding personnel must be properly trained and instructed in aseptic hand cleansing and garbing". The procedures have been outlined by organizations, such as the National Coordinating Committee on Large Volume Parenterals (NCCLVP), and The American Society of Health-System Pharmacists (ASHP). The Centers for Disease Control and Prevention (CDC) recommends following standard precautions, which includes hand washing and use of personal protective equipment or PPE. In addition, transmission precautions are important when performing aseptic manipulations. These include the following:

- Airborne—spread of small particles in the air
- Droplet—spread by coughing, sneezing, or talking
- Contact—spread by skin contact (touch) to the compounded sterile preparation (CSP) or contact with contaminated surfaces.

When preparing CSP's, all three of these must be considered. If the preparer does not use proper precautions, an infection can be spread.

HAND HYGIENE AND GARBING

According to the CDC, one of the most important ways to prevent contamination or transfer of an infection is proper hand washing (Procedure 4.1). This occurs in the ante room or Class 8 environment after garbing has been performed (Procedure 4.2) per the USP<797> chapter. This is the area outside of the clean room or buffer room, where the primary engineering controls (PEC), such as a laminar airflow system or LAFS, are placed, which will be discussed in Chapter 9.

Here are some key points to remember:
- Always remove loose jewelry or any item not easily cleaned.
   For example, personnel must:
- Remove personal outer garments, such as coats, scarves, and hats.
- Remove any loose powder-based cosmetics because they shed flakes and particles.

Procedure 4.1 Proper Hand Hygiene

GOAL: To learn to follow proper hand washing procedures to prevent the spread of infection.

EQUIPMENT AND SUPPLIES

- Facility-approved hand cleanser
- Nail brush or scrub sponge
- Nonshedding disposable towels or an electronic hand dryer
- Warm water
- Waterless alcohol-based hand rub

REMEMBER

- Personal electronic devices, such as cell phones or iPods and any associated attachments, must be removed before hand washing and should not be used in the sterile compounding area.

PROCEDURAL STEPS

1. Remove all visible jewelry and cosmetics before beginning the hand washing process.
   PURPOSE: To minimize the risk of bacterial contamination by minimizing the number of particles introduced into the sterile compounding area.
2. Wash the hands, nails, wrists, and forearms up to the elbows for at least 30 seconds with a brush and/or sponge, warm water, and a facility-approved cleansing agent.
   PURPOSE: To make certain all surfaces are clean and free from any residue. The cleansing agent should remain in contact with the skin for at least 30 seconds to complete the bactericidal activity.

Procedure 4.1   Proper Hand Hygiene—cont'd

3. Rinse thoroughly with the hands and forearms in an upright position, beginning with the fingertips down to the elbows.
   PURPOSE: To make certain contaminants flow away from the hands and all cleansing residue is removed.

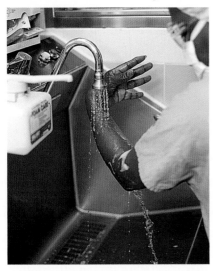

4. Dry the hands and arms with a non-shedding or lint-free cloth or with an electronic hand dryer.
   PURPOSE: To ensure that no contaminants are transferred from the towel to the clean hands. Remember to leave the water running, while you dry your hands and arms, and do not touch any part of the sink or dryer surfaces.*
5. After the hands and arms are completely dry, throw away damp towels and use a new towel to turn off the running water.
   PURPOSE: To ensure that clean hands and arms are not contaminated by touching any unclean surfaces.
6. Sanitize the hands by applying a waterless, alcohol-based hand rub and allow it to dry completely before putting on sterile gloves.
   PURPOSE: To prohibit regrowth of bacteria after hand washing.

*Touch is the most common source of contamination. Hands and gloves remain sterile only until they touch something.
Procedure and photo from Davis K, Guerra A: *Mosby's pharmacy technician*, ed 5, St Louis, 2019, Elsevier.

Procedure 4.2   Personnel Cleansing and Garbing Order

GOAL: To learn the steps required to cleanse and garb up, to properly prepare compounded sterile preparations

EQUIPMENT AND SUPPLIES

- Antiseptic hand cleanser
- Face mask or eye shield
- Head and facial hair cover
- Nonshedding gown
- Shoe covers
- Sterile powder-free gloves
- Surgical scrub

PROCEDURAL STEPS

1. Remove all personal outer garments.
   PURPOSE: Outer garments such as jackets or coats may have shedding fibers or hairs that could contaminate the compounding area.
2. Remove all cosmetics and jewelry (no artificial nails are allowed).
   PURPOSE: Cosmetics can flake off and jewelry and artificial nails can have dirt and other debris on and under the surface. These contaminants can be carried into the compounding area if not removed.

3. Put on personal protective equipment in the following order:
   Shoe covers
   Head and facial hair covers
   Face masks/eye shields

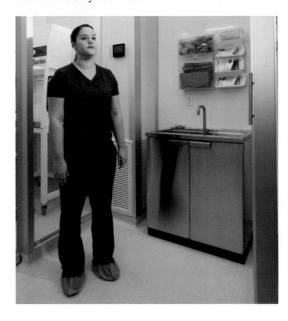

Continued

Procedure 4.2   Personnel Cleansing and Garbing Order—cont'd

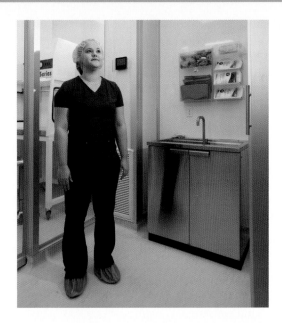

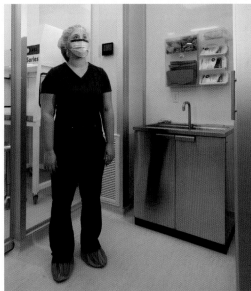

PURPOSE: Shoe covers help prevent any germs that may be on your shoes from entering the compounding area. Head and facial hair covers are used to keep any hairs from falling into the compounding area. Face masks and eye shields are used to protect the technician from exposure to medications that may splash or may accidentally spill during the compounding process.

4. Perform aseptic hand cleansing procedures with a surgical scrub.

   PURPOSE: Proper hand washing with a surgical scrub helps to lessen the bacteria found on the hands before beginning the compounding process.

5. Put on a nonshedding gown.

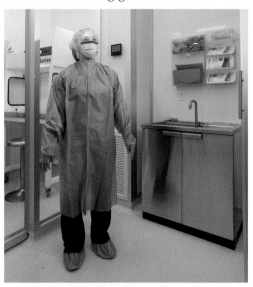

PURPOSE: Donning a nonshedding gown serves to prevent any contaminants that may be on the technician's clothes from getting into the compounding area. Most gowns are resistant to penetration by moisture, which helps protect the technician if a spill occurs.

6. Put on the sterile, powder-free gloves.

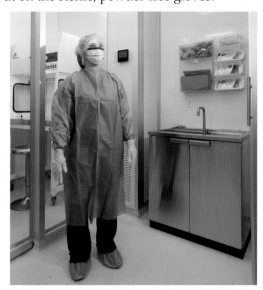

PURPOSE: Gloves protect the compounding area from skin that is constantly shedding from our hands. They also protect the technician from exposure to medications that may be used in the compounding process. Double gloving is recommended when compounding hazardous drugs or chemicals.

Procedure excluding photos from Davis K, Guerra A: *Mosby's pharmacy technician*, ed 5, St Louis, 2019, Elsevier.

- Remove all hand, wrist, and ear jewelry.
- Cover any markings or tattoos that cannot be removed.
- Keep natural nails clean and neatly trimmed to minimize particle shedding and avoid glove punctures. (No nail polish or artificial nails.)

Hand Hygiene Procedures Per USP<797>
After donning shoe covers, put on head and facial hair covers and face masks, and perform hand washing using unscented soap and water. Alcohol hand sanitizers alone are not sufficient. Brushes are not recommended because of the potential for skin irritation and increased bacterial shedding. Dry hands and forearms with either low-lint disposable towels or wipes. After hands are washed and dried, use an antiseptic agent before donning sterile gloves. Apply the product to dry hands only.
STEPS
- Wash hands and forearms up to the elbows with unscented soap and water for at least 30 seconds.
- Dry hands and forearms to the elbows completely with low-lint disposable towels or wipes.
- Immediately before donning sterile gloves, apply a suitable alcohol-based hand rub.
- Allow hands to dry thoroughly before donning sterile gloves.

 Tech Note!
Hand hygiene is required before initiating any compounding activities and when entering the ante area after a break in compounding activity.

Once proper hand washing is performed with all PPE on as described earlier, apply an alcohol-based hand rub and allow to dry before putting on sterile gloves.

Compounding personnel must be aware of the risks associated with the preparation of sterile medications and show diligence to ensure patient safety. This requires a personal responsibility along with USP<797> required testing and monitoring of skills and final products. Contamination can occur with the smallest error and result in significant harm or even death to the patient.

ENVIRONMENTAL CONTROLS
In addition to work practice controls, such as hand hygiene and proper garbing, the environment where sterile compounding takes place must be free of contamination. This requires specific cleaning procedures and documentation, as well as control and monitoring of temperature and humidity (to be discussed in Chapter 8) (Fig. 4.1).

WASTE MANAGEMENT
As part of infection control measures, waste management must be included. Expired, unused, or contaminated nonhazardous medications, such as IV bags, are

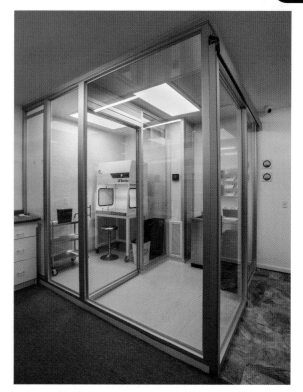
Fig. 4.1 Sterile compounding environment.

discarded in BLUE or BLUE and WHITE pharmaceutical waste containers. They are made of heavy plastic and are lined to prevent leakage of fluids. Needles and other sharp objects, such as broken ampules, are disposed of in RED biomedical plastic containers or bags. Supply packaging, gowns, and other PPE used in nonhazardous sterile preparation can be disposed of in the regular trash can.

Hazardous pharmaceutical waste and medications are to be disposed on in BLACK containers. This also includes the US Environmental Protection Agency (EPA)'s -P Listing of certain medications, as listed subsequently:
- Arsenic trioxide
- Nitroglycerin
- Phentermine
- Physostigmine
- Warfarin
- Empty containers of P-listed medications.

In addition, all chemotherapy medications are listed as U, and should be discarded in YELLOW containers. Dual waste (hazardous + infectious) goes into proper containers (PURPLE buckets), such as Live vaccines: Tetanus Toxoid, and Decavac (Fig. 4.2).

 Tech Note!
Do not flush down the toilet or pour down the sink any discarded medications, such as IV fluids. These medications may get into the water source and contaminate the environment.

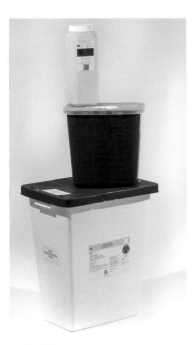

Fig. 4.2 Various sharps containers.

It is the responsibility of the preparer to ensure that proper techniques and disposal are followed in compounding sterile medications to ensure the safety of the healthcare staff, environment, and the receiving patient. Following industry standards, such as USP<797> guidelines for handwashing and garbing, is imperative to ensure a contamination-free sterile product is prepared.

REVIEW QUESTIONS

1. When discussing the chain of infection, this would be the term used to describe the interaction between the infectious agent and the host.
   A. Portal of entry
   B. Reservoir
   C. Portal of exit
   D. Mode of transmission
2. When preparing sterile compounds, it is important to remember, transmission methods include all the following, except:
   A. Germs
   B. Airborne
   C. Droplet
   D. Contact
3. In which of the following environment does handwashing take place?
   A. ISO Class 8
   B. ISO Class 7
   C. ISO Class 5
   D. Outside the LAFS
4. What is the proper order for garbing?
   A. Shoes, head cover, face mask, gown
   B. Gown, face mask, head cover, shoes
   C. Shoes, head cover, face mask, gloves, gown
   D. Gown, face mask, head covers, shoes, gloves

5. Nonhazardous IV bags with medication should be properly disposed of using the following method.
   A. Placed in a BLUE plastic disposal container
   B. Placed in a RED plastic disposal container
   C. Placed in a PURPLE disposal container
   D. Placed in a BLACK disposal container
6. A patient brings back a nitroglycerin bottle that has expired. Which would be the proper color of disposal container to use?
   A. RED
   B. BLACK
   C. PURPLE
   D. BLUE
7. Used PPE should be disposed of by which of the following methods?
   A. Placed in the regular trash
   B. Placed in a BLUE disposal container
   C. Placed in a YELLOW disposal container
   D. Placed in a PURPLE disposal container
8. Discarded chemotherapy medication vials should be placed in which of the following for disposal?
   A. BLUE container
   B. YELLOW container
   C. BLACK container
   D. PURPLE container
9. This organization requires all compounding personnel to be properly trained in hand washing and garbing.
   A. USP
   B. CDC
   C. NVVLP
   D. ASHP
10. This describes a compounder who may carry an infectious disease that could be transferred.
    A. Infectious agent
    B. Reservoir
    C. Susceptible host
    D. All of the above

CRITICAL THINKING

You are working in the IV room all week. When you wake up this morning, you feel like you have some respiratory problems. Describe how the infection you may have could be transferred through compounding, using the steps in the chain of infection.

BIBLIOGRAPHY

1. Blanchard, Loeb: *Nurse's handbook of I.V. drugs*, ed 3, Burlington, MA, 2009, Jones & Bartlett.
2. Delgin JH, Vallerand AH: *Davis' drug guide for nurses*, ed 11, Philadelphia, 2009, F.A. Davis Company.
3. Gahart BL, Nazareno AR: *2008 Intravenous medications*, ed 24, St Louis, 2007, Mosby Elsevier.
4. Phillips L: *Manual of I.V. therapeutics: evidence-based practice for infusion therapy*, ed 5, Philadelphia, 2010, F.A. Davis Company.
5. Trissel LA: *Handbook on injectable drugs*, ed 15, Bethesda, MD, 2008, American Society of Health-System Pharmacists.
6. U.S. National Library of Medicine: MedlinePlus: Drugs, Supplements, and Herbal Information. http://www.nlm.nih.gov/medlineplus/druginformation.html. Accessed March 1, 2013.

Calculations Used in Intravenous Preparations

Learning Objectives

1. Calculate the volume of an injectable solution and the quantity of drug in an injectable solution.
2. Calculate intravenous medications from a powder injectable.
3. Calculate intravenous flow rates for intravenous solutions.
4. Calculate a solution using the alligation method.

Terms & Definitions

Concentration Amount of medication per amount of fluid

Diluent Solution used to dilute a powder form of an injectable medication

Electrolytes Dissolved mineral salts, usually found in intravenous fluids, such as total parenteral nutrition or lactated Ringer's solution

Flow rate Amount of medication to be infused over a specific period of time

INTRODUCTION

When preparing intravenous (IV) admixtures, technicians must not only be careful to observe aseptic technique procedures but also be extremely cautious when calculating amounts of medications. These calculations are performed by pharmacists and technicians when the product is being prepared, as well as by the nurses who administer them. Special consideration should be taken with IV calculations, since this route of administration bypasses the alimentary canal and goes directly into the bloodstream. If an error occurs, there is no way to remove the medication from the blood and reverse the unwanted effects. In this chapter, we will discuss calculating medication dosages, as well as common units of measurements and IV flow rates.

Medications given intravenously require special calculations. An intramuscular (IM) injection is given into the skeletal muscle in an aqueous form, and drugs that are water-based are absorbed quickly. If given subcutaneously (Sub-Q), the medication goes into the fatty layers of tissue and is absorbed quickly. An IV medication is given into the vein. All of these routes of administration are most often ordered in milligrams, and these can be administered at home, in the hospital, or in the office.

CALCULATIONS INVOLVING INJECTABLE MEDICATIONS

When calculating the volume of an injectable medication, ratio and proportion is the most common method used. Medication labels will indicate the amount of medication in each unit, such as mg/mL. This information can then be used to calculate the amount of drug needed according to the physician's order or prescription.

IV medications are most often supplied in vials and ampules, which are glass containers. The amount of medication in a particular volume of fluid, such as microgram (mcg), milligram (mg), or gram (g) of medication in each milliliter (mL), will be on the label as the concentration. This will be used to determine how much should be dissolved in the appropriate liquid, such as normal saline (NS) or dextrose. The medication label may also use amounts of medication either in mg, unit (U), milliequivalent (mEq), or millimolar (mM) in a particular volume of fluid. Units are used for vitamins and chemicals, while mEq and mM are measurements for *electrolytes*, such as sodium and potassium and certain drugs. The physician's order will either state the amount of volume needed or the amount of medication needed. With the amount of drug in a specific amount of fluid (*concentration*), a ratio and proportion calculation can determine the correct amount of drug to be used.

 Did You Know?

Because of the recent medication errors with heparin, new safety verification processes have been implemented, such as new product labeling, double checks for medication pulled from inventory by two pharmacy personnel, and verifications for dosages involving one or more technicians, pharmacists, or nurses.

Example 1

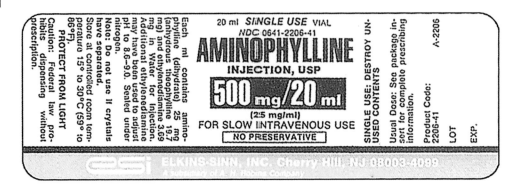

How many milliliters of aminophylline would be required to provide 1500 mg of medication?

$$Answer: \frac{500 \text{ mg}}{20 \text{ mL}} = \frac{1500 \text{ mg}}{X} \, X \, mL =$$

$$\frac{20 \text{ mL} \times 1500 \text{ mg}}{500 \text{ mg}} = 60 \text{ mL}$$

The ratio and proportion method can also be used to determine the amount of drug in an injectable solution.

Example 2

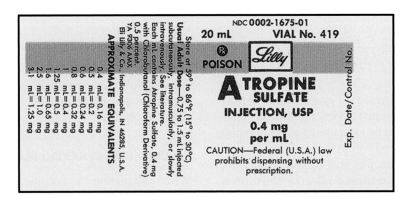

How many milligrams are in 3 mL of atropine?

$$Answer: \frac{0.4 \text{ mg}}{1 \text{ mL}} = \frac{X}{3 \text{ mL}} \, X \, mg =$$

$$\frac{3 \text{ mL} \times 0.4 \text{ mg}}{1 \text{ mL}} = 1.2 \, mg/3 \text{ mL}$$

Example 3

Heparin (Fig. 5.1) and insulin are considered high risk medications and involve additional checks. Heparin comes in several concentrations and the labels are very similar.

 Tech Note!

Inventory management to reduce the possibility of errors can include using special stickers (stop sign here) or placement on the shelves.

Let us look at some typical IV orders that involve units, such as insulin and heparin:

1. Order for heparin 12,000 units in NS 500 mL every (q)8h. How many milliliters of heparin will be needed to prepare one bag?

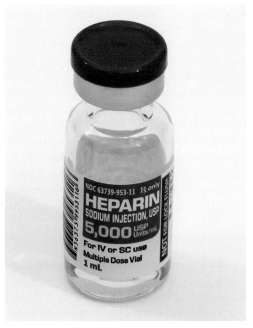

Fig. 5.1 Heparin is considered a high-risk medication and involves additional checks.

Choose the stock vial with the concentration of medication as close as possible to the desired concentration ordered. Since there are 10,000 units in each milliliter of the stock vial of medication, this would be the most appropriate, because the order calls for just a little over 10,000 units of medication to be used.

$$Answer: \frac{10{,}000 \text{ units}}{1 \text{ mL}} = \frac{12{,}000 \text{ units}}{X \text{ mL}} \times \text{mL} =$$

$$\frac{1 \text{ mL} \times 12{,}000 \text{ units}}{10{,}000 \text{ units}} = 1.2 \text{ mL of heparin}$$

2. Order for heparin 5500 units in NS 250 mL q8h. How many milliliters of heparin will be needed to prepare one bag?

   Choose the stock vial with the concentration of medication as close as possible to the desired concentration ordered. Since there are 1000 units in each milliliter of the stock vial of medication, this would be the most appropriate, because the order calls for just a little over 5000 units of medication to be used.

$$Answer: \frac{1000 \text{ units}}{1 \text{ mL}} = \frac{5500 \text{ units}}{X} =$$

$$\frac{1 \text{ mL} \times 5500 \text{ units}}{1000 \text{ units}} = 5.5 \text{ mL}$$

3. An order reads for heparin sodium 600 units subcutaneously stat.

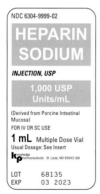

NDC 6304-9999-02

HEPARIN SODIUM

INJECTION, USP

1,000 USP Units/mL

(Derived from Porcine Intestinal Mucosa)
FOR IV OR SC USE

1 mL Multiple Dose Vial
Usual Dosage: See Insert

Knowledge Pharmaceuticals St. Louis, MO 63043 USA

LOT   68135
EXP   03 2023

(Label from Beale E: *Math calculations for pharmacy technicians*, ed 3, St Louis, 2019, Elsevier.)

   a. What volume of medication should be withdrawn from the vial?

$$Answer: \frac{1000 \text{ units}}{1 \text{ mL}} = \frac{600 \text{ units}}{X \text{ mL}} =$$

$$\frac{600 \times 1}{1000} = 0.6 \text{ mL}$$

   b. What size syringe would be most appropriate?
   Answer: **1-mL syringe**

4. An order calls for Humulin R (Fig. 5.2) 15 units each arm.
   a. How many mLs in each dose?

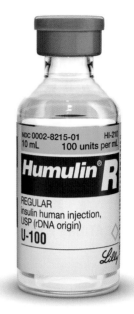

NDC 0002-8215-01   HI-210
10 mL   100 units per mL

Humulin® R

REGULAR
insulin human injection,
USP (rDNA origin)
U-100

Lilly

Fig. 5.2 Insulin vial and label. (Courtesy Eli Lilly and Company, Indianapolis, IN.)

$$Answer: \frac{100 \text{ units}}{1 \text{ mL}} = \frac{15 \text{ units}}{x \text{ mLs}} = \frac{15 \times 1}{100} = 0.15$$

   b. How many vials will they need for 30-days supply?
   Answer: 0.15 × 30 days = 4.5 mLs so one vial of 10 mL is dispensed

> 💬 **Tech Note!**
>
> Insulin vials are not dispensed in partials. Calculate to closest amount needed and dispense whole vials

5. An order calls for Humulin R 32 units at each meal.

$$Answer: \frac{100 \text{ units}}{1 \text{ mL}} = \frac{32 \text{ units}}{x \text{ mLs}}$$

$$\frac{32 \times 1}{100} = 0.32 \text{ (each dose) there are 3}$$

   Answer: 0.32 × 3 = 0.96 × 30 days = 28.8 mLs so 3 vials of 10 mL each are needed.

6. An order reads, "Add 44 mEq of sodium chloride (NaCl) to an IV bag." Using a stock label of 4 mEq/mL, how many milliliters of sodium chloride will be needed for this order?

$$Answer: \frac{4 \text{ mEq}}{1 \text{ mL}} = \frac{44 \text{ mEq}}{X \text{ mL}} \times \text{mL} =$$

$$\frac{44 \text{ mEq} \times 1 \text{ mL}}{4 \text{ mEq}} = 1 \text{ mL}$$

7. A hospice patient has been ordered a morphine drip. The order reads:
   Give morphine 10 mg per hour × 24 hours. Mix in D5W. How much morphine should be provided

to make a 24-hour supply? Note: Use a stock label of morphine 15 mg/mL.

$$Answer: \frac{15 \text{ mg}}{1 \text{ mL}} = \frac{10 \text{ mL}}{x \text{ mL}} = \frac{10 \times 1}{15} =$$
$$0.66 \text{ mL per hour}$$

0.66 mL × 24 (for each hour) = 16 mL needed for the day

*withdraw and add morphine 16 mL to the D5W bag

SPECIAL CONSIDERATIONS FOR PARENTERAL MEDICATIONS

POWDER VOLUME

Vials of medication can contain either a solution or a powder (Fig. 5.3). If it is in powder form, then it is made in a freeze-dried state and placed in a sterile container. To create a solution from this and be able to draw up the contents in a syringe, the powder must be reconstituted by adding a solution, such as bacteriostatic water, sterile water, or saline, known as a *diluent*. The correct type and amount of diluent can be found in drug references, such as the package insert or the *Handbook on Injectable Drugs* by Trissell.[9] It is very important to use the manufacturer's recommended solution to dilute the powder because each drug and patient is different.

> ### Tech Note!
> Bacteriostatic water for injection USP is a nonpyogenic preparation of water injection containing 0.9% of benzyl alcohol as a bacteriostatic preservative (www.drugs.com). Since benzyl alcohol is toxic in neonates, it cannot be used as a diluent for IV dilution in this population.

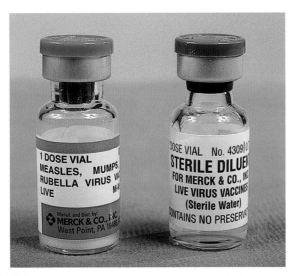

Fig. 5.3 Vials, powdered form. (From Bonewit-West K: *Clinical procedures for medical assistants,* ed 8, St Louis, 2012, Elsevier Saunders.)

This space that the powder occupies is known as *powder volume (PV)*. It is equal to the difference between the final volume (FV) and the volume of the diluting agent.

Formula

$$\text{powder volume (PV)} = \text{final volume (FV)} - \text{diluent volume (DV)}$$

Example 4 A powder antibiotic known as nafcillin sodium needs to be reconstituted for use. You must follow the manufacturer's reconstitution directions and then prepare an IV bag.
1. How much diluent will be used?
   Answer: 6.6 mL
2. What will the resulting powder volume be?
   Answer: 8 mL (FV) - 6.6 mL (DV) = 1.4 mL (PV)
3. What is the amount of medication in each milliliter?
   Answer: 250 mg

Example 5 You have an order for a medication that requires you to reconstitute 1 g of a dry powder. The label states to add 9.3 mL of diluent to make a final solution of 100 mg/mL. What is the powder volume?
Step 1. Calculate the final volume by starting with the fact that 1 g is the same as 1000 mg of powder. Using the information, calculate the final volume using the ratio and proportion method:

$$\frac{1000 \text{ mg of powder}}{X \text{ mL}} = \frac{100 \text{ mg}}{1 \text{ mL}} = 10 \text{ mL (FV)}$$

Step 2. Using the **calculated** final volume, use the formula to determine the powder volume.

$$Remember: \text{ powder volume (PV)} = \text{final volume (FV)} - \text{diluent volume (DV)}$$
$$PV = 10 \text{ mL} - 9.3 \text{ mL} = 0.7 \text{ mL}$$

CALCULATION EXAMPLES FOR INTRAVENOUS MIXTURES

PREPARING INTRAVENOUS MEDICATIONS FROM A POWDER INJECTABLE

Example 6
Miss Davis has penicillin (Pfizerpen) 400,000 units/NS 100 mL ordered for a severe infection. After reading the dilution directions, you add 75 mL of diluent to the powder vial. Based on this information, how many milliliters will need to be added to the bag of NS 100 mL for the order?
250,000 units in each milliliter is the amount of drug in each milliliter according to the label if 75 mL of diluent was added.

$$\frac{250,000 \text{ units}}{1 \text{ mL}} = \frac{400,000 \text{ units}}{X \text{ mL}} =$$
$$250,000 \text{ units} \times X \text{ mL } 400,000 \text{ units} \times 1 \text{ mL} = 1.6$$

Answer: The technician will now draw up 1.6 mL of Pfizerpen and add it to the bag of normal saline 100 mL.

Example 7

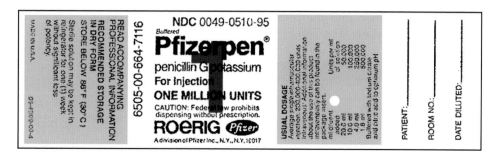

Using the same medication as earlier, add 11.5 mL of diluent to the vial of penicillin (Pfizerpen) and answer the following questions concerning the following order for Mr. Brown:

Pfizerpen 6,000,000 in NS 100 mL immediately (STAT).
1. How many units of medication is in each milliliter if 11.5 mL of diluent was added?
    Answer: 1,000,000 units/mL.
2. How many milliliters of Pfizerpen will need to be added to the bag for a dose of 6,000,000 units?

$$Answer: \frac{1{,}000{,}000 \text{ units}}{1 \text{ mL}} = \frac{6{,}000{,}000 \text{ units}}{X \text{ mL}} = 6 \text{ mL}$$

CALCULATING INTRAVENOUS ADMIXTURE FLOW RATES

An IV admixture order contains the IV fluid to be given, any additives, and the rate at which it should be infused. This *flow rate* is written as the amount of drug that is infused over a time period. This could be written as milliliters per hour (mL/h) or drops per minute (gtt/min). Administration sets come in a variety of sizes and are measured by a drop factor. This is the number of drops in a milliliter. Often the order will require the drug to be administered with a pump or IV infusion set for drops per minute (gtt/min). The appropriate amount of medication must be given over a certain period of time to ensure that the therapeutic response is achieved. As a pharmacy technician, there are often times that you will have to determine how many bags to make in a batch to last 24 hours.

Example 8

517410	DX: dehydration
05/04/55	ALLERGIES: NKA
K. Davis	
Rm: 433	
08/11/13	
1 L D5W with 20 mEq KCl added at 125 mL/h	

NKA, No known allergies.

In the aforementioned example, this bag will last 8 hours.

$$\text{Time the bag will last} = \frac{\text{volume of fluid}}{\text{flow rate}}$$

$$1 \text{ L} = 1000 \text{ mL} \quad \frac{1000 \text{ mL}}{125 \text{ mL/h}} = 8 \text{ hours to infuse}$$

A new bag will be needed every 8 hours for this order. As a technician making a 24-hour supply of IV fluids for this patient, you would determine that three bags should be sent to the floor using the subsequent formula:

$$\frac{24 \text{ hours}}{8 \text{ hours to infuse}} = 3 \text{ bags needed to last for 24 hours}$$

> **! Tech Alert!**
>
> Round down the duration of therapy to the whole hour. This will ensure that the nurse will hang the new bag before the old one is completely out.

Example 9

If an IV is running at 125 mL/h and three 1 liter (L) bags are sent to the floor, how long will these bags last?

1 L = 1000 mL × 3 = 3000 mL total volume

$$Answers: X \text{ hours} = \frac{3000 \text{ mL (3L)}}{125 \text{ mL/h}} = 24 \text{ hours}$$

If the order specifies a certain amount of medication to be given over a specific time period, this can also be determined.

Example 10

Medication: hydrocortisone sodium succinate (Solu-Cortef) 300 mg
Fluid volume: 250 mL
Time of infusion: 4 hours
What volume of fluid is to be given per hour, and what amount of drug is given per hour?
Determine the volume of fluid given by hour:

$$\frac{250 \text{ mL}}{4 \text{ hours}} = 62.5 \text{ mL/h}$$

The amount of drug per hour:

$$\frac{300 \text{ mg}}{4 \text{ hours}} = 75 \text{ mg/h}$$

Pumps are infusion devices, which are often used to deliver the IV therapy at home and in the hospital because they can ensure a predetermined flow rate. The amount of fluid can be programmed into the pump and then delivered to the patient safely (Fig. 5.4).

> **Tech Note!**
>
> Errors usually occur in the programming and all calculations should be double-checked. Since there are many types of pumps, special training is also involved, and caution is mandatory.

Drop sets are used to manually adjust the flow at the drop chamber or set the IV pump at the patient's bedside (Fig. 5.5). This setting can be determined by using mL/h or gtts/mL, depending on the patient and the medication. The larger the diameter of the tubing where it enters the drip chamber, the bigger the drop will be. An IV set is identified by the number of drops it takes to make 1 mL.

Common sets include:

- 10 gtt/mL: Macro set commonly used for 125 mL/h or more
- 15 to 20 gtt/mL: Macro set commonly used for 125 mL/h
- 60 gtt/mL: Often referred to as the minidrip or microdrip set and generally used for delivering amounts of fluids per hour 50 mL/h or less to critically ill or pediatric patients who are being given medication that is very specific in its dosing.

To determine a flow rate using gtts/min, the following formula should be used.

$$X \, gtt/min = \frac{(volume \, of \, fluid/delivery \, time) \times (set \, drop \, rate)}{60 \, min/h}$$

Example 11

If an IV is running at 60 mL/h, what is the rate in gtt/min using a 15 gtt/mL set?

Volume of fluid: 60 mL

Fluid delivery time: 1 hour

Drop rate of administration set: 15 gtt/mL

$$Answers: X \, gtt/min = \frac{(60 \, mL/1 \, h) \times (15 \, gtt/mL)}{60 \, min/h}$$
$$= 15 \, gtt/min$$

Example 12

You are to prepare an IV of 750 mg of medication in 75 mL to be infused over 30 minutes using a 10 gtt/mL set. How many drops per minute will that be?

Volume of fluid: 75 mL

Fluid delivery time: 30 minutes or 0.5 hours

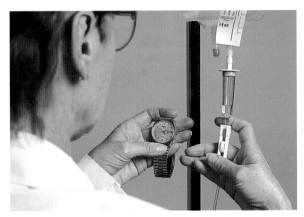

Fig. 5.5 Intravenous (IV) drop sets. (From Macklin D, Chernecky C, Infortuna MH: *Math for clinical practice*, ed 2, St Louis, 2011, Mosby Elsevier.)

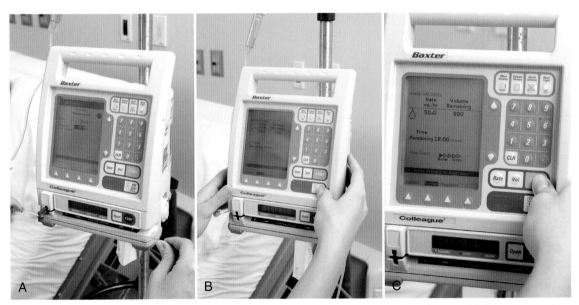

Fig. 5.4 Baxter infusion pump. (A) Insert intravenous tubing into chamber of control mechanism. (B) Select rate and volume to be infused. (C) Press start button. (From Perry AG, Potter PA, Elkin MK: *Nursing interventions and clinical skills*, ed 4, St. Louis, 2007, Elsevier Mosby.)

Drop rate of administration set: 10 gtt/mL

$$\text{Answers: } X \text{ gtt/min} = \frac{(75 \text{ mL}/0.5 \text{ h}) \times (10 \text{ gtt/mL})}{60 \text{ min/h}}$$
$$= 25 \text{ gtt/min}$$

 Tech Alert!

Flow rates are rounded to the nearest whole gtt. This will ensure that the bag will not empty before the next one is hung.

When a microdrip set is used, the flow rate in gtt/min is exactly the same as the volume in mL/h to be infused because there are 60 minutes in an hour and 60 drops in a minute.

Example 13
120 mL/h using a microdrip set = 120 gtt/min
80 mL/h using a microdrip set = 80 gtt/min
To determine the flow rate using gtt/mL, you must first determine the mL/h that it is running. Then, convert that number to mL/min, and calculate the gtt/min.

Example 14 An IV of 2500 mL is ordered to infuse in 24 hours using a 20 gtt/mL microdrip set.

1. $\dfrac{2500 \text{ mL}}{24 \text{ hours}} = 104 \text{ mL/h}$

2. $\dfrac{104 \text{ mL}}{60 \text{ mins}} = 1.7 \text{ mL/min}$

3. $\dfrac{20 \text{ gtt}}{1 \text{ mL}} = \dfrac{X \text{ gtt}}{1.7 \text{ mL}} = 34 \text{ gtt/min}$

A simpler way to show this is as follows:

$$\frac{(2500 \text{ mL}/24 \text{ h}) \times 20 \text{ gtt}}{60 \text{ min}} = 34.7 \text{ or } 34 \text{ gtt/min}$$

CALCULATING DILUTIONS USING ALLIGATIONS*

Alligation is a method of calculating mixtures of solutions that each have different percentage strengths. This requires determining a final strength from calculating the two initial stock medications. It is most commonly seen in total parenteral nutrition compounds as stock solutions, such as dextrose 10% or 70%, may be in stock, but the order requires a final solution of 20%.

To begin alligation alternate, think of preparing a box for playing tic-tac-toe to allow the numbers to be placed in the four corners and in the center box.

Steps and examples in this section are from Fulcher RM, Fulcher EM: *Math calculations for pharmacy technicians: a worktext*, ed 2, St Louis, 2013, Saunders.

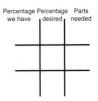

Step 1—Prepare the graph.
Step 2—Place the strength to be calculated in the center box.
Step 3—Place the highest percentage concentration in the left upper corner.
Step 4—Place the lowest percentage concentration in the lower left corner.
Step 5—Subtract the center square from the left upper square and place in the lower right square to reveal the parts of the lowest percentage concentration to be used in the new mixture.
Step 6—Subtract the lower left square from the center box and place in the upper right corner to reveal the parts of the highest percentage concentration to be used in the new mixture.
Step 7—Add the calculated parts together to find the total parts of the two ingredients in the compound.
Step 8—When the total quantity of the mixture is included in the prescription, then the parts of the mixture are placed into two ratio and proportion equations to calculate the exact amount of each ingredient to use. The total number of calculated parts is placed in the first ratio with the total amount of compound. The second ratio set in the proportion is the calculated number of parts of the stock ingredients to the unknown total compound amount. This step must be calculated for each part of the compound.

Example 15 Prepare 1 L solution of 70% alcohol from 50% alcohol and 95% alcohol.
Step 1—Draw the graph for calculating alligation.

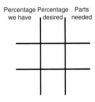

Step 2—Place the strength to be calculated in the center box.

Step 3—Place the highest percentage concentration in the left upper corner.

Step 4—Place the lowest percentage concentration in the lower left corner.

Percentage Percentage Parts
we have / desired / needed

95%

70%

50%

Step 5—Subtract the center square from the left upper square and place in the lower right square to reveal the parts of the lowest percentage concentration to be used in the new mixture.

Percentage Percentage Parts
we have / desired / needed

95%

70%

50%   25 parts

Step 6—Subtract the lower left square from the center box and place in the upper right corner to reveal the parts of the highest percentage concentration to be used in the new mixture.

Percentage Percentage Parts
we have / desired / needed

95%   20 parts

70%

50%   25 parts

Step 7—Add the parts of the concentration to find the total parts in the compound.

Percentage Percentage Parts
we have / desired / needed

95%   20 parts

70%

50%   25 parts
       45 parts

To prepare this solution, mix 20 parts of 95% alcohol with 25 parts of 50% alcohol.

Remember, this is a proportional amount that must be used to find the exact part amounts when the total weight or volume of the compound is indicated.

Step 8—Using the previous example, the total amount of the solution is 1 L of 70% alcohol.

The total number of compound parts as calculated using the alligation graph is 45 parts in 1000 mL (1 L) of solution.

First, calculate the number of milliliters of 95% alcohol (stock solution).

45 parts :1000 mL :: 20 parts : x
45 parts × x = 20 parts ×1000 mL
45 parts × x = 20 parts ×1000 mL
45x = 20,000 mL
x = 444.4 mL of 95% alcohol or 444 mL of 95% alcohol

Second, calculate the total number of milliliters of 50% alcohol (stock solution).

45 parts :1000 mL :: 25 parts : x
45 parts × x = 1000 mL × 25 parts
45 parts × x = 1000 mL × 25 parts
45x = 25,000 mL
x = 555.6 mL of 50% alcohol or 556 mL or 50% alcohol

Now check your calculations:

444 mL of 95% alcohol + 556 mL of 50% alcohol = 1000 mL of 70% alcohol

Therefore the calculations are correct.

Example 16 Prepare 1L of Dextrose 50% from 70% and 20%.

Percentage Percentage Parts
we have / desired / needed

70%   30 parts

50%

20%   20 parts
       50 parts

30 parts 70%
20 parts 20%
50 parts : 1000 mL = 20: x
50 parts × x = 20 parts × 1000
50 parts × x = 20 parts × 1000
50x = 20,000
Answer: x = 400 mL of 20%
50 parts : 1000 mL = 30 : x
50 parts × x = 30 parts × 1000
50 parts × x = 30 parts × 1000
50x = 30,000
Answer: x = 600 mL of 70%

PAIN CONTROLLED ANALGESIA

Often, patients require pain medications intravenously and medications, such as morphine, may be ordered to be infused by patient-controlled analgesia (PCA). PCAs are portable pumps designed for the patient to be able to give themselves a dose on demand.

Example 17 The order would be written as follows: The morphine concentration used is 1 mg/mL per 30-mL vial. What is the pump setting in mL/h?
Answer: 1 mg/10 minutes, 4-hour limit is 30 mg

Example 18

The hydromorphone (Dilaudid) concentration is 1 mg/mL per 30-mL vial. What is the pump setting in mL/h?
Answer: 0.2 mg/15 min, 4-hour limit is 2 mg

Pediatric and elderly patients may need smaller volumes of fluids and medications than young adults. The physician may order the medication based on the recommended adult dose for milligrams per kilogram for 24 hours. Calculations will be determined by using the weight of the patient in kilograms.

Use the following formula:

$$mg/kg/day\,(24\,h)$$

Example 19

Ampicillin 900 mg intravenous piggyback (IVPB) q6h is ordered for a 75-pound patient. How many milligrams per kilogram per 24 hours is the patient receiving?

Convert pounds (lbs) to kilograms using the conversion of 1 kg = 2.2 lbs.

1 kg = 2.2 lbs = x kg/75 lbs

Cross multiply to get weight: 75 lb = 34.1 kg

900 mg × 4 doses = 3600 mg/24 h (24 hours divided by every 6 hours = 4 doses a day).

Calculate the dose using mg/kg/day:

$$Answers: \frac{(3600\,mg/24\,h)}{34.1\,kg} = 105.6\,mg/kg/day$$

The recommended dose is 100 to 200 mg/kg/day administered every 6 to 8 hours, so this would be an appropriate dose for this patient. Anything ordered between 100 to 200 mg/kg/day is within the range.

REVIEW QUESTIONS

1. The label of a 4 g vial states that you are to add 11.7 mL to get a concentration of 250 mg/mL. What is the powder volume?
2. The physician has ordered 2800 mL to be given every 24 hours. At what rate should the pump be set to in milliliters per hour?
3. If a patient is given 60 mg of medication in 75 mL over 45 minutes, what is the flow rate in mL/h?
4. For the aforementioned problem, how many milligrams of medication will the patient receive?

5. An IV rate is set for 10 mL/h. If a 10-gtt set is used, what will the rate be in gtt/min?
6. A physician orders 7500 units of heparin IV STAT. Using a vial concentration of 10,000 units per mL, calculate the amount needed to be withdrawn.
   A. 13 mL
   B. 0.75 mL
   C. 1.03 mL
   D. 3 mL

7. A patient has been ordered Vistaril 35 mg IM q 4–6 PRN itching. Using the subsequent label, calculate the amount to be prepared in a syringe for delivery.

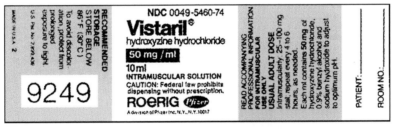

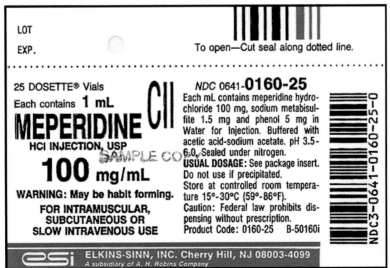

A. .7 mL
B. 0.15 mL
C. 15 mL
D. 0.66 mL

8. An order has been sent for meperidine 60 mg IM q6h PRN pain. Using the aforementioned label, how much medication should be withdrawn for one dosage?
   A. 1.6 mL
   B. 1.7 mL
   C. 0.6 mL
   D. 6 mL
9. Using the aforementioned label, calculate how much would be needed for a 24 hour period?
   A. 2.4 mL
   B. 1.8 mL
   C. 4.8 mL
   D. 6.4 mL

CRITICAL THINKING

1. A postoperative patient has an order for lactated Ringer's solution (LR) 1 L to be infused over 10 hours 3 days. How many milliliters per hour should the IV pump be programmed to deliver this order? How many bags should the technician prepare for a 24-hour period?
2. A pediatric patient has been ordered vancomycin 220 mg q6h IV using a syringe pump. He weighs 48 pounds, and the recommended manufacturer dosage is 40 to 60 mg/kg/24 h q6h. How many mg/kg/24 h is the child receiving? Is this dose appropriate?

BIBLIOGRAPHY

1. 2000–2019 Drugs.com: *Drug Information Online.* www.drugs.com. Accessed April 9, 2019.
2. Fulcher, Robert and Eugenia: *Math calculations for pharmacy technicians. A worktext.* ed 2, 2013, Elsevier.
3. Lacher BE: *Pharmaceutical calculations for the pharmacy technician,* Baltimore, MD, 2008, Lippincott Williams & Wilkins.
4. Pickar GD, Abernethy AP: *Dosage calculations,* ed 9, Clifton Park, NY, 2012, Delmar Cengage Learning.
5. Powers MF, Wakelin JB: *Pharmacy calculations,* ed 2, Englewood, CO, 2005, Morton Publishing Company.
6. Trissel LA: *Handbook on injectable drugs,* ed 15, Bethesda, MD, 2008, American Society of Health-System Pharmacists.

Medication Administration

Learning Objectives

1. Identify the types of parenteral medications and nutrition, and name at least three situations in which it would be beneficial to use a parenteral dose form.
2. Describe two types of intravenous (IV) administration and give an example of each.
3. Name two advantages and two disadvantages of administering IV medications.
4. Discuss the types of parenteral medications and supplies used in both health-system IV administration and home infusion therapy, as well as explain the technician's integral role in preventing medication errors when considering administration of parenteral medications.

Terms & Definitions

Bolus Also known as *direct injection* or *intravenous push (IV push; IVP)*; small amount of medication injected into a port, usually in an existing IV line

Epidural injection Injection into the epidural space

Intraarterial injection Injection into an artery

Intracardiac (IC) injection Injection into the cardiac muscle or heart

Intradermal (ID) route Injection into the dermal layer of the skin

Intramuscular (IM) injection Injection into the muscle

Intrathecal (IT) route Injection into the spinal canal

Intravenous (IV) injection Injection into the vein

IV push (IVP) Also known as *bolus*; small amount of medication injected into a port usually in an existing IV line

Lactated Ringer's solution (LR) Sterile isotonic intravenous fluid used for electrolyte or fluid replacement

Normal saline (NS) Sterile intravenous solution, also known as *sodium chloride*, used as a source of water or for fluid replacement

Subcutaneous route of administration Injection just below the skin into the subcutaneous fat layer

INTRODUCTION

Pharmacy technicians must have a good understanding of routes of administrations for parenteral medications. Certain drugs are available in limited forms and require special considerations when mixing with fluids and performing aseptic technique. In some cases, there are even medications that can only be administered one way and require special equipment that must be included with the prepared admixture. In this chapter, we will discuss patient considerations, some advantages and disadvantages of parenteral therapy, and types of infusions to avoid potential errors that may occur if not considered.

PARENTERAL MEDICATIONS AND NUTRITION

Medications that are given intravenously bypass the digestive processes. These medications reach the bloodstream almost immediately and can be useful in emergency situations where fluid replacement is needed and another dosage form is not appropriate. A parenteral dosage form may be administered in several ways, including methods such as intravenous (IV), intramuscular (IM), intracardiac (IC), and intrathecal (IT), but the most common is intravenously (Fig. 6.1).

IV injection medications are administered directly into the bloodstream through a vein. It is the most common parenteral route, and it has rapid effects. Injections can be via a syringe and needle, or in some cases, through a pump or programmable machine, such as for pain or diabetes control. This route is administered either through a peripheral line or a central line. A peripheral line goes into the extremities, such as the arm, hands, and feet.

Peripheral veins are smaller, which allows medication to be injected more easily. This is the most common method of administration. A central line is used for a weak patient or for one who has weak peripheral veins. Medications, such as total parenteral nutrition (TPN) or chemotherapy, are usually too concentrated for peripheral veins and are given centrally through an implanted port because there is more blood volume running through these larger veins.

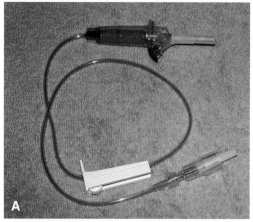

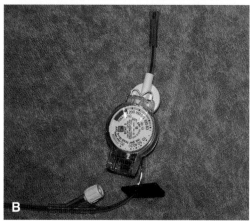

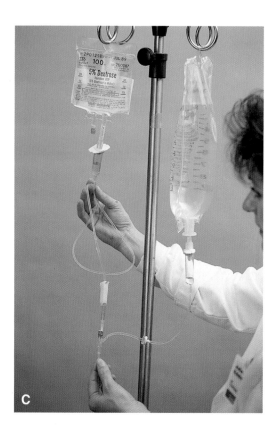

Fig. 6.1 (A) Primary infusion set showing drip chamber, tubing, and roller clamp. (B) Primary infusion set for IV piggyback (IVPB) additions. (C) IVPB being added to a primary line. (A and B, From Brown M, Mulholland JM: *Drug calculations: process and problems for clinical practice*, ed 8, St. Louis, Mosby, 2008. C, From Potter P, Perry A: *Fundamentals of nursing*, ed 8, St. Louis, 2013, Mosby.)

IM injections, such as hormones, vaccinations, and some antibiotics, are given directly into the muscle (Fig. 6.2).

IC injection medications are usually used in emergencies and 2013, are typically found on emergency or crash carts. These medications, such as epinephrine, are often used quickly to resuscitate a patient and are therefore packaged in prefilled disposable syringes with attached needles.

The ID route is used to inject medications in the capillary rich layer below the epidermis, such as in a skin test for tuberculosis (Fig. 6.3).

The IT route is used for injections directly into the space surrounding the spinal cord. Meningitis patients often receive injections through the IT route when a spinal tap is performed. All medications given through this route are preservative-free because the body may not be able to break them down, which could cause permanent paralysis.

Intraarterial injections may be used to inject anesthesia medications or dyes into an artery during a procedure, such as a heart catheterization.

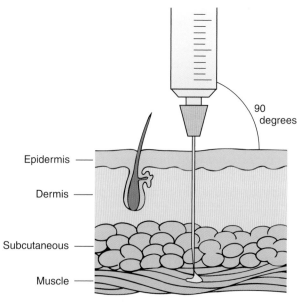

Fig. 6.2 An intramuscular (IM) injection. (From Clayton BD, Stock YN, Cooper SE: *Basic pharmacology for nurses*, ed 15, St Louis, 2010, Mosby Elsevier.)

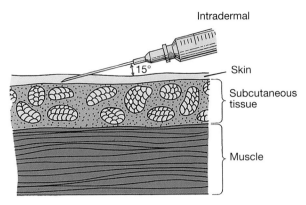

Fig. 6.3 Intradermal needle tip inserted into dermis. (From Perry AG, Potter PA, Elkin MK: *Nursing interventions & clinical skills*, ed 5, St Louis, 2012, Mosby.)

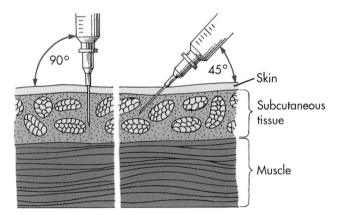

Fig. 6.4 Subcutaneous injection. Angle and needle length depend on thickness of skin fold. (From Perry AG, Potter PA, Elkin MK: *Nursing interventions & clinical skills*, ed 5, St Louis, 2012, Mosby.)

The subcutaneous route of administration is used for slowly absorbed medications, like insulin or heparin (Fig. 6.4).

! Tech Alert!

The abbreviation SQ or SC should not be used for subcutaneous because it could be mistaken for SL or sublingual and increase the chance of an error. You can find a list of "DO NOT USE ABBREVIATIONS" on The Joint Commission website at *http://www.jointcommission.org/assets/1/18/Do_ Not_Use_List.pdf*.

A direct injection, often called a bolus or IV push (IVP), is a small amount of medication in a syringe injected directly into a port in an existing IV line over 5 to 15 minutes, such as a pain medication. Pain or nausea medications for a hospital patient may be injected through the IV line for patients who already have an IV line inserted. This type of injection allows the patient to receive necessary medications, without the additional "stick" or puncture (Fig. 6.5).

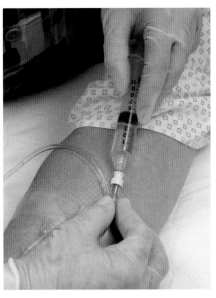

Fig. 6.5 Connecting the syringe to IV line with needleless blunt cannula tip. (From Perry AG, Potter PA, Elkin MK: *Nursing interventions & clinical skills*, ed 5, St Louis, 2012, Mosby.)

Epidural injections are given into the epidural space, such as anesthesia medication during labor.

Oral dosage forms must pass through the digestive processes to reach the bloodstream and be distributed to the organs and tissues.

Some drugs, such as heparin (an anticoagulant), are broken down completely by stomach acids and, for this reason, must be given parenterally. Therefore much of what determines the best route of administration results from the drug's effectiveness. There are also diseases or conditions that lead to the inability of a patient to be able to take an oral dose form, such as a tablet or an oral solution. These may include patients who are:
- Unconscious
- Experiencing extreme nausea and vomiting
- Unable to swallow a tablet, such as a child or elderly patient
- Uncooperative because of illness, such as psychiatric disorders
- Experiencing a life-threatening situation, such as blood loss, where immediate replacement intervention is required
- Unable to absorb medication through the gastrointestinal (GI) tract because of disease
- Extremely dehydrated.

INTRAVENOUS ADMINISTRATION

There are different types of IV administration. An IV injection can be a small amount of medication in a syringe injected directly into the vein through the skin, such as a pain medication. This method is called *IVP*. Sometimes these are injected directly into a port in an existing IV line to avoid an additional puncture in the skin. If a larger amount of medication is needed, it

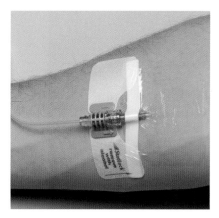

Fig. 6.6 Catheter stabilization device in place. Image © 2019 BD. Used with permission.

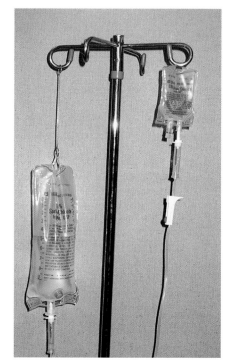

Fig. 6.7 A set of piggybacks. (From Brown M, Mulholland JL. *Drug calculations: process and problems for clinical practice*, ed 8, St Louis, 2007, Mosby.)

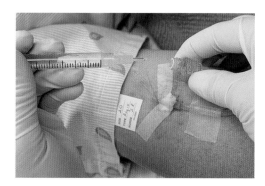

Fig. 6.8 Push; a small amount of medication injected directly into a vein, such as with pain medication. (From Ogden SJ, Fluharty LK. *Calculation of drug dosages: a worktext*, ed 9, St Louis, 2012, Elsevier Mosby.)

may be given as an IV infusion. This is designed to allow the medication to flow into the bloodstream over a longer period of time, such as in a blood transfusion or antibiotic treatment, which takes about 30 minutes. An IV catheter is inserted into the patient, with tubing that connects to the bag(s) (Fig. 6.6).

IV medications may be given continuously or intermittently. This is usually in the form of a large volume parenteral (LVP) between 250 and 1000 mL and over 2 to 24 hours. The orders will determine a rate of infusion, which is the amount of fluid that should enter the body over a certain period of time. This is often regulated with an infusion pump or electronic device. Examples of IV injections include hydration fluids, blood products, or drugs that need to be maintained at a constant or steady level for the patient.

Secondary infusions can be given along with a continuous infusion if they are compatible with the use of special multiple line tubing. This could be an antibiotic that is given 4 or 6 times daily over a short period of time, while a larger bag of fluid is being given continuously for hydration.

Intermittent infusions are volumes of fluid from 25 to 250 mL and are often infused from 15 to 90 minutes at specific intervals. These drugs can be given in between a continuous infusion and often through the existing tubing, so long as there are no compatibility issues with the drugs themselves. Examples include an antibiotic ordered at 6 hours over 30 minutes. This drug would be mixed in a small amount of fluid, such as dextrose or sodium chloride, and administered at specific intervals. These are often antibiotics, which are mixed in bags referred to as *Piggybacks* and can be given in between another IV that is running continuously. There is only one needle entry in the body, which allows for a single administration line in the patient (Fig. 6.7).

IVP method of administration (Fig. 6.8) is often referred to as *direct administration* and is used to administer high concentrations of medications, such as those needed for pain. This route is prepared aseptically and packaged in a syringe for administration. The dose is injected directly into the skin, but can often be given through an existing port in the person's IV tubing. This is a way to prevent another needle puncture for the patient and decrease the risk of infection and additional pain.

ADVANTAGES OF INTRAVENOUS MEDICATIONS

All medications must reach the blood and be distributed before they can be beneficial. Since parenteral doses of medication do not have to be processed through the digestive system, they are able to reach their intended organ or tissue rapidly. This is the greatest advantage, and for this reason IV injection is often used in emergency situations. Even antibiotics are given this way if there is a necessity to prevent the spread of infection quickly.

Other advantages of IV injections include:
- Drugs, such as insulin and heparin, that normally would be destroyed in the stomach can be administered
- There is a rapid onset of action, which means the medications take effect and begin to work fast (for example, relieving a high fever in a child)
- Patients receiving treatment therapy, such as dialysis, surgery, chemotherapy, or epidurals, can receive medications parenterally.

 Tech Note!

Since heparin is available in 10 units/mL, 100 units/mL, 1000 units/mL, and 10,000 units/mL and is considered a "high alert" drug, it is extremely important to double check all dosages through either a second person or other protocol established by your facility.

DISADVANTAGES OF INTRAVENOUS MEDICATIONS

Since drugs pass through a normal body's protective barrier and go directly into the bloodstream, there can be many complications. There is a significant risk of infection because of the entrance of a needle into the skin. This opening to the outside of the body allows a place for microbes to enter and cause an infection. Common adverse reactions to IV therapy include *phlebitis* and infiltration. Phlebitis is an inflammation of the vein and can cause symptoms, such as burning, redness, pain, and stinging. Infiltration can also occur, which is when the fluid goes into the tissue surrounding the vein at the injection site. Both of these conditions must be considered when administering IV medications (Fig. 6.9).

 Tech Note!

The opening in the skin created by the puncture needle presents significant risk for an infection, such as phlebitis.

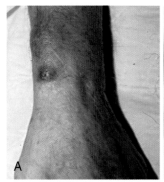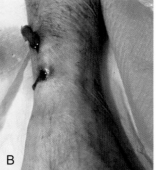

Fig. 6.9 Phlebitis from a peripheral intravenous line. (From Roberts JR, et al: *Roberts and Hedges' clinical procedures in emergency medicine and acute care*, ed 7, Philadelphia, 2019, Elsevier.)

There is always the "fear of being stuck by a needle" to consider and pain that accompanies IV medication therapy.

The effects of an error in parenteral medications are also a disadvantage. If an error or an interaction with the drug occurs, it is impossible to remove the medication immediately from the body because it is in the bloodstream. This often means that the patient will have to wait for the effects to wear off.

The cost of IV therapy is also a consideration. As discussed previously, these medications must be prepared aseptically by trained personnel and often require administration by home health nurses or hospitalization.

HEALTH-SYSTEM INTRAVENOUS ADMINISTRATION

IV therapy can be given in the hospital, in long-term care facilities (such as nursing homes), during emergency transport, in hospice, and in doctor's offices.

Medications can include anesthesia, hydration infusion, antibiotic therapy, nutritional therapy, pain management, and chemotherapy. Often a pump or electronic device is used to administer these fluids to regulate the infusion safely and accurately. Pumps used for pain therapy anesthesia, or diabetes management can be portable or even implantable (Fig. 6.10).

HOME INFUSION THERAPY

The supplies, including the pump, for IV therapy are delivered along with the IV medication. In general, technicians are responsible for maintaining these devices and supplies.

Some of the supplies needed include:
- IV start kits (Fig. 6.11)
- IV tubing
- Syringes and needles
- Alcohol swabs
- Sharps container
- Gloves
- Batteries.

 Tech Note!

Remember that patients who are receiving therapy at home are at a higher risk of acquiring an infection at the site because of the nonsterile conditions outside of a hospital environment.

All of these supplies are provided as part of the infusion delivery, and patients or family members can often administer these with nursing support. In long-term care or hospice, the nurse or a trained caregiver administers these IV medications, once they are prepared by a technician or pharmacist, using aseptic technique. It is imperative that a

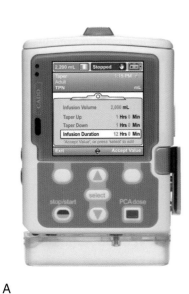

A

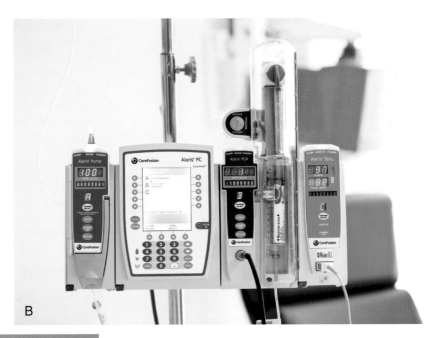

B

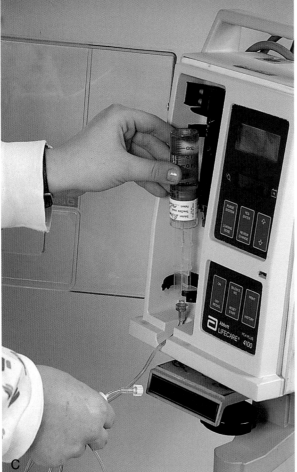

C

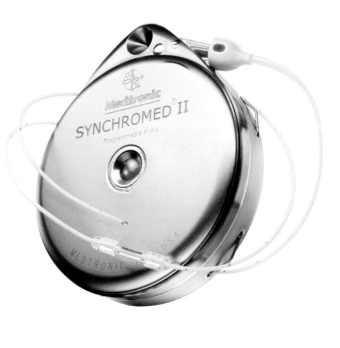

D

Fig. 6.10 Electronic infusion devices. (A) CADD®-Solis VIP ambulatory battery-operated infusion device used for IV parenteral nutrition. (B) Medley™ Medication Safety System. (C) Nurse using a patient-controlled analgesia (PCA) electronic infusion device. (D) Synchromed implantable pump. (A, Courtesy of Smiths Medical ASD, Inc. B, Courtesy of CareFusion, San Diego, California. C, From Potter PA, Perry AG. *Fundamentals of nursing*, ed 6, St Louis, 2005, Mosby. D, Reprinted with the permission of Medtronic, Inc. ©.)

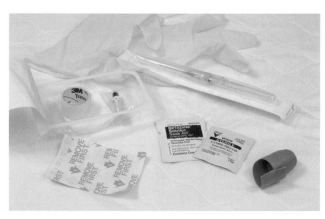

Fig. 6.11 Intravenous start kit. (From Perry AG, Potter PA, Elkin MK. *Nursing interventions & clinical skills*, ed 5, St Louis, 2012, Mosby.)

technician include all the supplies, such as pumps or tubing, needed to administer the medication so that the nurse or caregiver has what they need. Without the proper additional supplies (such as tubing, syringes, needles, and solutions used to flush the IV tubing), the nurse cannot administer the medication properly, and the patient will be unable to receive treatment.

The pharmacy technician or preparer must consider the route of administration to be used and the setting where it will be given when preparing parenteral medications. Whether the medication is to be given continuously, intermittently, or via IVP requires certain packaging and preparation methods. The healthcare team, starting with the preparer and ending with the patient, must consider IV therapy complications, such as phlebitis. Infection control begins with good aseptic technique and is the first step in quality management. Familiarity with the drugs, their preparation, and routes of administration are all factors in preventing medication errors and ensuring the patient is safe.

REVIEW QUESTIONS

1. Which of the following is an advantage of IV administration?
   A. The effects of the medication are rapid
   B. The effects of the medication are slow
   C. The patient experiences little discomfort with IV medications
   D. The patient can receive IV medication through an injection
2. Which of the following does NOT describe the IM injection route?
   A. The administration requires a catheter through a vein for administration
   B. The medication is compounded and delivered in a syringe
   C. The injection is sometimes referred to as an *IVP*
   D. The patient must be hospitalized to receive this route

3. This route of administration is usually used in emergencies, such as with a heart attack
   A. Intradermal (ID)
   B. Subcutaneous
   C. Intrathecal (IT)
   D. Intracardiac (IC)
4. The following must be given parenterally because of destruction by stomach acids if taken orally.
   A. Anesthesia medications
   B. Insulin for diabetes
   C. Antibiotics
   D. Chemotherapy
5. Which of the following is a condition that can occur from the administration of IV medications and that is characterized by redness and swelling?
   A. Phlebitis
   B. Paralysis
   C. Toxicity
   D. Muscle damage
6. This route of administration would be used to administer a tuberculosis skin test.
   A. Subcutaneous
   B. ID
   C. IT
   D. IV
7. This route of administration would be most appropriate to deliver medications to a patient through the spinal cord space.
   A. ID
   B. IT
   C. IV
   D. IC
8. The peripheral IV line can be placed in the following places in the body, except:
   A. Arm
   B. Hand
   C. Foot
   D. Buttock
9. When a heart catheterization is performed; dye is injected into the body by what route of administration?
   A. Intraarterial
   B. IC
   C. ID
   D. IM
10. An intermittent infusion is given of which of the following periods of time?
    A. 15–90 minutes
    B. 5–10 minutes
    C. Over 24 hours
    D. Over 2 hours

CRITICAL THINKING

For the following orders, determine what type of infusion they are considered to be and why:
1. The order reads:
   Give ampicillin 500 mg in NS 100 mL over 15 minutes every 6 hours.

2. The order reads:
   Give dextrose 1000 mL IV every 12 hours for 3 days.
3. The order reads:
   Give 25 mg promethazine (Phenergan) IV for nausea and vomiting stat.

4. The order reads:
   Give LR 1000 mL × 1 for dehydration.

LAB ACTIVITY

Order 1	
512333 OB-1	Diet _____WT __ /__ HT ____
05/26/05	Diagnosis _____gestational diabetes_____
Davis, Karen	Drug Allergies _____NKA_____
Dr. Davis	
05/28/13	
Obstetric	
05/28/13 0600	Admit pt, consult Debbie for diabetic teaching
	Ampicillin 1 g IV q8h 1st dose now
	LR c̄ 20 mg KCL at 125 mL/h
	Toradol 30 mg IVP q6h
	Repeat CBC and potassium level in AM
	Vitals q4h while awake
	1800 cal diet
	V/o Dr. Davis/ Mrs. Jones

CBC, Complete blood count; *IVP*, IV push; *KCL*, potassium chloride; *LR*, lactated Ringer's solution; *NKA*, no known allergies; *pt*, patient; *V/o*, vocal order.

Order 2	
512333 OB-1	Diet _____WT __ /__ HT ____
05/26/05	Diagnosis _____Pre-op_____
Davis, Karen	Drug Allergies _____NKA_____
Dr. Davis	
05/04/13	
PACU	
05/05/13 0700	Admit pt to PACU
	Give Narcan 0.4 mg immediately
	Toradol 30 mg IVP on arrival to PACU and repeat q6h for a total of 3 doses prn pain
	Ancef 1g IV q6h
	Phenergan 25 mg IV or IM q6h prn for itching
	LR @125 mL/h
	Vitals q4 while awake
	V/o Dr. Davis/ Mrs. Jones

IM, Intramuscular; *IV*, intravenous; *IVP*, IV push; *LR*, lactated Ringer's solution; *NKA*, no known allergies; *PACU*, post-anesthesia care unit; *prn*, as needed; *pt*, patient; *V/o*, vocal order.

Using the physician's aforementioned order, answer the following questions:
1. List the IV medications prescribed.
2. Which IV medication is a continuous infusion?
3. Which IV medication is an antibiotic? What type of infusion is this?
4. Are there any medications that could be given as IV push? If so, which ones, and what are they for?

BIBLIOGRAPHY

1. Pharmaceutical compounding-sterile preparations (general information chapter 797). In: *The United States Pharmacopeia,* *27th rev. and The National Formulary*, ed 22, pp. 2350–70, Rockville, MD, 2004, The United States Pharmacopeial Convention.
2. Wallace L: *Basics of aseptic compounding technique video training program*, ed 1, Bethesda, MD, 2006, American Society of Health-System Pharmacists.
3. Davis K, Sparks J: *Getting started in non-sterile compounding video training program*, ed 1. Bethesda, MD, 2007, American Society of Health-System Pharmacists.
4. The Joint Commission: Facts About the Official "Do Not Use" List. http://www.jointcommission.org/assets/1/18/Do_Not_Use_List.pdf. Accessed March 1, 2013.

United States Pharmacopeia USP<797>: Pharmaceutical Compound-Sterile Preparations

7

Learning Objectives

1. Explain the history of USP<797>.
2. Discuss types of sterile compounds and who must adhere to USP<797> guidelines.
3. Identify risk categories, their beyond-use dates (BUDs), and characteristics associated with each.
4. Discuss documentation and records management related to USP<797>.

Terms & Definitions

Batch More than one unit of a product compounded in a single process

Beyond-use date (BUD) The date and time at which a compound-sterile preparation (CSP) must be discarded and cannot be used any longer

Category 1 CSP This is a CSP which has been assigned a BUD of 12 hours or less at room temperature or 24 hours or less refrigerated

Category 2 CSP: This is a CSP which has been assigned a BUD of greater than 12 hours at room temperature or greater than 24 hours refrigerated.

Certificate of Analysis (COA) A report provided by manufacturer or supplier to indicate specifications and results of testing for the item

Disinfectant Chemical agent used to destroy bacteria, fungi, and viruses

Media fill test A process simulating compounding processes or products to ensure that microbial growth is not present

Preservative A substance used to prevent microbial growth

Pyrogen-free A substance that lacks fever inducing toxins

Release testing Testing that ensures a product meets required quality characteristics

Segregated unclassified compounding area (SCA) A designed space, (area or room) that contains a primary engineering control (PEC) where category 1 compounds can be prepared

Sporicidal A concentrated agent that destroys bacterial and fungal spores when used in a specific time period

Stability The time that a CSP retains physical and chemical properties throughout its assigned BUD

Verification Confirmation of a process, method, or system that occur under normal conditions

INTRODUCTION

USP is a nonprofit science-based organization that has developed quality standards for compounded sterile products. In addition to chapter 797, the organization publishes other standards associated with pharmacy. Understanding the associated risks and environmental requirements of sterile compounds is provided to ensure patient safety, and information is provided with regard to any public health concerns. With the millions of compounds being made each year; facilities and compounding personnel must understand the contamination or incorrect dosing that can occur if not properly trained.

HISTORY OF USP

The USP has more than 2000 chapters. Chapters 1 through 999 are considered requirements and are therefore enforceable by the US Food and Drug Administration (FDA). Chapters 1000 through 1999 are informational and include additional nonenforceable recommendations. Chapters 2000 and later apply to nutritional supplements. Chapter 797 will be covered extensively here, but there are also other subsequent chapters that will be referred to later:

- 1 Injections
- 71 Sterility Tests
- 85 Bacterial Endotoxin Test
- 795 Pharmaceutical Compounding—Nonsterile
- 797 Pharmaceutical Compounding—Sterile Preparations
- 800 Hazardous Drugs-Handling in Healthcare Settings
- 825 Radiopharmaceuticals—Preparation, Compounding, Dispensing, and Repackaging
- 1072 Disinfectants and Antiseptics
- 1075 Good Compounding Practices
- 1160 Pharmaceutical Calculations
- 1191 Stability Considerations in Dispensing
- 1211 Sterilization and Sterility Assurance.

As a compounding technician, the other chapters may provide additional information, such as stability of products, calculations, or practices considered "good" for industry standards.

The USP<797> general chapter discussed here identifies responsibilities, training, and testing of compounding personnel and facilities, as well as labeling, storage, and testing of compounded products. The newest revision was released June 1, 2019. This chapter was provided to the public for comments and suggestions in July 2018. Beginning in December 2019, the chapter was published as the current version for industry.

Pharmacy technicians must have a good understanding of this chapter as state boards of Pharmacy and facilities adhere to these standards and require personnel to follow the chapter's guidelines to ensure the compound-sterile preparations (CSPs) released are sterile.

TYPES OF STERILE COMPOUNDS

The CSPs affected by this chapter include several types of sterile compounds. The practices and guidelines are designed to prevent contamination through practices and environmental quality and ensure sterility of the final CSPs made. These may be for human or animal use and the most common form is injectable, but there are also the following forms:

- (Water–based) aqueous-bronchial inhalations
- Live organ baths and soaks
- Ophthalmic medications
- Internal body cavity irrigations.

The common thread for all of these is "internal" or those medications which enter the body through direct openings, such as the eyes, or directly into the bloodstream. As discussed earlier, the body's natural defense mechanism against bacteria is bypassed if a medication enters and bypasses the digestive system, and so these CSPs are considered sterile. Other routes, such as those administered orally or topically, are considered nonsterile and are absorbed through the skin. The USP 795 Pharmaceutical Compounding—Non-Sterile general chapter covers the guidelines for nonsterile compounding, such as ointments, creams, and lozenges.

PERSONNEL AND FACILITIES

Any person who compounds, such as a pharmacist, technician, nurse, veterinarian, or doctor, must adhere to the chapter guidelines. Facilities where this takes place can include hospitals, community pharmacies, long-term care facilities, infusion pharmacies or specialty centers, or veterinary offices. Regardless of the environment, the guidelines for ISO standards must apply and management must ensure that the facility and personnel are tested for quality and meet certification standards.

RISK CATEGORIES

There are three categories of sterile compounds in the current revision of USP<797>. The characteristics and guidelines associated with each vary and will be discussed here.

CATEGORY 1 CSP

The CSPs considered to be in this category must meet a particular set of criteria and be prepared in the proper environment. The beyond-use date (BUD) is assigned with a maximum of 12 hours at room temperature and less than 24 hours if kept in refrigerator. This allows for a short-term shelf-life and quick delivery if a facility sends the final CSP to an outside facility. The facility may receive orders daily and, if in a hospital, can make what is needed for a group of patients for a 24-hour period.

The environmental controls for category 1 can be compounded in a segregated compounding area (SCA) or a classified area that includes a separated ISO class 7 and 8 area. The SCA must be located away from regular traffic flow and any unsealed windows or outside doors. The area must contain a ISO Class 5 primary engineering control [PEC], where the CSPs are prepared and requirements for testing and personnel are still mandatory.

Personal Hygiene and Protective Equipment

Personnel preparing category 1 CSPs must adhere to the requirements for garbing and handwashing. This is a visual check performed at least quarterly. See Table 7.1 for the requirements of personal protective equipment (PPE) to be used for category 1 compounding. In an

Table **7.1**	Garb and Glove Requirements (USP<797>) Proposed Standards.	
CSP CATEGORY	**PEC TYPE**	**PPE**
Category 1	All	Noncotton, low-lint disposable gown, head cover, mask, and shoe covers. Sterile gloves and sterile sleeves *if sterile gown is used, no sleeves required.
Category 2	LAFS or BSC	Noncotton, low-lint disposable gown, hair, face, and shoe covers. Sterile gloves and sterile sleeves *if sterile gown is used, no sleeves required. *Eye shield is optional.
Category 2	RABS (CAI, CACI)	Noncotton, low-lint disposable gown, shoe and hair covers, and sterile gloves.

BSC, Biological safety cabinet; *CACI, CAI*, compounding aseptic isolator or compounding aseptic containment isolator; *CSP*, compound-sterile preparation; *LAFS*, laminar airflow workbench or system; *PEC*, primary engineering control; *PPE*, personal protective equipment; *RABS*, restricted access barrier system.

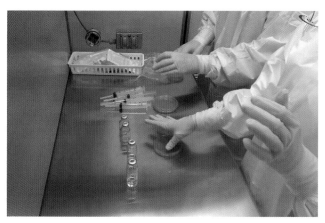

Fig. 7.1 Gloved fingertip/thumb sampling inside the ISO Class 5 primary engineering control must also be performed at least every 6 months at the end of medial fill testing. (Courtesy CriticalPoint, LLC, Totowa, New Jersey.)

SCA, the sink must be located at least 1 meter from the PEC. The process of garbing and handwashing should not interfere with the air quality surrounding the PEC. Gloved fingertip/thumb sampling inside the ISO Class 5 PEC must also be performed quarterly. If a restricted access barrier system (RABS), isolator, or compounding aseptic isolator (CACI) is used, the sampling must be taken from sterile gloves placed over the gauntlet gloves. This is done with completion of three separate testings before initial compounding (Fig. 7.1). Once this has been accomplished, this must be completed quarterly, beginning with full garbing and handwashing. Both gloved hands are sampled by lightly pressing the tips of the fingers and thumb into two agar plates, one for each hand, with media growth material. Sampling occurs inside the PEC, followed by recording the date, time, and personnel information and then incubating and watching for growth. Control of materials, such as medication vials and supplies used to compound, must be away from the PEC, and only trained personnel should enter the SCA.

Environment
Before a facility can begin compounding, it must be certified by an independent, qualified person for a certain set of quality and design specifications. Measurements of air quality and presence of microbials in the PEC (ISO Class 5), within the SCA, must be certified by an approved outside organization at least every 6 months. This includes:
- Airflow testing
- High-efficiency particulate air (HEPA) filter integrity
- Total particle counts
- Smoke studies.

Surface Sampling
Sampling of the interior of the PEC in a SCA is required monthly. This is performed by using a contact sampling device or plate with a growth media, such as trypticase soy agar (TSA) with lectin and polysorbate 80. The plate

is then inverted and placed in an incubator for 7 days at 20°C to 25°C followed by and additional 2 to 3 days at 30°C to 35°C. The plates should be observed daily during work hours and the number of microbes recorded. If the PEC sample exceeds the recommendations set by USP, a corrective action plan must be implemented. This may require additional cleaning, retraining of personnel, or verification of storage or expiration dates of the testing materials used.

CATEGORY 2 CSP
The CSPs considered to be in this category are considered a higher risk level for possible contamination than category 1 and must also meet a particular set of criteria and be prepared in the proper environment. The BUD is assigned with greater than 12 hours at room temperature or greater than 24 hours if kept in a refrigerator.

The CSPs in category 2 must be prepared in a PEC, which is placed in a classified area that includes an ISO Class 8 or ante area, an ISO Class 7 or buffer area, and the ISO Class 5 or PEC. These designated areas must adhere to air quality that increases, as movement is made through the operational areas, with the ISO Class 5 PEC being the highest quality.

Unlike category 1, which can be prepared in the PEC located within a SCA; when preparing category 2 compounds, the PEC, such as a laminar airflow workbench (LAFW), must be located within a restricted buffer area with an ISO Class 7 or better environment. The ISO Class 7 area must contain a ISO Class 5 (PEC) where the CSPs are prepared; requirements for testing and personnel are still required.

Personal Hygiene and Protective Equipment
Personnel preparing category 2 CSPs must also adhere to the requirements for garbing and handwashing, but this process takes place in a designated space known as the *ante area* or *ISO Class 8 area*. This is a visual check performed at least quarterly. See Table 7.2 for the requirements of PPE to be used for category 2 compounding. The sink must be located in the ante area to allow for garbing and handwashing before entering the buffer area where the PEC is located. The process of garbing and handwashing should not interfere with the air quality surrounding the PEC. Gloved fingertip/thumb sampling must also be performed quarterly. This is done with completion of three separate testings before initial compounding. Once this has been accomplished, this must be completed quarterly, beginning with full garbing and handwashing. Both gloved hands are sampled by lightly pressing the tips of the fingers and thumb into two agar plates, one for each hand, with media growth material. Sampling occurs inside the PEC followed by recording the date, time, and personnel information and then incubating and watching for growth. Control of materials, such as medication vials and supplies used to compound, must be away from the PEC, and only trained personnel should enter the designated areas.

Table 7.2 Summary of Requirements for Category 1 and 2 CSPs.

CSP CATEGORY	CATEGORY 1 CSPS	CATEGORY 2 CSPS
Visual observation hand washing and garbing	Quarterly	Quarterly
Gloved fingertip thumb sampling (Procedure 7.1)	Quarterly	Quarterly
Media fill testing (Procedure 7.2)	Quarterly	Quarterly
PECs	Not required to be in an ISP classified area	IS required to be in an ISO classified area
Recertification by approved outside	Every 6 months	Every 6 months
Viable airborne sampling	Monthly	Monthly
Surface sampling (Procedure 7.3)	Monthly	Monthly
Physical inspection of CSPs for release testing	Required	Required
Sterility testing of CSP	Not required	Not required
Endoxin testing of CSP	Not required	Only if NON-sterile ingredients were used in compounding
BUD	Less than 12 hours room temperature or 24 hours refrigerated	More than 12 hours room temperature or 24 hours refrigerated

BUD, Beyond-use date; *CSP*, compound-sterile preparation, *PEC*, primary engineering control.

Procedure 7.1 Performing Gloved Fingertip/Thumb Sampling per USP Standards

EQUIPMENT AND SUPPLIES
Sterile gloves
Two plates filled with nutrient agar containing neutralizing agents (e.g., lecithin and polysorbate 80) in a size range of 24- to 30-cm^2

STEPS
1. Perform garbing and handwashing in the Ante room before entering the buffer area (see Chapter 4).
   PURPOSE: When entering the SCA or segregated compounding area, personnel must avoid the introduction of pathogens. This is because patients receiving intravenous medications have compromised immune systems and may be more susceptible to infection from contamination or transfer of germs from the compounding person to the product.
   Note: Sampling must occur inside the ISO Class 5 PEC area. Do not disinfect gloves with alcohol or any other disinfectant before sampling.
   PURPOSE: Touch contamination is the most likely source for microorganisms. Compounding

personnel must be evaluated regularly to show compliance with proper handwashing, garbing, and techniques.
2. Collect a gloved fingertip and thumb sample from both hands by lightly pressing each fingertip into the agar. Use a separate plate for each hand.
   PURPOSE: If microorganisms are present on the finger tips or thumbs, this shows improper handwashing or garbing techniques.
3. Cover and record date, time, right or left hand, and person identifier on each plate.
   PURPOSE: The results should be reviewed with the person and documentation kept to show compliance with USP standards for evaluators and outside agencies. These records are maintained at the facility to demonstrate that personnel are properly trained and evaluated.
4. Invert the plates and incubate the contact sampling devices at 20°C to 35°C for 5 days.
   PURPOSE: The warm environment will promote bacterial growth if present.

Procedure 7.2 Performing Media Fill

Goal: To learn the steps for performing media fill testing per USP standards

EQUIPMENT AND SUPPLIES
Media fill kit (commercially available)
Incubator

STEPS
1. Perform garbing and handwashing in the ante room before entering the buffer area (see Chapter 4)
   PURPOSE: When entering the SCA or segregated compounding area, personnel must avoid the introduction of pathogens. This is because

Procedure 7.2   Performing Media Fill—cont'd

patients receiving intravenous medications have compromised immune systems and may be more susceptible to infection from contamination or transfer of germs from the compounding person to the product.

Note: Use the most challenging compounding procedures for the facility. Do not interrupt the test once it begins.

2. Using the commercial kit, follow the instructions in the laminar airflow workbench (LAFW) using aseptic techniques.

   PURPOSE: All compounding personnel must be tested to ensure their techniques do not contain or transfer bacteria to a prepared sterile compound.

3. Incubate the media-filled vials at 20°C to 35°C for a minimum of 14 days. If two temperatures are used for incubation of media-filled samples, incubate the filled containers for at least 7 days at the lower temperature (20°C–25°C) followed by 7 days at 30°C to 35°C.

PURPOSE The warm temperature will allow bacteria to grow if present.

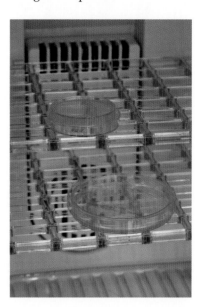

Procedure 7.3   Performing Surface Sampling per USP Standards

Goal: To learn the steps for performing surface sampling per USP standards

EQUIPMENT AND SUPPLIES

Contact sampling device, such as paddles, slides, or plates with a size range of 24 to 36 cm
Sterile swabs wetted with sterile water
Incubator

STEPS

1. Perform garbing and handwashing in the ante room before entering the buffer area (see Chapter 4)

   PURPOSE: When entering the SCA or segregated compounding area, personnel must avoid the introduction of pathogens. This is because patients receiving intravenous medications have compromised immune systems and may be more susceptible to infection from contamination or transfer of germs from the compounding person to the product.

2. Remove the cover of the contact sampling device aseptically and press firmly to the surface being

sampled. Cover the contact material back up.

   PURPOSE: The contact media will be exposed to the surface and allow bacteria to grow on it if bacteria is present.

3. Invert the plates and incubate the contact sampling devices at 20°C to 25°C for 5 to 7 days and then at 30°C to 35°C for 2 to 3 additional days.

   PURPOSE: The warm environment will promote bacterial growth if present.

4. Examine the sampling devices for growth daily during normal business hours, and record the observed count at each time point. At the final time point, record the total number of discrete colonies of microorganisms (CFU/sample) on the environmental sampling record based on sample type, sample location and sample date.

   PURPOSE: The contact device used should be free of bacteria to show proper cleaning and environmental controls, such as temperature and humidity, are being maintained.

Environment

Before a facility can begin compounding, it must be certified by an independent, qualified person for a certain set of quality and design specifications. Measurements of air quality and presence of microbials in the PEC (ISO Class 5), within the classified areas, must be certified by an approved outside organization at least every 6 months. This not only includes the ISO Class 5 or PEC area, but airflow adequacy in the ISO Class 7 and 8 rooms must be evaluated. These two

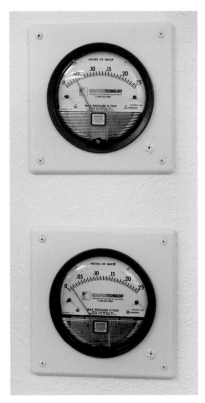

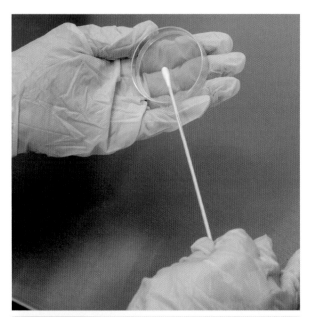

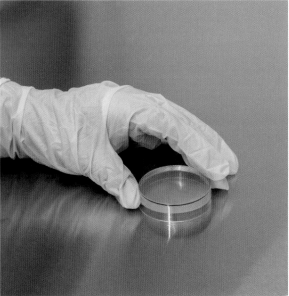

Fig. 7.2 The pressure gauges located between the ante area and the general environment.

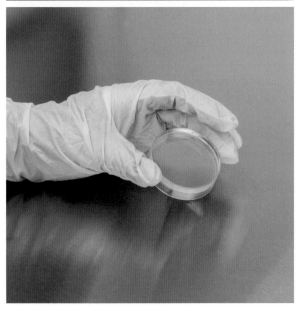

areas or rooms must be separated by walls and doors between them. The air in the lower quality area (ISO Class 8 or ante room) must not flow to the higher quality area (buffer area or ISO Class 7). Movement of materials and personnel should be limited so as to not stir dust or create disruptions in the airflow. Air must be introduced via the HEPA filters located in the ceiling of the buffer area (where the PEC is located) and returns should be mounted on the wall. This allows for the cleanest air to flow in a downward motion.

In addition to certification of the PEC, airflow adequacy of the ISO-classified areas is required every 6 months. The filtered air must measure an air exchanges per hour (ACPH) that is not less than 30. To prevent the poorer quality air from moving from one area to another that is of higher quality; a differential positive pressure reading is required from a 0.02-inch water column. A pressure gauge located between the ante area and the general environment is placed and results recorded at least daily (Fig. 7.2).

Surface Sampling

Sampling of the interior of the ISO classified areas are required monthly. This is performed by using a contact sampling device or plate with a growth media, such as TSA with lectin and polysorbate 80. Use a sterile swab to touch the flat work surface in the PEC and place the sample on the device or plate (Fig. 7.3). If the sample is taken in a crevice or hard-to-reach place, a sterile swab may be used to collect the sample (Fig. 7.4).

Fig. 7.3 Surface sampling.

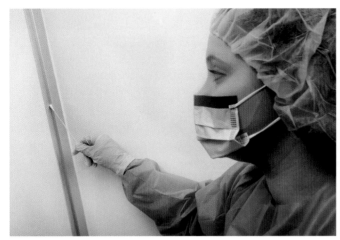
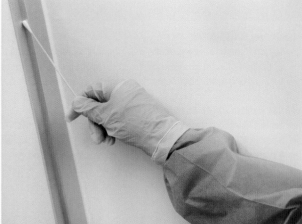

Fig. 7.4 Surface sampling in a crevice.

The plate is then inverted and placed in an incubator for 7 days at 20°C to 25°C, followed by an additional 2 to 3 days at 30°C to 35°C. The plates should be observed daily during work hours, and the number of microbes should be recorded. If the PEC sample exceeds the recommendations per USP<797>, compounding of category 2 CSPs must cease immediately, and a corrective action plan must be implemented. Once an investigation occurs to determine the cause of the failure, a cleaning and retesting of facility must occur before resuming compounding.

URGENT USE CPSS

The third category of CSPs includes compounds that may be needed in an emergency situation, such as cardiopulmonary resuscitation, or if a patient would suffer additional risks from a delay. If the time is not available for preparation in a category 1 or 2 environment, and it is for a single patient, the compound can be prepared using aseptic technique and must be administered immediately following completion. The entire amount of time from the beginning of the compounding procedure cannot exceed 1 hour.

Cleaning and Disinfectant Tools

Surfaces in the compounding areas are a major source of contamination when compounding CSPs. USP<797> provides a cleaning and disinfecting schedule (see Chapter 8). The most common type of disinfectant is 70% Isopropyl alcohol or IPA.

 Tech Note!

Always allow the disinfectant (IPA 70%) to dry before manipulation or use of object.

Sporicidal agents are also used weekly in all ISO classified areas, as well as SCA. USP<1072> *Disinfectants and Antiseptics* describes these products. An example of a sterile industrial sporicidal and disinfectant Environmental Protection Agency (EPA)-registered cleaner is PeridoxRTU.

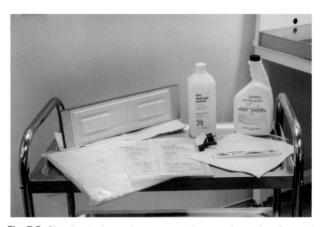

Fig. 7.5 Cleaning tools, such as mops, wipes, and mop heads, must be sterile and low lint.

Cleaning tools, such as mops, wipes, and mop heads, must be sterile and low lint. They should be dedicated to the ISO classified areas only and discarded based on the condition of the material. Disposal should be in a sealed bag outside the SCA or ISO classified areas (Fig. 7.5).

Products used in the cleaning and disinfecting of compounding areas should have a *certificate of analysis or (COA)*. This report from the manufacturer provides written description and analysis of ingredients and should be kept on file in the facility (Fig. 7.6).

Cleaning logs should be maintained with signature, date, and product used. In addition to the scheduled times, cleaning and disinfecting must be repeated if there is a spill, a known contamination, or a visible soiled surface.

In addition, the product will have a safety data sheet or SDS to provide any hazards associated with the product and actions that should be taken upon exposure. For example, if there is a hazard for eye irritation, the SDS will list this and describe first aid measures, such as flushing the eyes with water. The facility should maintain an eye wash station to cleanse the eyes (Fig. 7.7). It is important for personnel performing the cleaning tasks to review the product COA and SDS information for the products and supplies being used before use.

Text continued on page 64

Executive Summary / Testing Criteria

Room Pressurization Test
- Tested in accordance with the most current versions of ISO-14644 and USP<797>.
- Specifications are compliant with IEST recommended practices, CETA CAG and/or customer supplied specifications.
- Each area is tested by measuring pressure differential across each doorway using a NIST traceable calibrated manometer.

Airflow Volume and Air Changes Per Hour Test
- Tested in accordance with the most current versions of ISO-14644 and USP<797>.
- Specifications are compliant with IEST recommended practices, CETA CAG and/or customer supplied specifications.
- Airflows are measured using a NIST traceable calibrated air data multimeter and a flow hood / velgrid to capture total airflow. Calculations for the room air changes per hour are noted. Sterile compounding cleanrooms are typically dilutioncontrol (turbulant airflow.)

HEPA Filter Leak Test
- Tested in accordance with the most current versions of ISO-14644 and USP<797>.
- Specifications are compliant with IEST recommended practices, CETA CAG and/or customer supplied specifications.
- Leak testing was performed by introducing hot or cold PAO generated aerosol into the upstream side of the HEPA filters. The downstream side of the HEPA was scanned for less than 0.01% leakage of the upstream challenge using a NIST traceable calibrated aerosol photometer.

Non-Viable Particle Count Test
- Tested in accordance with the most current versions of ISO-14644 and USP<797>.
- Specifications are compliant with IEST recommended practices, CETA CAG and/or customer supplied specifications.
- Particle counts were taken 42" above the floor or 6" above the work surface with a NIST tracable particle counter. All counts 0.5 microns and larger were recorded at each location. Grid patterns were conducted with the most current version

Smoke Pattern Test
- Tested in accordance with the most current versions of ISO-14644 and USP<797>.
- Specifications are compliant with IEST recommended practices, CETA CAG and/or customer supplied specifications.
- In situ air pattern analysis via smoke studies are conducted at the critical area to demonstrate unidirectional airflow and sweeping action over and away from the product to support aseptic conditions. Additonal smoke studies are conducted to demonstrate correct airflows around doorways, pass throughs, corners and edges. A visible source of smoke using a glycol based fog generator is used. Testing conducted under dynamic conditions.

Viable Particle Counts
- Tested in accordance with the most current version of ISO-14644 and USP <797> & <1116>.
- Specifications are compliant with IEST recommended practices, CETA CAG and/or customer supplied specifications.
- The number of discrete colonies of microorganisms are reported as colony forming units (and documented on the microbial lab report. USP <797> states the recovery of any mold, yeast, coagulase-positive Staphylococcus or gram-negative rod is not in compliance and immediate investigation and remediationinto the cause must be conducted. Testing conducted with a NIST traceable calibrated spinner under dynamic conditions.

xxxx	**Testing Conducted By:**	**Customer Information:**
	xxx	Pharmacy Name
		City, ST ZIP
	Test Date:	**Control ID:**
	Test Date: 16MAY2016	CID- 051616V1.0

Fig. 7.6 Certificate of analysis (COA). (Courtesy Dennard Drugs Pharmacy, Soperton, Georgia.)

Compliance Summary Cleanroom

Room Pressurization

Location	ΔP Required	ΔP Actual	Compliant / Non-Compliant
Ante Room to Exterior	> 0.02"	0.0451"	Compliant
Positive Buffer Rm to Ante Rm	> 0.02"	0.0375"	Compliant
Negative Buffer Rm to Ante Rm	> – 0.01"	– 0.0181"	Compliant
Comments: N/A			

Room Air Exchange Rate

Location	Supply Volume	Room Volume	ACPH Required	ACPH Actual	Compliant / Non-Compliant
Ante Room	642	1110	30	34.7	Compliant
Positive Buffer Room	1425	2601	30	32.9	Compliant
Negative Buffer Room	372	292	30	35.8	Compliant
Comments: N/A					

HEPA Filter Leak Test

Location	# of HEPA Filters	# Passed	# Failed	Compliant / Non-Compliant
Cleanroom	5	5	0	Compliant
Comments: N/A				

Non-Viable Particle Count Test

Location	# of Counts	Avg Count	High Count	Class Limit	Required ISO Class	Compliant / Non-Compliant
Ante Room to Exterior	5	76	118	10,000	ISO 7	Compliant
Positive Buffer Rm to Ante Rm	8	153	301	10,000	ISO 7	Compliant
Negative Buffer Rm to Ante Rm	5	274	391	10,000	ISO 7	Compliant
Negative Buffer Rm to Ante Rm	5	0	0	100	ISO 5	Compliant
Negative Buffer Rm to Ante Rm	5	0	0	100	ISO 5	Compliant
Comments: N/A						

Fig. 7.6, cont'd

Compliance Summary Cleanroom

Smoke Pattern Test

Location	Test Criteria	Compliant / Non-Compliant
LFH SN-90645329	Air pattern analysis was conducted under dynamic conditions at the critical area to demonstrate unidirectional airflow and sweeping action over and away from the product and provides adequate unidirectional airflow to support aseptic operations.	Compliant
BSC SN-2CH-15-CH-1234	Air pattern analysis was conducted under dynamic conditions at the critical area to demonstrate unidirectional airflow and sweeping action over and away from the product and provides adequate unidirectional airflow to support aseptic operations.	Compliant
Positive Buffer Room	Air pattern analysis was conducted under dynamic conditions at the critical area to demonstrate correct airflow pattern around the edges, doorways, pass throughs and corners of the room to support operations.	Compliant
Negative Buffer Room	Air pattern analysis was conducted under dynamic conditions at the critical area to demonstrate correct airflow pattern around the edges, doorways, pass throughs and corners of the room to support operations.	Compliant
Ante Room	Air pattern analysis was conducted under dynamic conditions at the critical area to demonstrate correct airflow pattern around the edges, doorways, pass throughs and corners of the room to support operations.	Compliant

Comments: N/A

Bioaerosol Sampling for Bacterial & Fungal Analysis

ID#	Location	Volume	Total Count	Action Level	Compliant / Non-Compliant
A	Negative Control	N/A	0	Growth	Compliant
B	Positive Control	N/A	0	No Growth	Compliant
1	BSC SN-2CH-15-CH-1234	1000	0	>1	Compliant
2	LFH SN-90645329	1000	3	>1	Compliant
3	Positive Buffer Room	1000	0	>10	Compliant
4	Negative Buffer Room	1000	0	>10	Compliant
5	Ante Room	1000	0	>10	Compliant

Comments: N/A

Fig. 7.6, cont'd

Non-Viable Particle Counts (0.5µm and Larger) Positive Buffer Room

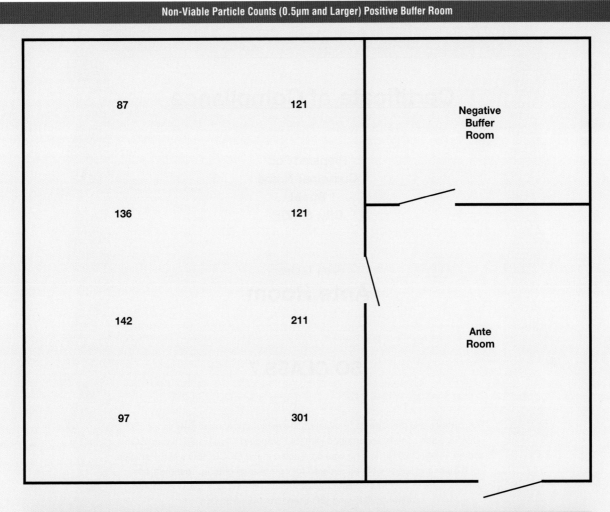

Particle Count Summary		
	m³	**ft³**
Average	5,399	153
High Count	10,630	301
Class Limit	352,000	10,000
Room Area ft²	**Room Area m²**	**Required Counts**	**Counts Taken**
275	25.5	7	8
Meets ISO Class 7		
Test Conditions: "Operational" and probe height 42" above the floor.		

Fig. 7.6, cont'd

Certificate of Compliance

Prepared For:
Customer Name
Street
City, ST ZIP

Area Tested:

Ante Room

ISO CLASS 7

This certifies this area meets or exceeds the minimum requirements for an ISO CLASS clean zone in accordance with ISO Standard 14644-1:2015 and ISO Standard 14644-2:2015. Testing was conducted in the OCCUPIED state. Particles of 0.5 µm and larger were considered for compliance criteria. Test methods utilized were in accordance with ISO Standard 14644-1:2015, ISO Standard 14644-2:2015 and ISO Standard 14644-3:2015.

Fig. 7.6, cont'd

Certificate of Compliance

Prepared For:

Customer Name
Street
City, ST ZIP

Area Tested:

BSC SN 2CH-15-CH-1234

ISO CLASS 5

This certifies this area meets or exceeds the minimum requirements for an ISO CLASS clean zone in accordance with ISO Standard 14644-1:2015 and ISO Standard 14644-2:2015. Testing was conducted in the OCCUPIED state. Particles of 0.5 μm and larger were considered for compliance criteria. Test methods utilized were in accordance with ISO Standard 14644-1:2015, ISO Standard 14644-2:2015 and ISO Standard 14644-3:2015.

Certificate Issued By:

Fig. 7.6, cont'd

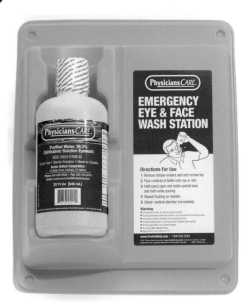

Fig. 7.7 Eye and face wash station.

 Tech Note!

Remember: Compounding personnel performing cleaning and disinfecting MUST be garbed and perform handwashing in every instance.

Equipment, such as automated compounder devices or ACDs used to make total parenteral nutritions (TPNs), must be sterilized and depyrogenated using USP guidelines and calibrated for accuracy on a daily basis. These processes remove **pyrogens** (fever-producing agents) or endotoxins by use of dry heat or steam, depending on the equipment.

HANDLING, STORAGE, AND TRANSPORTING OF CSPs

A process for storing, handling, packaging, and delivery must be described in standards of operating procedures (SOPs). The storage area must be checked for proper room temperature once daily. Temperature fluctuations, for instance, can affect the **stability** of a compound. This also includes the refrigerator, and values should be recorded on a log.

 Tech Note!

If refrigerated: any compound that exceeds the warmest labeled limit or temperatures exceeding 40°C for more than 4 hours should be discarded.

Proper packaging of CSPs should be selected to ensure the packaging will maintain sterility, prevent damage or leakage, and maintain stability of the product. If the product requires refrigeration for instance, a cooler with sufficient cooling should be used in the transport process. If it is light-sensitive, light-resistant packaging must be used.

Personnel, including delivery drivers, must be trained to understand the importance of maintaining the CSPs integrity and sterility. If special instructions, such as DO NOT SHAKE, are needed, then the compounding personnel must ensure this is addressed. Use of tamper proof seals on prepared bags and syringes will serve two purposes: first, to prevent outside contamination through the port or syringe hub and second, to provide evidence of any tampering that may have occurred.

BUD ASSIGNMENT FOR CSPs

Determining the BUD for CSPs should include consideration of the time that passes between the actual compounding and administration to the patient. Compatibility of the container is also a consideration, as medication may degrade over time because of stage conditions.

Category 1 CSPs must be assigned BUDs of a maximum of 12 hours at room temperature and less than 24 hours if kept in a refrigerator. Category 2 CSPs adhere to BUDs of greater than of 12 hours at room temperature or greater than 24 hours if kept in a refrigerator. Compounding facilities must adhere to guidelines for sterile compounding and show SOPs and proper records of **release testing** of products. Both CSP 1 and 2 categories prepared with sterile ingredients must be prepared using aseptic techniques, and sterility testing is not required for release. A visual inspection, using a white and black background box of the product, is required however to include checks for cloudiness, particulate matter, leakage, or container compromise. If there is an indication of compromise, the compound should be immediately discarded or isolated and a determination of what and how it occurred should be investigated.

DOCUMENTATION AND RECORDS

USP<797> requires each facility to maintain SOPs for all compounding and establish a formal quality assurance (QA) and quality control (QC) program to ensure that high-quality CSPs are prepared. Processes to ensure techniques and activities demonstrate that all aspects of USP<797> guidelines are met and include a **verification** of completion for each. All personnel must be trained in each SOP and are responsible for ensuring they are followed. Competency in performing the procedures is validated periodically and documentation is kept as part of a QA and QC program. This will be discussed in more detail in Chapter 16.

REVIEW QUESTIONS

1. The sampling of the interior of the ISO class 5 PEC in an SCA is required _____.
   A. weekly
   B. bimonthly
   C. monthly
   D. biweekly

2. The time that a CSP retains physical and chemical properties throughout the assigned BUD is called:
   A. stability
   B. beyond-use date (BUD)
   C. verification
   D. preservative

3. If refrigerated: any compound that exceeds the warmest labeling limit or temperature exceeding 40 degrees for more than _____ should be discarded.
   A. 3 hours
   B. 2 hours
   C. 30 minutes
   D. 4 hours

4. The date and time at which a CSP must be discarded and cannot be used any longer is called:
   A. release testing
   B. stability
   C. beyond-use date (BUD)
   D. verification

5. Which CSP has been assigned a BUD of 12 hours or less at room temperature or 24 hours or less refrigerated?
   A. sporicidal
   B. Category 1 CSP
   C. batch
   D. Category 2 CSP

6. Measurements of air quality and presence of microbials in the PEC (ISO class 5) within the SCA must be certified by an approved outside organization at least every _____.
   A. 6 months
   B. 2 years
   C. 3 months
   D. 1 year

7. Proper packaging of CSPs should be selected to ensure the packaging will maintain the following, except:
   A. prevent damage or leakage
   B. sterility
   C. light resistant
   D. stability of the product

8. Gloved fingertip/thumb sampling inside the ISO class 5 PEC must be performed _____.
   A. monthly
   B. quarterly
   C. weekly
   D. bimonthly

9. The CSP that has been assigned a BUD of greater than 12 hours at room temperature or greater than 24 hours refrigerated is called _____.
   A. batch
   B. media fill test
   C. Category 1 CSP
   D. Category 2 CSP

10. In emergency situations, such as cardiopulmonary resuscitation or if a patient would suffer additional risk from a delay, a third category CSP can be made. The entire amount of time, starting at the beginning of the compound procedure, cannot exceed _____.
    A. 30 minutes
    B. 45 minutes
    C. 1 hour
    D. 2 hours

BIBLIOGRAPHY

1. General Chapter 797 Pharmaceutical Compounding-Sterile Preparations. http://www.usp.org/compounding/general-chapter-797. Retrieved January 15, 2019.
2. General Chapter 1072 Disinfectants and Antiseptics (website): Retrieved January 23, 2019 from http://www.uspbpep.com/usp31/v31261/usp31nf26s1_c1072.asp.
3. American Society of Health-System Pharmacists: ASHP Guidelines on Quality Assurance for Pharmacy-Prepared Sterile Products. http://www.ashp.org/s_ashp/docs/files/BP07/Prep_Gdl_QualAssurSterile.pdf. Accessed August 26, 2018.

The Sterile Environment

8

Learning Objectives

1. Discuss USP<797> standards related to building and facilities construction and design.
2. Discuss both the ante room, or ISO Class 8, and buffer area, or ISO Class 7, environments.
3. Identify the various parts of an ISO Class 5 environment.
4. Describe USP<797> specific guidelines for garbing, cleaning and disinfecting the environment, and testing and surface sampling in the compounding environment.

Terms & Definitions

ACPH Air changes per hour

Ante area International Organization for Standardization (ISO) Class 8 area where personal hand hygiene, garbing, and staging of components, order entry, labeling, and high particulate activities are performed before entering the buffer area

Biological safety cabinet (BSC) Special hood where air flows downward through a HEPA filter; used for chemotherapy preparation

Buffer area ISO Class 7 area where LAFW or other PECs are physically located and aseptic manipulations of compounded sterile preparations (CSPs) occur

CACI, CAI Compounding aseptic isolator or compounding aseptic containment isolator

Contamination Introduction of pathogens or microbes into or on normally clean or sterile objects, surfaces, or spaces

Critical area ISO Class 5 environment where aseptic manipulations take place

Critical site Area to never touch (such as needle tips, tops of vials, and syringe plunger) to avoid cross-contamination during aseptic manipulations

First air Direct flow of air exiting the HEPA filter inside the PEC, which should never be interrupted and is essentially particle-free

Garbing Apparel or clothing that should be worn during aseptic preparation of CSPs

High-efficiency particulate air (HEPA) filter Special filter used in the LAFW designed to remove 99.97% of particles that are 0.3 microns or larger. This creates a bacteria-free environment in which to perform aseptic technique manipulations.

Isolator Type of PEC that provides isolation from outside areas, while maintaining a Class 5 environment required to prepare CSPs

Laminar airflow workbench or system (LAFW, LAFS) Also known as the "*hood*." This area is designed to be used to perform aseptic technique because it uses a HEPA filter to create an environment that produces sterile air

Personal protective equipment (PPE) Equipment, including shoe and hair covers, beard covers, gowns, masks, and gloves

Piggyback (PB) Containers of sterile solution used to administer medications through a secondary set or intermittent infusion; usually 50 to 250 mL in volume

Primary engineering control (PEC) ISO class 5 or higher areas located in the buffer area where all CSPs must be prepared. Examples include LAFWs, CACIs, BSCs, and RABS

Restricted Access Barrier system (RABS) ISO class 7 or higher area that uses glove ports to separate the surrounding areas to allow aseptic manipulations to take place inside

Segregated compounding area (SEC) Unclassified area separated from a facility's main workflow areas where category 1 CSPs may be compounded

Trypticase soy agar (TSA) General microbiologic growth medium that supports bacterial and fungi growth used to perform sampling

INTRODUCTION

Aseptic technique involves strict guidelines, and its primary goal is to prevent the spread of microbial contaminates. Technicians who prepare intravenous (IV) preparations must understand the importance of maintaining sterility and preventing medication errors.

To safely prepare IV medications and avoid errors, the processes, guidelines, and proper handling of equipment is essential. In this chapter, we will discuss United States Pharmacopoeia Chapter 797 (USP<797>) guidelines for the building and facilities required in the sterile compounding of compounded sterile preparations (CSPs), as well as monitoring, cleaning, and disinfecting requirements.

BUILDING AND FACILITIES CONSTRUCTION AND DESIGN

The designated areas where sterile compounding must occur should be designed to allow for movement of personnel, supplies, and operations to be completed without disruption of air flow that allows for possible contamination (Fig. 8.1). USP<797> outlines the areas and placement of equipment to decrease the risks associated with preparing CSPs aseptically. The chapter also discusses the environmental controls that must be in place to maintain the sterility of these areas.

Using the International Classification of Particulate Matter in Room Air (ISO) is the accepted standard for determining the risk of contamination in the air. Each class has a particle count of microbes found in the air and certain areas must adhere to these standards.

ISO CLASS	PARTICLE COUNT/m³	AREA(S)
Class 5	3,520	PECs
Class 7	352,000	Buffer area
Class 8	3,520,000	Ante area

Based on the previous chart, these are the main areas for the facilities used in sterile compounding. The highest air quality is found in Class 5, which is where all compounding must take place. The Class 7 environment or buffer area is where the Class 5 or primary engineering controls (PECs) are kept, while the Class 8 or ante area is where handwashing,

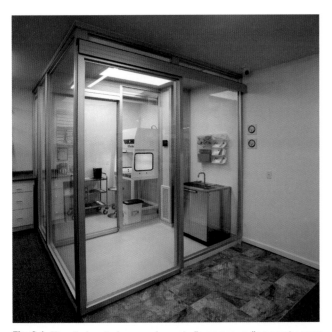

Fig. 8.1 The designated areas where sterile compounding must occur should be designed to allow for movement of personnel, supplies, and operations to be completed without disruption of air flow that allows for possible contamination.

garbing, and preparation before entering the buffer area occurs.

These guidelines, along with the American Society of Health-System Pharmacists (ASHP) guidelines and the National Coordinating Committee on Large Volume Parenterals (NCCLVP) guidelines of practice, are designed to identify air quality standards that will prevent harm (or even death) to patients that results from contamination.

This cleanroom space or segregated compounding area (SEC) layout consists of a designated ante area, buffer area, and a PEC (Fig. 8.2). The ante and buffer areas should be separated by a permanent door and wall to ensure proper air quality. Air is introduced through HEPA filters in the buffer room ceiling and returns are low on the wall to create a top-down flow of air (Fig. 8.3).

Always ensure the pass-through doors between the buffer and ante area are NEVER opened at the same time.

ANTE ROOM OR ISO CLASS 8 ENVIRONMENT

The *ante room*, or ISO Class 8 environment, is the outermost ring of the three areas (Fig. 8.4). USP<797> defines this environment as the area for handwashing, garbing, gathering of components needed, order entry, labeling, and other activities that may "stir up dust." This area is located directly outside of the buffer area, where the handwashing and garbing procedure should be performed. The air in this room, or area, is considered an ISO Class 8 environment, which means that the air contains 100,000 particles of 0.5 microns per cubic meter or less. Cartons and packaged compounded supplies (such as needles, syringes, IV bags, and tubing sets) should be unpacked and wiped down with sterile 70% alcohol before passing on to the buffer area. This room must be separate from the ISO class 7 or buffer room with its own controls to prevent the flow of lower air quality into the more controlled area (buffer or ISO Class 7 area. The doors separating these areas should never be opened at the same time; instead, open one door at a time to prevent flow of less quality air entering the buffer area. Personnel must be limited to authorized personnel only.

Temperature and humidity in the ISO Class 7 are also controlled through heating systems, ventilation, and heating, ventilation and air-conditioning (HVAC) to prevent the growth of bacteria. This area must be maintained at 68°F or cooler with less than 60% humidity. Documentation and monitoring these parameters are part of a daily routine (Fig. 8.5).

 Did You Know?

A sneeze contains droplets of bacteria or viruses that can travel as far as 3 feet before landing on a surface.

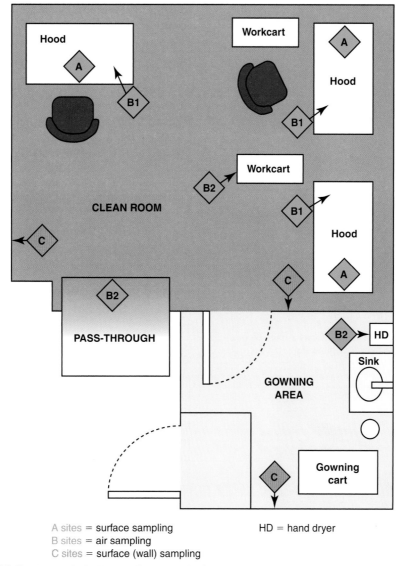

A sites = surface sampling   HD = hand dryer
B sites = air sampling
C sites = surface (wall) sampling

Fig. 8.2 The layout of a buffer area (clean room). (Courtesy of CriticalPoint, LLC, Totowa, New Jersey.)

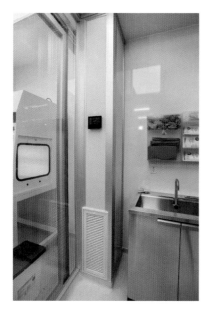

Fig. 8.3 Air is introduced through high-efficiency particulate air (HEPA) filters in the buffer room ceiling and returns are low on the wall to create a top-down flow of air.

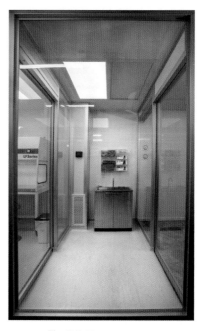

Fig. 8.4 The ante room.

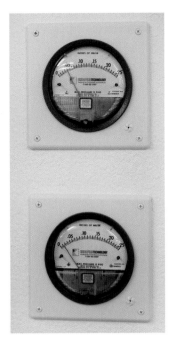

Fig. 8.5 Temperature and humidity in the ISO Class 7 must be maintained at 68°F or cooler with less than 60% humidity.

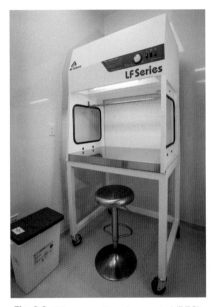

Fig. 8.6 Primary engineering control (PEC).

BUFFER AREA (CLEAN ROOM) OR ISO CLASS 7 ENVIRONMENT

The buffer area is the main compounding area where PEC are located (Fig. 8.6). This area is where the actual aseptic manipulations of CSPs take place, and it should be located out of the flow of traffic and have limited personnel access. The opening of cartons and boxes or supplies should take place before entering this area to reduce the amount of dust particles and ensure a clean product. If items are brought into the buffer area, they should be cleaned and disinfected first. The buffer area is known as an *ISO Class 7 environment*, which means that the air contains no more than 10,000 particles of 0.5 microns per cubic meter or less.

PEC OR ISO CLASS 5 ENVIRONMENT

The most common types of PECs are commonly referred to as *"hoods."* All CSPs must be prepared in a PEC and these include the **laminar airflow workbench, LAFW** or *LAFS,* the **biologic safety cabinet (BSC), Restricted access barrier systems (RABS)**, and isolators.

> 📝 **Tech Note!**
>
> The most common form of contamination is touch contamination.

LAMINAR AIRFLOW WORKBENCH OR LAMINAR AIRFLOW SYSTEM

The LAFW area provides an ISO Class 5 environment for CSP preparation inside the buffer area. LAFWs should be placed out of the traffic flow and are the cleanest work surface in the system. The most important part of this "hood," as it is sometimes referred to, is the special filter known as a **high-efficiency particulate air (HEPA) filter**. The filter should never be touched, cleaned, or sprayed with alcohol. The air is unidirectional and smooth, which provides a constant flow of first air for compounding.

> 🦉 **Did You Know?**
>
> High-efficiency particulate (HEPA) filters can remove 99.97% of particles that are less than 0.3 micron or larger, which are about the size of most airborne microorganisms.

Sitting in front of the LAFW is like sitting in front of a fan blowing wind in your face. The air, known as *critical air*, enters the prefilter at the front of the hood, travels through the HEPA filter at the back, where bacteria and other air contaminants are removed, and then flows horizontally across the work surface (Fig. 8.7). This allows purified air to circulate from the back to the front constantly in parallel lines. This is where exposure to uninterrupted HEPA-filtered air, or **first air**, occurs when preparing aseptic preparations. **Critical sites** (such as the tops of vials and needle surfaces) should always be exposed to first air to avoid contamination from particles allowed to linger in the air. Surfaces (such as needles, syringe plungers, or vial tops) should be exposed to first air at all times.

Observe the following guidelines when working in the LAFW:

- Always perform all manipulations at least 6 inches inside the hood
- Remember first air: Never interrupt the airflow between the HEPA filter and sterile objects

Horizontal Hood

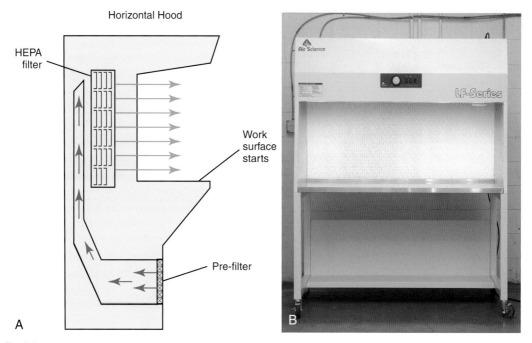

Fig. 8.7 (A) Diagram of airflow direction. (B) Hood with horizontal airflow. (B, Courtesy Air Science, Fort Myers, Florida.)

- Avoid spraying or wiping the HEPA filter
- The hood should be turned on at least 30 minutes before use.

> **Tech Alert!**
>
> One of the most important elements to aseptic technique is not allowing any interruption between the HEPA filter and a sterile object. First air is the cleanest air!

BIOLOGICAL SAFETY CABINET

This PEC is used for hazardous compounding of CSPs located inside the ISO Class 7 area (buffer). It uses inward and downward air flow (vertical) rather than the LAFW's horizontal flow (Fig. 8.8). The placement must be out of traffic patterns and air flow currents. Chapter 14 discusses the cleaning and operation guidelines as described in USP<800>.

RESTRICTED ACCESS BARRIER SYSTEMS

These include the compounding aseptic isolator (CACI) or compounding aseptic containment isolator (CAI) as environments, which provide an ISO Class 5 inside the ISO Class 7 area (buffer) by use of glove ports that physically separate the outside area from the inside compounding area. Every opening or port must be documented and recovery time allowed to regain the ISO Class 5 area inside (Fig. 8.9).

ISOLATORS

A completely closed system uses transfer ports to move supplies, medications, and other items from outside to inside the isolator. Pressure and decontamination are

maintained as part of the system controls to continuously meet ISO Class 5 conditions.

> **Tech Note!**
>
> If an isolator maintains an ISO Class 5 environment, it can be placed in an ISO Class 8 area or ante area.

GARBING

USP<797> also has specific guidelines for the apparel or clothing that should be worn during aseptic manipulations, as well as cleaning and disinfecting tasks. There is a certain order for donning **personal protective equipment (PPE)**, such as gloves, gowns, and hair covers. PPE is designed to prevent the spread of infectious diseases during aseptic preparation and cleaning (Fig. 8.10).

Before entering the ante room, personnel shall remove outer garments (such as jackets, sweaters, or hats), all cosmetics, and any visible jewelry or piercings that interfere with garb. Personnel should don garb beginning with shoe covers, then hair nets and beard covers, followed by face shields or masks. In general, the order should be dirtiest to cleanest (for example, shoe covers before head covers). Hospitals may have slight variations for this procedure because of room layout and facility protocols.

Perform hand cleansing in the ante area, (see the handwashing procedure described in Chapter 4). Don a nonshedding gown that fits snugly around the wrists and neck. Upon entering the buffer area, perform antiseptic hand cleansing with antiseptic waterless

Vertical Hood

HEPA filter
(exhaust)

HEPA filter
(air supply)

Glass shield

Intake

Blower

A

B

Fig. 8.8 (A) Diagram of airflow direction. (B) Hood with vertical airflow. *HEPA*, High-efficiency particulate air. (B, Courtesy Air Science, Fort Myers, Florida.)

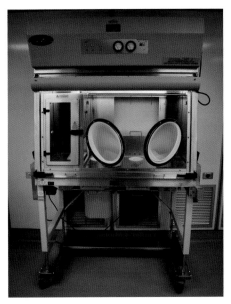

Fig. 8.9 One type of restricted access barrier system (RABS), specifically a Compounding Aseptic Containment Isolator (CACI). (Courtesy CriticalPoint, LLC, Totowa, New Jersey.)

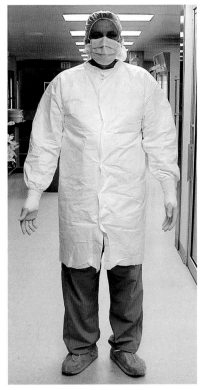

Fig. 8.10   A technician in full personal protective equipment (PPE). (Courtesy CriticalPoint, LLC, Totowa, New Jersey.)

alcohol-based surgical hand scrub, and then don sterile gloves. Only compounding personnel trained to clean should be in this area. Outside environmental workers or cleaning personnel are not permitted to clean the sterile environment.

 Tech Note!

If the gloves become contaminated by touching a nonsterile surface, you can reapply 70% alcohol to the surface area of the gloves and let them dry thoroughly.

When exiting the buffer area, the gown may be reused during the same work shift if it remains in the buffer area and is not soiled. However, shoe covers, masks, and gloves need to be replaced, and hand-washing needs to be performed if the buffer area is reentered.

In addition, only stainless-steel shelving, carts, and nonporous surfaces are allowed in the ISO Class 7 environment (buffer area), where the PECs are located. Items, such as computers, carts, and nonessential containers should not be stored or kept in this room. Staging of items and calculations should take place before entering the LAFW (clean room), and only immediate necessary items, not cases of fluids, should be in this room because cardboard will cause excessive dust and contamination.

CLEANING AND DISINFECTING THE ENVIRONMENT

Compounding personnel performing cleaning must garb and gown first. The order should be in the direction of cleanest area to the dirtiest (Box 8.1). Start with cleaning the PEC with 70% sterile alcohol and lint-free wipes. Next, using a disposable lint-free mopping system, clean the ceiling and walls of the buffer area. If there are hard-to-reach corners, use wipes to clean where the mop will not reach. Wipe down all surfaces, such as tables, carts, trash cans, and sharps containers. Mop the floor from inside to outside and then repeat this same process in the ante area, including the sink. This allows the cleanest area to be done first, working outward to the ante area, so as to bring the dirt out (Fig. 8.11). USP<797> provides the environment cleaning and disinfecting schedule as follows:

DAILY SCHEDULE

Floors, counters, and easily cleanable work surfaces in the ante area and buffer area should be cleaned and

---

Box 8.1   Cleaning Procedure of the PEC (Hood)

The PEC (except for the isolator) must be cleaned before each shift, before a batch, and no longer than 30 minutes following a previous cleaning when compounding is occurring. In addition, it should be cleaned any time there is a suspected contamination, such as a spill.

SUPPLIES FOR CLEANING THE LAMINAR AIRFLOW WORKBENCH (LAFW)
Lint-free cloth
Sterile 70% isopropyl alcohol (IPA)
Begin by soaking a stack of cloths with the alcohol

CLEAN IN THE FOLLOWING ORDER
(Note: Garbing will be performed before any cleaning activities.)
1. Clean walls in an up-and-down motion, working outward from back to front.
2. Work surface from back to front in long strokes. Start at the back corner and go across in parallel lines, working your way to the front while being careful to overlap and cover every area of the work surface. As the cloths get dirtied, discard them. Allow the area to dry before beginning aseptic manipulations. *Note*: Be sure to overlap slightly when wiping to prevent any areas of the surface from being missed. Never clean the **high-efficiency particulate air** (HEPA) filter!

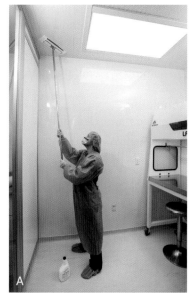

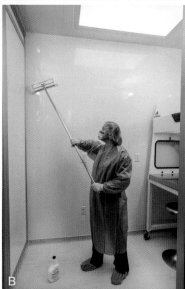

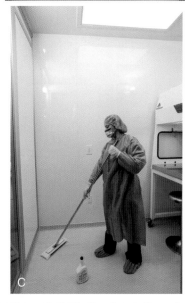

Fig. 8.11 Cleaning and disinfecting the sterile environment should be started in the cleanest area and ended in the dirtiest area: ceiling (A), walls (B), and floor (C).

disinfected daily when no aseptic operations are in progress. This includes the sink and all contact surfaces.

Supplies Needed for Cleaning (Fig. 8.12):
- Disinfectant solution, such as diluted bleach
- Microfiber cleaning system (alternative to mop).

Cleaning Techniques
- Clean all counters and cleanable work surfaces in the buffer area with disinfectant.
- Mop the floor, starting at the wall opposite the room entry door.
- Mop in even strokes toward the operator, moving carts as needed.
- In the ante room, clean the sink and contact surfaces, and clean the floor as described earlier.

MONTHLY SCHEDULE
Wall, storage shelving, and ceilings should be cleaned and disinfected monthly with a germicidal detergent-soaked, lint-free wipe and then followed with 70% isopropyl alcohol (IPA). This includes wiping the inside of trash cans, emptying storage bins, and cleaning chairs in the buffer area.

See Box 8.2 for a summary of what items should be cleaned and how often. Document all environmental values and cleaning procedures; include who performed the activities along with dates and times and include these records as part of the quality assurance program for the facility (Figs. 8.13 and 8.14).

See Procedure 8.1 for the steps to cleaning the LAFW and hood.

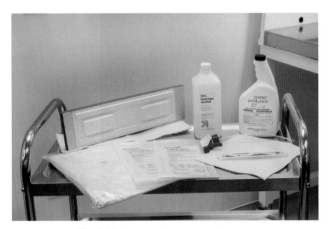

Fig. 8.12 Supplies needed for cleaning.

Box 8.2　**Cleaning Schedule for the Compounding Areas (Environment) From USP<797>**

SITE	FREQUENCY
PEC (except isolator)	at beginning of each shift before each batch at least every 30 minutes during on-going compounding after a spill or known contamination occurs
Isolator	clean and contaminate after each time it is opened
Work surfaces (ante and buffer areas)	daily
Floors	daily
Walls	monthly
ceilings	monthly
storage shelving	monthly

PEC, Primary engineering controls.
chartper USP<797> proposed standards, at
http://www.usp.org/compounding/general-chapter-797.

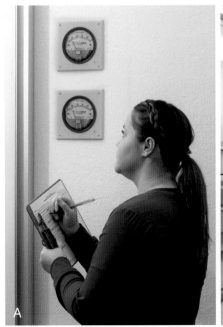

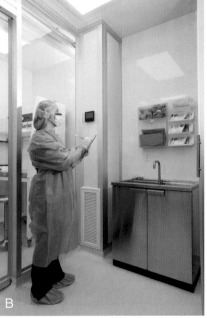

Fig. 8.13 Document all environmental control values (A) and cleaning procedures (B).

Sample Pharmacy

Daily/Monthly Cleaning Log for Controlled Sterile Compounding Environments & Adjacent Areas

Month: _____   Year: _____   Key: CA: EPA reg one-step bactericidal disinfectant cleaner   SA: EPA reg one-step sporicidal disinfectant cleaner   DA: decontamination agent   sIPA: sterile 70% IPA

	Activity	1	2	3	4	5	6	7	8	9	10	11	12	13	14	15	16	17	18	19	20	21	22	23	24	25	26	27	28	29	30	31
Daily HD Buffer Room (BR)	BSC1: DA➡CA/SA➡sIPA																															
	BSC2: DA➡CA/SA➡sIPA																															
	Empty trash																															
	All horizontal surfaces																															
	High touch surfaces																															
	All floors																															
Daily NH Buffer Area (BA) /Anteroom	LAFW1: CA/SA ➡sIPA																															
	LAFW2: CA/SA➡sIPA																															
	LAFW3: CA/SA ➡ sIPA																															
	Empty trash																															
	All horizontal surfaces																															
	High touch surfaces																															
	All floors																															
Monthly HD BR (+ daily)	All surfaces of ceiling																															
	Walls/all surfaces pass thru																															
	All surfaces furniture, trash bins, outside surfaces PECs																															
	Storage bins																															
Monthly NHD BA/Ante (+daily)	All surfaces of ceiling																															
	Walls/all surfaces pass thru																															
	All surfaces furniture, trash bins, outside surfaces PECs																															
	Storage bins																															
Monthly Other (+ daily)	General Prep Area																															
	Refrigerators/Freezers																															
	Incubator/Autoclave																															
	Other:																															

Note: Perform cleaning per SOP-304. Staff performing cleaning task to initial appropriate box. Write N/A and draw arrow through any task not due or required by SOP-304. Circle if CA or SA used. Mark an asterisk (*) next to initials to designate that a three-time clean was performed; see additional documentation of Three-Time Clean Form, F-304.c

Fig. 8.14 Daily/monthly cleaning log for controlled sterile compounding environments and adjacent areas. (©1997–2019 CriticalPoint, LLC All rights reserved. Portions of this information and these forms are proprietary to and subject to copyright ownership of, CriticalPoint, LLC and have been modified by [Sample Pharmacy] under license and for limited

Procedure 8.1 Cleaning a LAFW

GOAL: To learn the steps for properly cleaning a Laminar Airflow Workbench (LAFW).

EQUIPMENT AND SUPPLIES
- Lint-free cloths (5–6)
- Sterile 70% IPA (isopropyl alcohol)

PROCEDURAL STEPS

1. Perform nonhazardous garbing and handwashing in the ante room before entering the buffer area (see Chapter 4).
   PURPOSE: When entering the SCA or segregated compounding area, personnel must avoid the introduction of pathogens. This is because patients receiving intravenous medications have compromised immune systems and may be more susceptible to infection from contamination or transfer of germs from the compounding person to the product.

2. Arrange the lint-free wipes in a stack within 6 inches of front of hood edge.
   PURPOSE: All work inside the LAFW must be within 6 inches of the edges and sides of the hood to avoid air turbulence.

3. Pour alcohol on the stack, soaking through to the bottom one.
   PURPOSE: The cloths should be soaked, but not dripping, for the cleaning process.

4. Pull the first cloth off the stack and wipe the ceiling using side-to-side, overlapping strokes starting at the back and moving outward from back to front. Discard when done.
   PURPOSE: Cleaning should start at the top and back of the LAFW to bring contaminants forward, and eventually out of the LAFW.

5. Pull the second wipe and clean the pole and hooks, if applicable. Discard the wipe.
   PURPOSE: The pole is next highest in the hood area and any loose materials, if present, will fall down and be cleaned last.

6. Pull the third wipe from the stack and clean a side. Start in the back top corner, using overlapping strokes from top to bottom and working outward (back to front). Discard.

7. Repeat the same on the other side.
   PURPOSE: The sides should be cleaned from back to front to bring contaminates outward.

8. Use remainder of the stack of cloths to clean the work surface. Start at the back corner, working in overlapping strokes side to side, cleaning from back to front. Discard the cloths.
   PURPOSE: Cleaning the work surface last will ensure that any loose material has been caught from previous areas, and moving from back to front will bring all contaminates out without pushing material into the hood.

TESTING AND SURFACE SAMPLING

The compounding environment itself in the ISO Classes 5, 7, and 8 must be certified no less than every 6 months by an approved organization from the Controlled Environment Testing Association (CETA) National Board of Testing Registered Cleanroom Certification. Certification includes airflow testing, HEPA filter integrity testing, total particle counts, and smoke studies. Each organization should include an environmental monitoring program in its standards of operations or SOPs. Results must be recorded and maintained (Fig. 8.15).

One of the most important aspects of aseptic technique is understanding the ways the environment ensures a sterile medication for the patient. Contamination can occur at many levels throughout the preparation of sterile medications, as well as during cleaning and disinfecting. Technicians should be aware of the potential dangers in these processes, as well as the consequences of improper environmental controls. Along with proper training and equipment, the environment should be maintained and checked periodically according to UPS<797> standards by using a quality assurance program. This will be discussed in Chapter 17.

REVIEW QUESTIONS

1. How often must the floors be cleaned in the ISO Class 7 area?
   A. Daily
   B. Weekly
   C. Monthly
   D. Before each batch

2. How often must the walls and ceilings be cleaned in the ISO Class 8 area?
   A. Daily
   B. Monthly
   C. Weekly
   D. Before each batch

3. What four types of hoods are found in the ISO Class 5 compounding area?
   A. LAFW, BSC, CACI, RABS
   B. LAFW, BSC, PTCB, TPN
   C. CACI, RABS, ASHP, BSC
   D. CACI, RABS, TPN, RABS

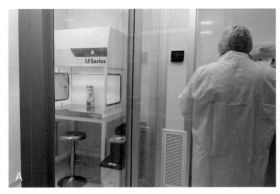 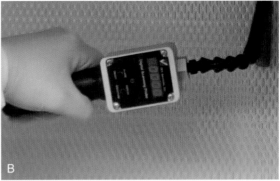

Fig. 8.15 Each organization should include an environmental monitoring program in its standards of operations. Results must be recorded and maintained.

4. Which organization must certify the ISO Classes 5, 7, and 8 areas no less than every 6 months?
   A. USP
   B. CETA
   C. ASHP
   D. NVVLP

5. Performance of handwashing and garbing should take place in which of the following environments?
   A. Ante room
   B. Buffer room
   C. Segregated compounding area
   D. PEC

6. Which of the following has the highest air quality?
   A. ISO Class 5
   B. ISO Class 7
   C. ISO Class 8
   D. SEC

7. Which of the following areas are considered critical sites?
   A. Needle tips, tops of vials, and syringe plunger
   B. Needle tips, syringe tip, alcohol swab
   C. Needle cap, syringe package, IV container
   D. Needle package, syringe, vial top

8. Which critical site must be swabbed with a sterile alcohol swab before use?
   A. IV seal
   B. Vial top
   C. Syringe plunger
   D. Needle tip

9. Temperature and humidity in the ISO Class 7 are also controlled through heating systems, ventilation, and HVAC to prevent growth of bacteria at which of the following temperatures?
   A. 60% humidity, 68°F
   B. 68% humidity, 60°F
   C. 68% humidity, 68°C
   D. 60% humidity, 60°C

10. A LAFW should only be turned on a minimum of _____ before use.
   A. 1 hour
   B. 24 hours
   C. 30 minutes
   D. 15 minutes

CRITICAL THINKING

1. You are assigned to the IV room for the week and you have a new externship student assigned to you. The student asks, "Is it really necessary to be so clean when preparing an antibiotic for a patient? Won't the medication kill any germs on the bag while it is fighting the patient's infection?" What would you say? Explain aseptic technique and why it is important to the patient.

2. Why is touch contamination the easiest form of contamination? Explain how using proper aseptic technique can prevent this from occurring.

COMPETENCIES

EQUIPMENT AND FACILITIES (USP<797>) GUIDELINES FOR ASEPTIC COMPOUNDING

Evaluation Key: S = Satisfactory   NI = Needs Improvement

Name: _____   Quarter: _____   Date: _____

COMPETENCIES	STUDENT			INSTRUCTOR		
Student will be able to:	S	NI	Comments	S	NI	Comments
Define *aseptic techniques*.						
Discuss USP<797> and its primary goal.						
Identify common equipment used in aseptic compounding.						
Discuss environment and quality control for the aseptic compounding area.						
Identify common personal protective equipment (PPE) and why USP<797> garbing procedures are used.						
Explain cleaning procedures for the laminar airflow workbench (LAFW).						
List the common duties that can be performed in the ante area.						
List the common duties performed in the buffer area.						
List several USP<797> guidelines to follow when working in the buffer area.						
Discuss the daily and monthly cleaning procedures for the aseptic compounding area.						
Discuss garbing procedures according to the USP<797> guidelines.						

Review each concept to ensure that the learning objectives for the chapter have been met. Your instructor or supervisor will evaluate this as well.

BIBLIOGRAPHY

1. Pharmaceutical compounding-sterile preparations (general information chapter 797). In: *The United States Pharmacopeia, 27th rev. and The National Formulary*, ed 22, 2350–70, Rockville, MD, 2004, The United States Pharmacopeial Convention.

Equipment and Supplies

9

Learning Objectives

1. Identify the sizes of syringes and needles used in aseptic preparation.
2. Discuss alcohol, vials, ampules, and filter needles and straws.
3. Identify the various container types and sizes used for sterile compounding.
4. Discuss requirements for maintaining the critical sites of various supplies, as well as describe additional supplies used in compounding.

Terms & Definitions

Critical area ISO Class 5 environment where aseptic manipulations take place

Critical site Area to never touch (such as needle tips, tops of vials, and syringe tips and plunger) to avoid cross-contamination during aseptic manipulations

Docking procedure used to attach bag and vial used with proprietary bag and vial systems

Gauge (ga) Size of the needle shaft (thickness); the finer the needle, the higher the gauge number

Large volume parenteral (LVP) Containers of sterile solution used for intravenous medications; usually 500 to 3000 mL in volume

Personal protective equipment (PPE) Equipment, including shoe and hair covers, beard covers, gowns, masks, and gloves

Piggyback (PB) Containers of sterile solution used to administer medications through a secondary set or intermittent infusion; usually 50 to 250 mL in volume

Secondary set When a piggyback infusion is hung higher than the main IV solution, which allows it to run into the vein faster. An example would be an antibiotic that would be ordered to infuse in 30 minutes

Small volume parenteral (SVP) Containers of sterile solutions used for intravenous medications; usually 50 to 100 mL or less in volume

INRODUCTION

Performing aseptic technique involves strict guidelines and special equipment and supplies. Much of these are disposable to prevent the spread of microbial contaminates. Technicians who prepare intravenous (IV) preparations must understand how to use each piece of equipment or supply because this is essential to preventing contamination or errors. In this chapter, we will discuss the various supplies and common equipment used in performing aseptic technique.

SUPPLIES USED IN ASEPTIC PREPARATION

Supplies (such as syringes, needles, alcohol pads, solution containers, vials, ampules, and filters) are commonly used in IV preparations.

SYRINGES

Syringes come in several sizes and are used to draw up solutions or medications to be injected into a solution container. Sterile disposable syringes are packaged individually and should be discarded after one use.

Common sizes include: 60 mL, 30 mL, 20 mL, 10 or 12 mL, 5 or 6 mL, 3 mL, 1 mL, and 0.5 mL (Fig. 9.1).

They consist of two parts: the barrel and the plunger (Fig. 9.2).

 Tech Alert!

The plunger and the tip of a syringe are considered critical sites and should never be touched.

The plunger is a piston-type rod that is cone-shaped on one end and is inside the barrel of the syringe. The other end has flanges on it for hand placement. The barrel has graduations on it to indicate the volume of the solution held inside. Each size has its own graduations and varies from milliliters to fractions of milliliters. Insulin syringes known as *U-100* (or 100 units per mL/cc) have units indicated on them, as well as fractions of millimeters. This is because insulin orders are normally written as units, such as *50 units regular insulin qd* (Fig. 9.3). When very small doses are

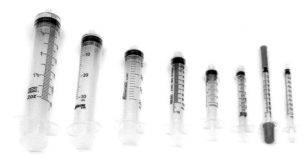

Fig. 9.1 Various sizes of syringes.

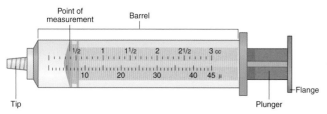

Fig. 9.2 Anatomy of a syringe. (From Hopper T: *Mosby's pharmacy technician: principles and practice*, ed 3, St Louis, 2011, Elsevier Saunders.)

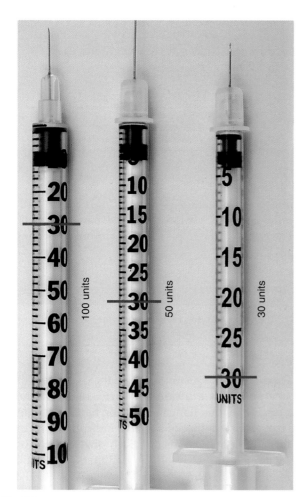

Fig. 9.3 From left to right: 30 units measured on a 100-unit syringe (each calibration is 2 units), a 50-unit syringe (each calibration is 1 unit), and a 30-unit syringe (each calibration is 1 unit). (From Macklin D, Chernecky C, Infortuna MH: *Math for clinical practice*, ed 2, St Louis, 2011, Mosby Elsevier.)

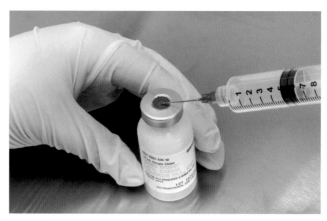

Fig. 9.4 The bevel of a needle is inserted face up into a vial stopper.

required, they are measured in tuberculin (TB) syringes, which are calibrated in hundredths.

Common Syringes and Measurements

60 mL	Each line indicates 1 mL or cc.
20 mL	Each line indicates 1 mL or cc.
10 or 12 mL	Each line indicates 0.2 mL or cc or two-tenths.
5 or 6 mL	Each line indicates 0.2 mL or cc or two-tenths.
3 mL	Each line indicates 0.1 mL or cc or tenths.
1 mL	Each line indicates 0.02 mL or cc or hundredths.
Insulin 1 mL or 0.5 mL	Each line indicates 0.02 mL or cc or hundredths.

NEEDLES

Needles consist of two basic parts: a shaft and a hub. The shaft or long hollow tube has a bevel on the end. The bevel is a flat cut part that is inserted face up into a vial stopper (Fig. 9.4).

The hub is where it attaches to the syringe. Hubs are often colored to indicate the **gauge (ga)**, or size, of the needle and range from 27 ga, which is the smallest or finest, to 13 ga, which is the largest. They also come in different lengths, ranging from ⅜ to 3½ inches (Fig. 9.5). The needle is attached to the syringe securely by a locking device, such as Luer-Lok. This allows the needle to attach more securely, because it is a circular collar that requires a half turn to lock the needle to the syringe. The needle can then be inserted into a container or vial, and fluid is drawn up into the barrel of the syringe. There are also vented needles that are used mainly for reconstituting a powder form of a medication. This process will be discussed in Chapter 10 (Fig. 9.6).

 Tech Alert!

Syringes and needles are disposable and should be discarded after one use

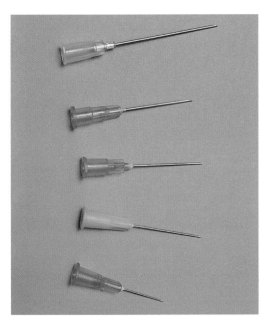

Fig. 9.5 From top to bottom: Needle sizes shown are 19, 20, 21, 23, and 25 gauge. (From Hopper T: *Mosby's pharmacy technician: principles and practice,* ed 3, St Louis, 2011, Elsevier Saunders.)

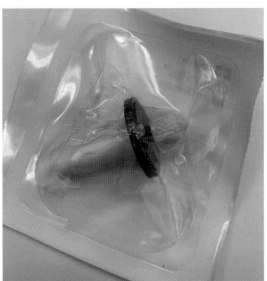

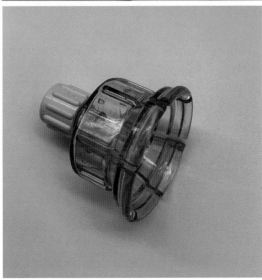

Fig. 9.6 Vented needles.

ALCOHOL

Sterile 70% isopropyl alcohol (IPA) in a spray or bottle form and lint-free wipes are used to clean the primary engineering controls (PEC)/laminar airflow workbench (LAFW), wipe down items entering the buffer area, and wipe down supplies upon entry into the PEC. Alcohol swabs come in commercial, individually foil-sealed packaging and should be used to wipe the tops of vials and ports of containers during sterile preparation (Fig. 9.7) The proper way to use the pads is very important when cleaning a critical site, such as a vial top. The pad should only be used once by swabbing across the surface and should then be allowed to dry completely before proceeding.

The process of the alcohol drying is when the dehydration of the bacteria cell occurs, which is necessary to kill it. If the alcohol is still "wet" during manipulations, it may allow microorganisms to be suspended in the fluid and cross over from one product to another during aseptic manipulations. In addition, 70% sterile IPA may be used to disinfect any work surfaces and *critical sites* including ampule necks, vial tops, and IV injection ports on bags.

> ### ⚠ Tech Alert!
> The tops of vials and ports on IV bags are both considered critical sites and must be disinfected with a 70% sterile alcohol swab before entry with a needle and syringe.

VIALS

Vials are plastic- or glass-closed containers that hold medication in solution or powder form. They have a rubber stopper for the needle to be inserted and fluid to be withdrawn. The contents can be various amounts of either crystallized powder or liquid and should be utilized as a one-time use unless the vial indicates it is a multidose vial (MDV) (Fig. 9.8).

An MDV allows for use of partial contents and reentry into the vial based on the manufacturer's recommendations for storage once opened (Fig. 9.9).

> ### 🗩 Tech Note!
>
>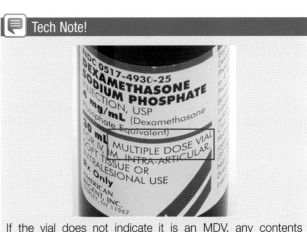
>
> If the vial does not indicate it is an MDV, any contents remaining after a single entry must be discarded.

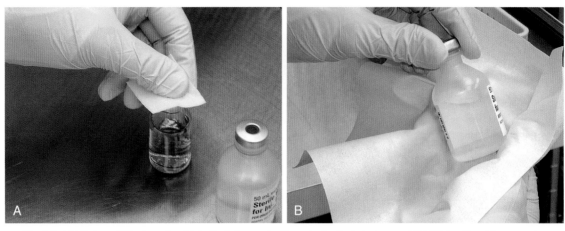

Fig. 9.7 (A) Wiping off the top of a vial (critical site area) with a sterile alcohol wipe, and (B) Wiping the vial upon entry into the laminar airflow workbench (LAFW, hood area). (Courtesy CriticalPoint, LLC, Totowa, New Jersey.)

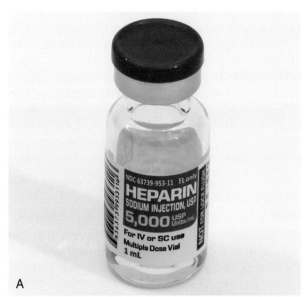

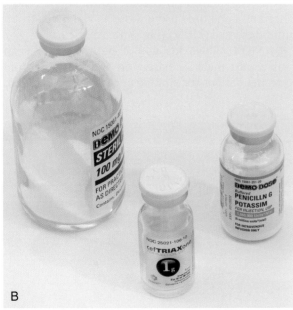

Fig. 9.8 (A) Vials containing solution. (B) Vials containing powder.

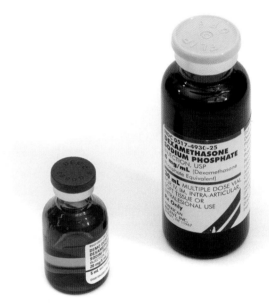

Fig. 9.9 Multidose vials.

AMPULES

Medication can also come in glass ampules, which are designed to be broken at the neck (Fig. 9.10). Fluid is withdrawn using a special filter needle to catch all the glass particles that remain in the fluid. Once the fluid is withdrawn from the ampule into the syringe, the filter needle is removed and discarded, a new needle is placed on the syringe, and the contents can be injected into the bag.

FILTER NEEDLES AND STRAWS

Special filters are often required when preparing medication from an ampule or when particles must be removed from a solution. Filter straws may be used when withdrawing the contents of an ampule, but they are not needles (Fig. 9.11).

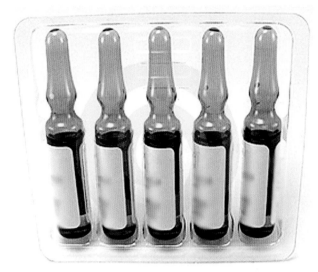

Fig. 9.10 Ampules. (Courtesy of CriticalPoint, LLC, Totowa, New Jersey.)

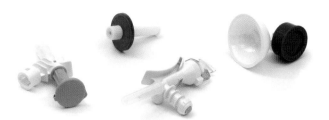

Fig. 9.12 Needleless systems.

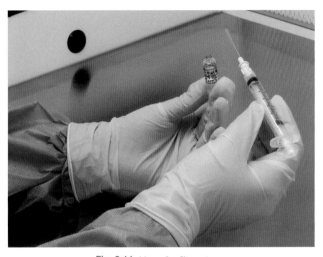

Fig. 9.11 Use of a filter straw.

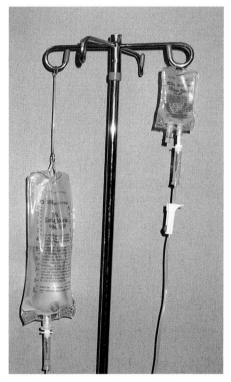

Fig. 9.13 An example of a large volume parenteral (LVP) and small volume parenteral (SVP) running together. (From Brown M, Mulholland JL: *Drug calculations: process and problems for clinical practice,* ed 8, St Louis, 2007, Mosby.)

They can be replaced by a standard needle, added to the syringe, and used to add the medication to an IV bag via the port. These devices filter particles of varying sizes and attach on the end of the syringe, sometimes as a separate device or a special needle, with the filtering mechanism inside the hub itself. These filter needles can range in size from 0.22 to 10 microns, depending on the medication to be filtered (Fig. 9.12).

CONTAINERS

Solution containers can vary in size and are usually plastic or glass. They have two ports on the end, one for adding medication, which is a critical site, with a needle and syringe and another rubber port used to connect IV tubing, such as a **secondary set** (Fig. 9.13).

Bags from 50 to 250 mL are known as **piggybacks (PBs)** or **small volume parenterals (SVPs)** and are generally used for antibiotics or small amounts of fluid. Bags from 500 to 1000 mL are known as **large volume parenterals (LVPs)** and can be used for fluid replacement and other types of medication therapy. There are special proprietary bag and vial systems, which are designed to be **docked** or put together by removing the seals and attaching the two components. The advantage of these systems are a longer shelf-life and no mixing of contents (solution and drug vial contents) until time of administration. This will be discussed further in Chapter 10. There are also 2000 to 3000 mL bags used for total parenteral nutrition (TPN) or irrigation (Fig. 9.14).

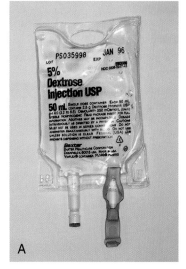

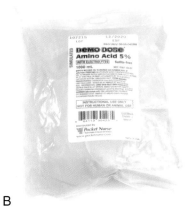

A   B

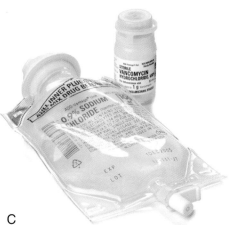

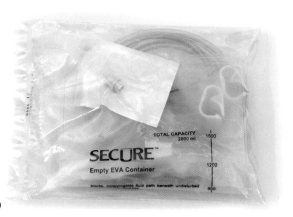

C   D

Fig. 9.14 (A) Piggyback or small volume parenteral (SVP). (B) Large volume parenteral (LVP). (C) Bag and vial system. (D) Used for total parenteral nutrition (TPN). (A, Brown M, Mulholland JL: *Drug calculations: process and problems for clinical practice*, St. Louis, 2007, Mosby Elsevier. C, Courtesy Hospira Inc., Lake Forest, IL.)

CRITICAL SITES

Critical sites, such as syringe plungers and tips, needle hubs, vial stoppers, and bag ports must always be exposed to *first air*. This is the high-efficiency particulate air (HEPA) filtered air that is uninterrupted. The surfaces of the vial stopper and bag ports must be swabbed with 70% IPA sterile alcohol pads and allowed to dry, while the other critical sites must never be touched.

ADDITIONAL SUPPLIES

Tamper-evident seals are used to cover the port once a medication has been added to an IV bag. This indicates that a medication has been added to a stock bag of fluid and ensures that there will be no breach of the sterile container before administration to the patient (Fig. 9.15).

Tamper proof caps are used to seal a syringe dose (Fig. 9.16). This may be required for an IV Push, an immunization, or a special medication that does not

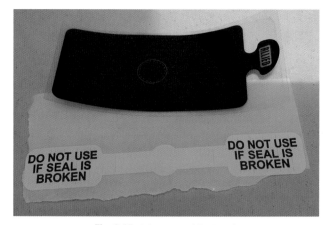

Fig. 9.15 A tamper-evident seal.

require the drug to be mixed in a bag. The cap is sterile and is added to the filled syringe by using aseptic technique. There may also be a "tamper proof" seal added to ensure that no other medication has been added to a prepared syringe.

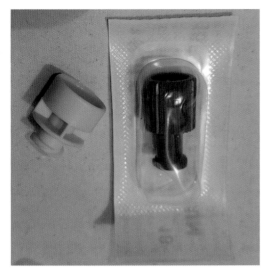

Fig. 9.16 Tamper-proof caps.

REVIEW QUESTIONS

Using a highlighter, identify the dosages measured on the following syringes by highlighting the measurement on the syringe.

1. 2.4 mL on a 3-mL syringe

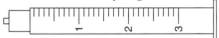

2. 10.6 mL on a 20-mL syringe

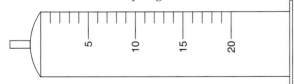

3. 30 U on a 1-mL insulin syringe

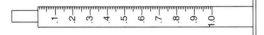

4. 10.4 mL on a 20-mL syringe

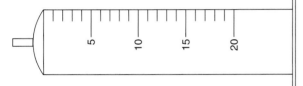

5. 12.5 cc on a 20-mL syringe

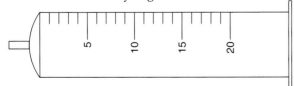

6. 1.5 cc on a 3-mL syringe

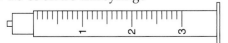

7. 0.06 mL on a TB syringe

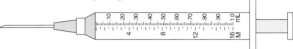

8. 0.15 cc on a TB syringe

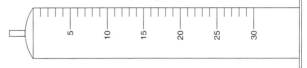

9. 32.5 mL on a 60-mL syringe

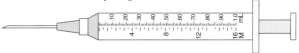

10. 19 mL on a 30-mL syringe

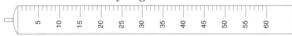

11. Which of the following needles listed subsequently has the largest bore?
    A. 19 ga
    B. 21 ga
    C. 23 ga
    D. 25 ga

12. Which of the following would be considered an LVP?
    A. IV bag of 1000 mL
    B. IV bag of 50 mL
    C. IV bag of 100 mL
    D. IV bag of 250 mL

13. When withdrawing medication from an ampule, which of the following best describes the withdrawal process?
    A. Withdraw contents from ampule using a filter straw, change to a regular needle to add contents to IV container
    B. Withdraw contents from ampule using a filter straw, change to a filter needle to add contents to the IV container
    C. Withdraw contents from ampule using a regular needle, change to filter straw to add contents to the IV bag
    D. Withdraw contents from ampule using a regular needle, change to filter needle to add contents to the IV bag

14. Which of the following should be used to disinfect the critical sites of a vial?
    A. Sterile IPA 70% alcohol
    B. IPA 90% alcohol
    C. hydrogen peroxide
    D. IPA 70% alcohol

15. When withdrawing fluid contents, use the following part of the syringe to place your fingers.
    A. Plunger
    B. Barrel
    C. Flange
    D. Tip

16. To prevent coring, which of the following best describes the best practice?
    A. Inserting the needle bevel down at a 45 degree angle
    B. Inserting the needle bevel up at a 45 degree angle
    C. Insert the needle quickly
    D. Insert the needle as straight up as possible
17. Which of the following special equipment can be used when reconstituting a powder vial?
    A. Filter needle
    B. Vented needle
    C. Filter straw
    D. Seal
18. What term is used to describe the fluid used to reconstitute a powder vial?
    A. Alcohol
    B. Water
    C. Sterile water
    D. Diluent
19. Which of the following terms describes the uninterrupted HEPA filtered air in the PEC?
    A. Critical air
    B. First air
    C. Horizontal air
    D. Vertical air
20. When preparing an IV Push dose for delivery, which of the following best describes the process?
    A. Replace the needle with a sterile cap and tamper seal
    B. Cover the bag port with a sterile seal
    C. Place the filled syringe and needle in a thick bag
    D. Leave syringe and needle attached and cover the end with a sterile cap and tamper seal

CRITICAL THINKING

1. You are assigned to the IV room for the week, and you have a new externship student assigned to you. The student asks, "Is it really necessary to be so clean when handling the supplies when preparing an antibiotic for a patient? Won't the medication kill any germs on the bag while it is fighting the patient's infection?" What would you say? Explain the parts of a needle and syringe that must not be touched and why.
2. Why is it necessary to use a filter needle or straw when withdrawing medication from an ampule?

BIBLIOGRAPHY

1. Pharmaceutical compounding-sterile preparations (general information chapter 797). In: *The United States Pharmacopeia, 27th rev. and The National Formulary*, ed 22, pp. 2350–70, Rockville, MD, 2004, The United States Pharmacopeial Convention.
2. Gahart BL, Nazareno AR. *2007 Intravenous medications*, ed 23, St Louis, 2007, Mosby.
3. Phillips LD: *Manual of I.V. therapeutics*, ed 4, Philadelphia, 2005, F.A. Davis Company.

Sterile Practice

10

Learning Objectives

1. Explain procedures for common aseptic manipulations, using the proper supplies and equipment.
2. Demonstrate the following procedures:
   a. Proper procedures used to prepare user and enter materials into the buffer area.
   b. "Staging" or preparing the admixture for the pharmacist to check.
   c. Transferring medication using a vial with powder.
   d. Transferring medication from an ampule using a syringe and filter needle.
   e. Adding medication to a plastic bag.
   f. Adding medications to a bottle.

Terms & Definitions

Closed system Used to describe a vial, which is a sealed container of solution, where air is not allowed to move freely in and out of the container

Reconstitution Used to describe the process of adding a sterile solution to a vial of powdered medication to make a liquid

Stage Term used to describe how the final preparation is prepared for the pharmacist check of a sterile compound

Vented needle A specialty needle used when compounding with vials of powdered medications that require reconstitution

INTRODUCTION

Aseptic technique requires sterile equipment and a sterile environment, but it also includes manipulations that ensure sterility. Areas known as critical sites should never be touched to prevent contamination. These include tips of syringes, hubs of needles, ports of bags, tops of vials, and ends of filters or dispensing pins. Good hand placement will ensure the avoidance of contact to these areas, as well as maintaining an open, direct path for first air in the laminar airflow workbench (LAFW) across these surfaces.

Before any manipulations can occur, certain tasks must be performed. Handwashing and garbing using the USP<797> guidelines are essential, as well as cleaning the LAFW (see Chapter 4 for procedures). Technicians must understand these procedures and follow them to prevent contamination and subsequently avoid harm to the patient. We will discuss various techniques used in aseptic preparation, as well as manipulation of the equipment, in this chapter.

All aseptic technique is performed in the Class 5 environment, or clean room. Once proper handwashing and garbing is completed, the preparer enters the buffer area and begins the process of aseptic technique in the primary engineering controls (PEC), such as an LAFW. The area where all aseptic manipulation takes place is the PEC. Items are sprayed down with 70% isopropyl alcohol (IPA) before entering into the buffer area. Only necessary items should be brought into the buffer area. No cardboard, excess packaging or wrapping is allowed. Once inside, the items can be staged on a nonporous surface and are placed in the PEC, one at a time, by using a specific procedure (Fig. 10.1).

First, only those items necessary should be placed in the PEC and excess paper items, such as alcohol pad paper and outer wrappers, are discarded on the outside. Each item used during aseptic manipulation, including syringes, needles, and medication vials, are sprayed with 70% IPA and wiped down at the edge of the LAFW. Sterile supplies are removed from their outer wrappings at the edge of the PEC, as they are introduced into the International Organization for Standardization (ISO) class 5 area environment (PECs) (Fig. 10.2). All items are spread out at least 6 inches apart to ensure that there is sufficient space to work between them, without disrupting the airflow or first air. In addition, items are kept at least 6 inches from the back and sides, and all manipulations are at least

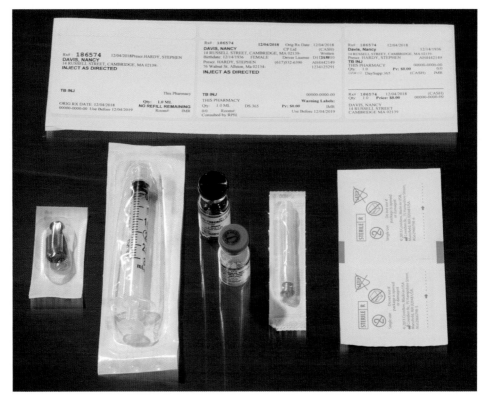

Fig.10.1 Items used for aseptic technique.

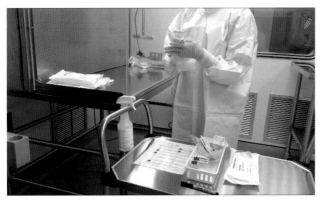

Fig.10.2 Sterile supplies are removed from their outer wrappings at the edge of the primary engineering controls (PEC), as they are introduced into the International Organization for Standardization (ISO) class 5 area environment. (Courtesy CriticalPoint, LLC, Totowa, New Jersey.)

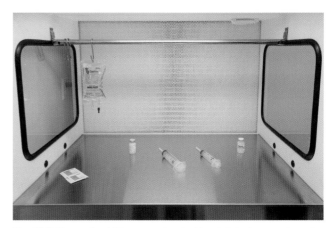

Fig. 10.3 Items should be spread out at least 6 inches apart on the primary engineering controls (PEC).

6 inches inside the hood. Leave a workspace, which is not directly over the components, left open for the actual manipulations to take place. This will ensure that first air is never interrupted by an item placed in the PEC. Stage or place items on either side of this open area to avoid disruption of airflow (Fig. 10.3).

 Tech Note!

Remember to think of the LAFW as clean air flowing toward the operator that has been filtered and should never be interrupted by hands or any object being used.

EQUIPMENT USED IN ASEPTIC MANIPULATIONS

Good hand placement is essential to proper aseptic technique. Not only must the technician ensure that the "first air" is not compromised, but there are critical areas of the equipment that must never be touched. For example, when working with a syringe, the plunger and tip should never be touched. Needle hubs should also never be touched. If these areas are touched or blocked from first air, they can become contaminated.

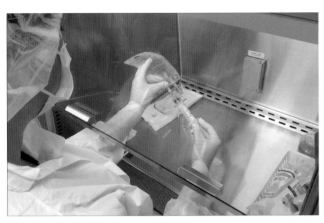

Fig. 10.4 When pulling back the plunger of a syringe, hold only the flat knob at the end, to avoid compromising the barrel of the syringe if it will be used for more than one withdraw. (Courtesy CriticalPoint, LLC, Totowa, New Jersey.)

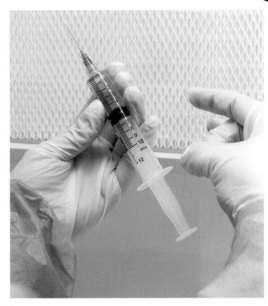

Fig. 10.5 Firmly tap the sides of the syringe to allow the bubble to move to the top.

To properly attach a needle to a syringe, remove the protective outer wrapping without compromising the critical areas. When pulling back the plunger of the syringe, hold only the flat knob at the end (Fig. 10.4).

 Tech Note!

Place all outer wrappings, paper, and excess garbage in the trash, if possible, or near the side of the hood. Do *not* place them in the PEC.

Ampule necks and vial tops should be disinfected with sterile 70% IPA swabs. This should be done by making one gentle stroke across the surface, disposing the swab, and allowing the area to dry. These surfaces are considered *critical sites* because they are a fluid pathway surface. They should be wet for at least 10 seconds and allowed to dry so that microorganisms are eliminated (discussed in Chapter 4). Equipment, such as needles, syringes, and tubing, is packaged in protective covering from the manufacturer and is disposable.

Many syringes are manufactured with a locking mechanism designed to connect to the needle. When you attach a needle to this Luer-Lok system, it requires a slight turn, and then the needle is "locked" into place. There are other syringes known as *slip-tip*, which just hold the needle on by friction.

REMOVING AN AIR BUBBLE

A common problem when using a syringe, to withdraw a solution from a vial, is that air bubbles can form in the barrel. These will prevent accurate measurements and must be removed.

First, hold the syringe upright and pull back the plunger slightly to allow a space for the bubble to go to the top. Firmly tap the sides of the syringe to allow the bubble to travel to the top. Expel the air in

the syringe by slowly pushing the plunger up until the fluid fills the barrel completely. Read the measurement by looking at the rubber end of the plunger aligned with the graduations on the barrel (Fig. 10.5).

A vial is a **closed system**, which means air is not free to go in and out of the container. Whenever a liquid is withdrawn from it, there must be an equal volume of air injected into it first. For example, if 3 mL of solution is needed, first inject 3 mL of air into the vial to replace this volume. This prevents a vacuum from forming and sucking the plunger back down, which will cause "spraying of the contents" upon withdrawal of the needle. If a **vented needle** is available, this procedure is not required because there will be no pressure build-up.

When inserting a needle into the rubber closure on a vial, the needle must never be "stabbed" into it. This can cause coring, which is when small pieces of the rubber closure get pushed into the solution and then possibly added to the bag. The needle should be placed at a 45-degree angle with the bevel up. This will force the pieces away from the bevel (Fig. 10.6).

Remember to ensure that first air is not interrupted, impeded, or diverted when setting up components in the PEC. Allow for approximately 6 inches between each item and 6 inches from the back of the hood. All supplies should be placed in the PEC, so that clutter is reduced and maximum efficiency of workflow can occur. Now that we have discussed equipment, let us put this all together and prepare some admixtures.

Before performing any aseptic manipulations, always perform proper handwashing and garbing in the ante area, and once in the buffer area, clean the LAFW.

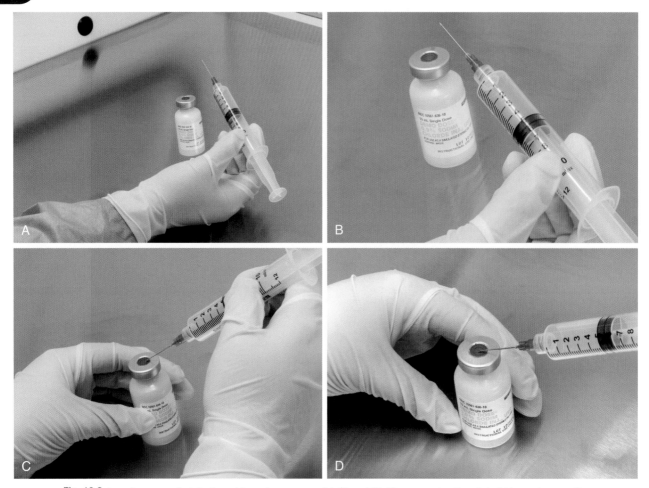

Fig. 10.6 Inserting a needle into the rubber closure on a vial. **(**A and B**)** After removing the air bubble, make sure the bevel is facing up. (C and D) Place the needle at a 45-degree angle.

MANIPULATIONS USED IN ASEPTIC PREPARATION

TRANSFERRING CORRECT MEDICATION FROM A LIQUID VIAL TO A BAG (CONTAINER)

See Procedure 10.1.

Ante Area

- Perform all calculations or research required to prepare the medication ordered.
- Gather necessary items required for compounding the preparation(s) and wipe down with alcohol.
- Perform proper hand hygiene, garbing, and gowning procedure.

Buffer Area

- Spray hands with 70% IPA or disinfectant, allow to dry, and don sterile gloves.
- Spray gloved hands with alcohol and allow to dry.
- Perform cleaning procedure for the LAFW.
- All supplies used in the PEC should be gathered and decontaminated by spraying or wiping the outer surface with sterile 70% IPA, or removing the outer packaging at the edge of the LAFW, as it is entered into the aseptic workspace. This will aid in removing dust particles and any other contaminates.
- Attach syringes to needles inside the PEC, without contact contamination or interruption of first air.
- Disinfect all critical sites using sterile 70% IPA alcohol wipes and wait at least 10 seconds before use.
- Withdraw the correct volume of medication from the vial by injecting an equal or less amount of air into it first. (For example, if 2 mL are required, inject 2 mL of air into the vial and then withdraw the 2 mL of fluid.) Use the see-saw method to allow fluid and air to swap from the vial to the syringe (Fig. 10.7).
- Replace the protective needle cover and remove any air bubbles by gently tapping on the syringe. Air bubbles will cause the reading on the syringe to be inaccurate because it allows the air to take up space, and it reflects in the final measurement.
- Recheck all calculations.

Procedure 10.1   Transferring Liquid Contents (Vial) to an Intravenous (IV) Container

EQUIPMENT AND SUPPLIES
Medication order
Pen
Calculator
CSP label (prepared)
Vial of medication (to be added)
IV container (fluid)
Syringe
Sterile seal (for bag)
Personal protective equipment (PPE)
Waste container
Sharps container

STEPS: PERFORM OUTSIDE OF ISO CLASS 7 OR 8 ENVIRONMENT

1. Complete any calculations needed and prepare label before entering the ISO class 8 ante area.
   PURPOSE: The ante area is considered a controlled environment and lose papers or excessive movement or equipment introduced can create dust or the introduction of unwanted microbes.

STEPS: PERFORM IN ANTE AREA (ISO CLASS 8)

1. Perform handwashing and garbing per USP<797> guidelines.
   PURPOSE: To ensure there is no contamination or transfer of infection from the compounder to the final compound

2. Ensure the laminar airflow workbench (LAFW) has been cleaned and turned on for at least 30 minutes.
   PURPOSE: The LAFW airflow must have time to circulate through the high-efficiency particulate air (HEPA) filter.

STEPS: PERFORM THE FOLLOWING IN BUFFER AREA (ISO CLASS 7)

1. Stage the medication, bag, label, and supplies needed on a (work surface) stainless-steel cart beside the LAFW.
   PURPOSE: Staging ensures there can be a review to ensure every item needed is there at arm' length; this allows less interruption once work starts inside the LAFW. Every time the compounder comes out of the primary engineering controls (PEC), there is a chance of introduction of contaminants that can be brought in from the ISO class 7 (buffer area) to the ISO class 5 environment (PEC).

2. Place items in the LAFW one a time, maintaining correct spacing of at least 6 inches, spraying each item with sterile isopropyl alcohol (IPA) 70%,

and removing outer packaging at the edge of the hood.
   PURPOSE: Each item is sprayed and unwrapped before entering the ISO class environment (PEC) to allow for less contaminants from outer wrappings or excess paper. ONLY what is needed should be in the ISO class 5 area.

3. Attach the needle and syringe without touching the critical site areas (needle hub or syringe tip) and lay to the side.
   PURPOSE: The needle and syringe are packaged separately, and attachment must take place in the ISO class 5 or LAFW.

4. Remove the plastic cap from the vial and wipe the top (critical site) with an alcohol swab.
   PURPOSE: The top of the vial is a critical site and must be disinfected before puncturing.

5. Wipe the port of the IV container.
   PURPOSE: The port of the container is a critical site that must be disinfected before puncturing.

6. Withdraw the appropriate contents from the vial using the seesaw method.
   PURPOSE: Using the seesaw method allows air to be entered in the closed system (vial) and the same amount of fluid to be released into the syringe. This prevents an excessive build up pressure in the vial, which can spew contents from the vial.

7. Replace needle and remove air bubbles.
   PURPOSE: Replacing the needle before removing air bubbles from the syringe, either by thumbing or striking the syringe, keeps excessive fluid from getting on the work surface. In addition, the correct amount of fluid is measured in the syringe, without any air space.

8. Inject the medication into the IV bag and affix a seal on the port of the bag.
   PURPOSE: After adding the medication to the bag per the ordered amount, the seal protects the port, which has been entered and also indicates to any person handling the bag has added contents in it.

9. Inspect the bag for leaks, cloudiness, or particulate matter.
   PURPOSE: A visual inspection can find incompatibilities or leaks before patient administration.

10. Remove from PEC and label.
    PURPOSE: Labeling the bag right outside of the LAFW (PEC) ensures that correct label goes with correct bag in case there are multiple bags to be made.

11. Remove needle from syringe used and draw back the amount injected into the container.
    PURPOSE: Once the bag is prepared and labeled, it will be checked by a Pharmacist. The needle

Continued

Procedure 10.1 Transferring Liquid Contents (Vial) to an Intravenous (IV) Container—cont'd

should be placed in the sharps inside the ISO class 7 area, before removing it to another area. This prevents a possible needle stick when items are being checked, possibly in another area in the Pharmacy.

12. Recheck calculations.

    PURPOSE: Always recheck calculations to ensure that the correct compound was prepared. Never assume or rely on the Pharmacist to find an error. When you are finished, consider it ready and correct, and consider the Pharmacist to be a validation or second check in the system.

13. Allow the Pharmacist to check with the syringe, medication, and labeled bag staged.

    PURPOSE: Create a "staged" layout so the Pharmacist can easily see how much you added per the syringe pulled back and the medication you used, and can verify that the container is labeled correctly.

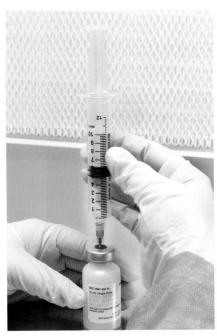

Fig. 10.7 Withdraw the correct volume of medication from the vial by injecting an equal or less amount of air into it first.

If a medication is to be dispensed in a syringe, use the previous steps to withdraw the contents and eliminate air bubbles. Attach a push-on or twist-on cap for delivery, and label (Fig. 10.8).

"STAGING" OR PREPARING THE ADMIXTURE FOR THE PHARMACIST TO CHECK

To "stage" the admixture for the pharmacist to check, follow these steps:

- Remove the needle from the syringe and place it in the sharps container.
- Lay the bag out with the stock bottle or vial of medication and the syringe drawn back to the amount of solution added to the bag.
- Initial the label, and check for a final time (Fig. 10.9).

TRANSFERRING MEDICATION USING A VIAL WITH POWDER

Transferring medication using a vial with powder requires an additional step known as **reconstitution**. The powder must be mixed into a solution first to withdraw it from the vial (Fig. 10.10). See Procedure 10.2.

Ante Area

- Perform all calculations or research required to prepare the medication ordered.
- Gather necessary items required for compounding the preparation(s) and wipe down with alcohol.
- Perform proper hand hygiene, garbing, and gowning procedure.

Buffer Area

- Spray hands with 70% IPA or disinfectant, allow to dry, and don sterile gloves.
- Spray gloved hands with alcohol and allow to dry.
- Perform cleaning procedure for the LAFW.
- All supplies used in the PEC should be gathered and decontaminated by spraying or wiping the outer surface with sterile 70% IPA or removing the outer packaging at the edge of the LAFW, as it is entered into the aseptic workspace. This will aid in removing dust particles and any other contaminates.
- Attach syringes to needles inside the PEC without contact contamination or interruption of first air.
- Disinfect all critical sites using sterile 70% IPA alcohol wipes and wait at least 10 seconds before use.
- Add the correct fluid (diluent) to the vial according to manufacturers' recommendations. (If a vented needle is available, it is not necessary to add the equal volume of air.) (Fig. 10.11).
- Swirl or shake the vial to mix the powder.
- Once the powder is dissolved completely, and using a needle and syringe, withdraw the required amount of solution from the vial and remove any air bubbles, as discussed earlier.
- Add the drug to the bag of fluid ordered and label.

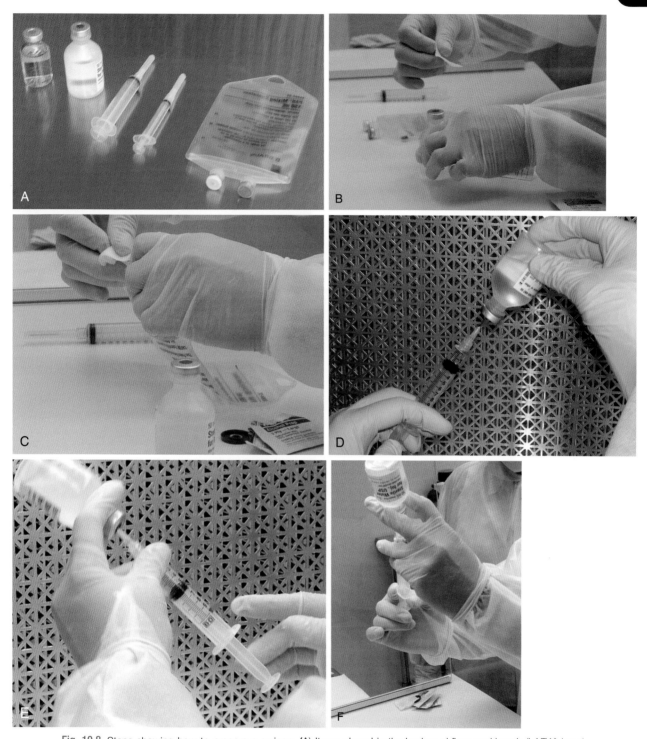

Fig. 10.8 Steps showing how to prepare a syringe. **(A)** Items placed in the laminar airflow workbench (LAFW) hood. (B) Clean vial top (critical area) with a sterile alcohol wipe. (C) Clean the port on bag (critical area) with a sterile alcohol wipe. (D) Add air to replace amount of fluid needed to withdraw. (E) Withdraw fluid from the vial. (F) Measure the amount needed in the syringe. (Courtesy CriticalPoint, LLC, Totowa, New Jersey.)

Did You Know?

Some medications, such as immune globulin, must not be shaken. Always refer to manufacturers' recommendations concerning preparation to find special mixing instructions about any medication.

TRANSFERRING MEDICATION FROM AN AMPULE USING A SYRINGE AND FILTER NEEDLE

See Procedure 10.3.

Ante Area

- Perform all calculations or research required to prepare the medication ordered.

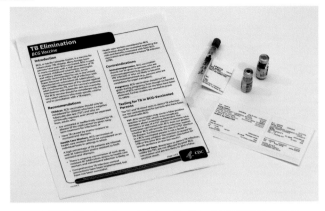

Fig. 10.9 Staging the admixture for the pharmacist to check.

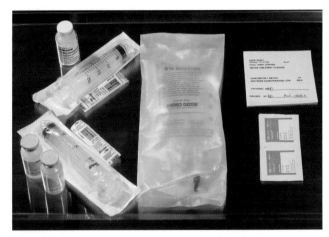

Fig. 10.10 Items needed for transferring medication using a vial with powder.

Procedure 10.2 Steps for Reconstituting a POWDER Vial and Transferring Liquid Contents to an Intravenous (IV) Container

EQUIPMENT AND SUPPLIES

Medication order
Pen
Calculator
CSP label (prepared)
Vial of medication (to be added)
Diluent vial
IV container (fluid)
Syringe
Sterile seal (for bag)
Personal protective equipment (PPE)
Waste container
Sharps container

STEPS: PERFORM OUTSIDE OF ISO CLASS 7 OR 8 ENVIRONMENT

1. Complete any calculations needed and prepare label before entering the ISO class 8 ante area.
   PURPOSE: The ante area is considered a controlled environment and lose papers or excessive movement or equipment introduced can create dust or the introduction of unwanted microbes.

STEPS: PERFORM IN ANTE AREA (ISO CLASS 8)

1. Perform handwashing and garbing per USP<797> guidelines.
   PURPOSE: To ensure there is no contamination or transfer of infection from the compounder to the final compound
2. Ensure the laminar airflow workbench (LAFW) has been cleaned and turned on for at least 30 minutes.
   PURPOSE: The LAFW airflow must have time to circulate through the high-efficiency particulate air (HEPA) filter.

STEPS: PERFORM THE FOLLOWING IN BUFFER AREA (ISO CLASS 7)

1. Stage the medication, bag, label, and supplies needed on a (work surface) stainless-steel cart beside the LAFW.
   PURPOSE: Staging ensures there can be a review to verify that every item needed is there at arm's length, which allows less interruption once work starts inside the LAFW. Every time the compounder comes out of the primary engineering controls (PEC), there is a chance of introduction of contaminants that can be brought in from the ISO class 7 (buffer area) to the ISO class 5 environment (PEC).
2. Place items in the LAFW one a time, maintaining correct spacing of at least 6 inches, spraying each item with sterile isopropyl alcohol (IPA) 70%, and removing outer packaging at the edge of the hood.
   PURPOSE: Each item is sprayed and unwrapped before entering the ISO class environment (PEC) to allow for less contaminants from outer wrappings or excess paper. ONLY what is needed should be in the ISO class 5 area.
3. Attach the needle and syringe without touching the critical site areas (needle hub or syringe tip) and lay to the side.
   PURPOSE: The needle and syringe are packaged separately, and attachment must take place in the ISO class 5 or LAFW.
4. Remove the plastic cap from the vials (diluent and powder vial) and wipe the tops (critical site) with an alcohol swab.
   PURPOSE: The tops of vials are critical sites and must be disinfected before puncturing.
5. Wipe the port of the IV container.
   PURPOSE: The port of the container is a critical site that must be disinfected before puncturing.

Procedure 10.2   Steps for Reconstituting a POWDER Vial and Transferring Liquid Contents to an Intravenous (IV) Container—cont'd

6. Withdraw the appropriate contents from the diluent vial using the seesaw method.
   PURPOSE: Using the seesaw method allows air to be entered in the closed system (vial) and the same amount of fluid to be released into the syringe. This prevents an excessive build up pressure in the vial, which can spew contents from the vial.

7. Replace needle and remove air bubbles.
   PURPOSE: Replacing the needle before removing air bubbles from the syringe, either by thumbing or striking the syringe, keeps excessive fluid from getting on the work surface. In addition, the correct amount of fluid is measured in the syringe without any air space.

8. Inject the powder vial with the diluent withdrawn to reconstitute, allowing pressure to escape. As you add liquid, there may be push back on syringe. Do not fight it.
   PURPOSE: Injecting a diluent into a vial of powder is reconstituting the powder, which can then be withdrawn. Fighting the pressure could allow small amounts of liquid to try to escape through the rubber stopper and contaminate the work surface.

9. Swirl the powder vial to mix contents well. Withdraw the calculated amount.
   PURPOSE: Swirling the vial mixes the powder and diluent and ensures that all of the drug is mixed well before withdrawing it, for the called amount needed.

10. Inject the medication into the IV bag and affix a seal on the port of the bag.
    PURPOSE: After adding the medication to the bag per the ordered amount, the seal protects the port, which has been entered and also indicates to any person handling it that the bag has added contents in it.

11. Inspect the bag for leaks, cloudiness, or particulate matter.
    PURPOSE: A visual inspection can find incompatibilities or leaks before patient administration.

12. Remove from PEC and label.
    PURPOSE: Labeling the bag right outside of the LAFW (PEC) ensures that the correct label goes with the correct bag, in case there are multiple bags to be made.

13. Remove the needle from the syringe used and draw back the amount injected into the container.
    PURPOSE: Once the bag is prepared and labeled, it will be checked by a Pharmacist. The needle should be placed in the sharps inside the ISO class 7 area, before removing it to another area. This prevents a possible needle stick when items are being checked, possibly in another area in the Pharmacy.

14. Recheck calculations.
    PURPOSE: Always recheck calculations to ensure that the correct compound was prepared. Never assume or rely on the Pharmacist to find an error. When you are finished, consider it ready and correct and consider the Pharmacist to be a validation or second check in the system.

15. Allow the Pharmacist to check with the syringe, medication, and labeled bag staged.
    PURPOSE: Create a "staged" layout so the Pharmacist can easily see how much you added per the medication and diluent displayed, with each perspective syringe used if different, and so that he or she can verify that the the container is labeled correctly.

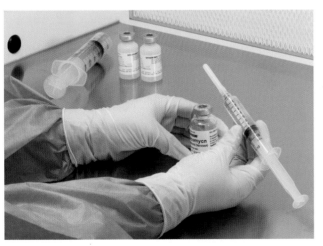

Fig. 10.11 When transferring medication using a vial with powder, add the correct fluid to the vial.

* Perform proper hand hygiene, garbing, and gloving procedure.

> **! Tech Alert!**
>
> You must ensure that first air is not interrupted, impeded, or diverted when setting up equipment in the LAFW. Allow for approximately 6 inches between each item and 3 inches from the back of the hood.

Buffer Area
* Perform cleaning procedure for the LAFW.
* All supplies used in the LAFW should be gathered and then decontaminated by spraying or wiping the outer surface with sterile 70% IPA, or removing the outer packaging at the edge of the LAFW,

Procedure 10.3   Steps for Withdrawing Contents From an Ampule and Adding Contents to an Intravenous (IV) Container

EQUIPMENT AND SUPPLIES

Medication order
Pen
Calculator
CSP label (prepared)
Ampule (medication)
Filter needle or straw
Regular needle
IV container (fluid)
Syringe
Sterile seal (for bag)
Personal protective equipment (PPE)
Waste container
Sharps container

STEPS: PERFORM OUTSIDE OF ISO CLASS 7 OR 8 ENVIRONMENT

1. Complete any calculations needed and prepare label before entering the ISO class 8 ante area.
   PURPOSE: The ante area is considered a controlled environment and lose papers or excessive movement or equipment introduced can create dust or the introduction of unwanted microbes.

STEPS: PERFORM IN ANTE AREA (ISO CLASS 8)

1. Perform handwashing and garbing per USP<797> guidelines.
   PURPOSE: To ensure there is no contamination or transfer of infection from the compounder to the final compound
2. Ensure the laminar airflow workbench (LAFW) has been cleaned and turned on for at least 30 minutes.
   PURPOSE: The LAFW airflow must have time to circulate through the high-efficiency particulate air (HEPA) filter.

STEPS: PERFORM THE FOLLOWING IN BUFFER AREA (ISO CLASS 7)

1. Stage the medication, bag, label, and supplies needed on a (work surface) stainless-steel cart beside the LAFW.
   PURPOSE: Staging ensures there can be a review to verify that every item needed is there at arm's length, which allows less interruption once work starts inside the LAFW. Every time the compounder comes out of the primary engineering controls (PEC), there is a chance of introduction of contaminants that can be brought in from the ISO class 7 (buffer area) to the ISO class 5 environment (PEC).

2. Place items in the LAFW one at a time, maintaining correct spacing of at least 6 inches, spraying each item with sterile isopropyl alcohol (IPA) 70%, and removing outer packaging at the edge of the hood.
   PURPOSE: Each item is sprayed and unwrapped before entering the ISO class environment (PEC) to allow for less contaminants from outer wrappings or excess paper. ONLY what is needed should be in the ISO class 5 area.
3. Wipe the port of the IV container.
   PURPOSE: The port of the container is a critical site that must be disinfected before puncturing.
4. Attach the filter needle or straw and syringe, without touching the critical site areas (needle hub or syringe tip) and lay to the side.
   PURPOSE: The needle and syringe are packaged separately, and attachment must take place in the ISO class 5 or LAFW.
5. Clean the ampule with an alcohol swab and break it on the score line. Place the glass top in the sharps container immediately.
   PURPOSE: The ampule is considered a sharps and should be discarded in the sharps container with other glass to prevent a stick.
6. Withdraw the appropriate contents from the ampule. There is no need to use seesaw method.
   PURPOSE: An ampule is an open system and no pressure is built up inside.
7. Replace filter needle or straw with a regular needle and remove air bubbles.
   PURPOSE: The filter needle or straw should collect any glass shards from the broken ampule. Replacing the filter needle or straw provides a clean way to inject medication into the IV container. Removing air bubbles ensure the correct amount of fluid is measured in the syringe without any air space.
8. Inject the medication into the IV bag and affix a seal on the port of the bag.
   PURPOSE: After adding the medication to the bag per the ordered amount, the seal protects the port, which has been entered and also indicates to any person handling it that the bag has added contents in it.
9. Inspect the bag for leaks, cloudiness, or particulate matter.
   PURPOSE: A visual inspection can find incompatibilities or leaks before patient administration.
10. Remove from PEC and label.
    PURPOSE: Labeling the bag right outside of the LAFW (PEC) ensures that the correct label goes with the correct bag in case there are multiple bags to be made.

11. Remove the needle from the syringe used and draw back the amount injected into the container.
    PURPOSE: Once the bag is prepared and labeled, it will be checked by a Pharmacist. The needle should be placed in the sharps inside the ISO class 7 area before removing it to another area. This prevents a possible needle stick when items are being checked, possibly in another area in the Pharmacy.

12. Recheck calculations.
    PURPOSE: Always recheck calculations to ensure that the correct compound was prepared. Never assume or rely on the Pharmacist to find an error. When you are finished, consider it ready and correct, and consider the Pharmacist to be a validation or second check in the system.

13. Allow the Pharmacist to check with the syringe, medication, and labeled bag "staged".
    PURPOSE: Create a "staged" layout so the Pharmacist can easily see how much you added per the syringe pulled back, the medication (ampule) you used, and can verify that the container is labeled correctly. *In some cases, they will want to see the filter straw or needle laid out to ensure it was used, so do **not** discard until you know.*

as it is entered into the aseptic workspace. This will aid in removing dust particles and any other contaminates.

- Attach a syringe to the filter needle or straw without contact contamination.
- Disinfect all critical sites using sterile 70% IPA alcohol wipes, and wait at least 10 seconds before use.
- Withdraw the correct volume of medication from the ampule by first holding the ampule upright and tapping the top to remove any solution from the head space.
- Swab the neck of the ampule with an alcohol swab and grasp it with the thumb and index finger of each hand.
- Quickly snap the neck, being careful to direct the spray away from the high-efficiency particulate air (HEPA) filter.
- Remove the correct amount of solution from the ampule by tilting the ampule to at least a 20-degree angle. Position the needle in the shoulder area of the ampule and pull the plunger back with the thumb and index finger of the opposite hand.
- Replace protective needle cover and remove any air bubbles.
- Remove the filter straw or filter needle and replace it with a standard needle before injecting the solution into a bag.
- Recheck all calculations (Fig. 10.12).

Tech Note!

Be careful at all times to not obstruct the first air with hand placement. Doing this will contaminate the surfaces of the critical sites and can cause infection in the patient.

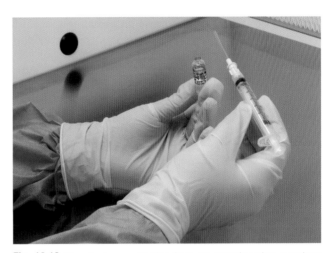

Fig. 10.12 Transferring medication from an ampule using a syringe and filter needle.

ADDING MEDICATION TO A PLASTIC BAG

Once the medication is drawn up into a syringe and the bag port is swabbed with sterile 70% IPA, inject the medication into the bag and cover the port with a foil seal. Inspect the bag for particulate matter, such as coring, or any evidence of incompatibility. This may be a color change, cloudiness, haze, or solid particles (Fig. 10.13).

Remove from the LAFW and label appropriately. Recheck all calculations. Once the admixture is ready, it should be labeled and "staged" with the needle removed, the syringe drawn back to the added amount, and the stock vial that was used all placed together. Multiple-dose vials should be initialed, dated, and sealed with a foil seal. Discard any glass or sharp equipment in a disposable sharps container. Outer wrappings may be discarded in the regular trash.

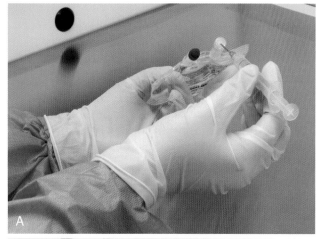

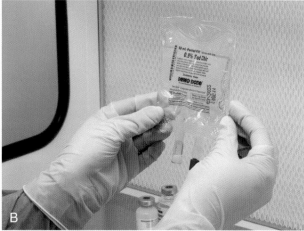

Fig. 10.13 (A) Once the medication is drawn up into a syringe and the bag port is swabbed with sterile 70% IPA, inject the medication into the bag and cover the port with a foil seal. (B) Inspect the bag for particulate matter, such as coring, or any evidence of incompatibility.

> **Tech Note!**
>
> Remember to always be aware of possible incompatibilities between medications that can occur. These can be found in reference material, such as the *Handbook on Injectable Drugs*, or on the package insert.

ADDING MEDICATIONS TO A BOTTLE

Some medications are packaged in a glass bottle, under a vacuum, and sealed by a rubber stopper.

Ante Area
- Perform all calculations or research required to prepare the medication ordered.
- Perform proper hand hygiene, garbing, and gloving procedure.

Buffer Area
- Perform cleaning procedure for the LAFW.
- All supplies used in the DCA should be gathered and then decontaminated by spraying or wiping

the outer surface with sterile 70% IPA, or removing the outer packaging at the edge of the DCA, as it is entered into the aseptic workspace. This will aid in removing dust particles and any other contaminates.
- Remove the foil seal from the bottle, wipe with a 70% alcohol swab, and allow to dry.
- Insert the medication into the bottle using a slight angle to prevent coring. The contents will be drawn in because of the vacuum effect.

Technicians preparing intravenous medications must use proper aseptic technique and environmental controls to ensure that products are safe for patients. Manipulations must be performed inside the PEC and airflow should not be disrupted. If a critical area is touched or first air is impeded, the technician must restart the process to ensure a safe and sterile product for the patient.

REVIEW QUESTIONS

1. All the following are considered critical sites EXCEPT:
   A. Syringe plunger
   B. Needle tips
   C. Syringe tip
   D. Syringe flange
2. All aseptic technique must take place in which of the following environments?
   A. ISO class 7
   B. ISO class 8
   C. ISO class 5
   D. SEC
3. When placing items in the PEC, how must space should be kept between each item?
   A. 8 inches
   B. 12 inches
   C. 6 inches
   D. 3 inches
4. A vial, which is not considered a multidose vial, is considered which of the following systems?
   A. Closed, single use container
   B. Closed, multiple use container
   C. Open, single use container
   D. Open, multiple use container
5. Which of the following would result in touch contamination during aseptic compounding?
   A. Forgetting to swab the vial top before entering
   B. Forgetting to swab the needle hub before use
   C. Forgetting to swab the syringe tip before use
   D. Forgetting to swab the dispensing pin top before use
6. In what environment should all calculations take place?
   A. Ante area
   B. Buffer area
   C. PEC
   D. LAFW

7. Before leaving the PEC, and following the injection of medication into a port of an intravenous container, which step should be performed?
   A. Cover the port with a sterile seal
   B. Inspect for leaks
   C. Inspect for cloudiness
   D. Label the bag appropriately
8. Preparing a labeled bag, with syringe drawn back and medication container for a final Pharmacist check is known as which of the following?
   A. Staging
   B. Reconstitution
   C. Garbing
   D. Aseptic compounding
9. When withdrawing medication using a needle from a liquid vial, which of the following best describes the first step?
   A. Inject an equal or slightly less amount of air than the amount of fluid to be withdrawn
   B. Inject slightly more air than the amount of fluid to be withdrawn
   C. Do not inject air before withdrawing fluid
   D. Inject twice the amount of air than the amount of fluid to be withdrawn
10. Disinfect all critical sites using sterile 70% IPA alcohol wipes and wait at least _____ seconds before use.
    A. 20
    B. 30
    C. 5
    D. 10

CRITICAL THINKING

1. You have just prepared a stat order for a vancomycin IV. You have it "staged" and ready to be checked by the pharmacist, when you overhear a nurse at the window requesting it. The tech from the front comes and asks when it will be ready? You reply, "I am waiting on the pharmacist to check it. So, it will be a few minutes." The tech insists that you made it correctly and that you should just let her have the bag. What would you say and why? Would a stat order override the need to make her wait for a pharmacist check? Explain your answer.
2. You have just prepared a large volume bag of normal saline (NS) with 4 mEq of sodium phosphate. The pharmacist on the floor has asked you to get it to him as quickly as possible. When you are staging the preparations for the pharmacist to check, you notice that one of the bottles is actually sodium acetate. Explain in detail what you would do and why?

BIBLIOGRAPHY

1. Trissel LA: *Handbook on injectable drugs*, ed 20, Bethesda, MD, 2008, American Society of Health-System Pharmacists.

Packaging, Labeling, and Documentation of CSPs

11

Learning Objectives

1. Define the characteristics associated with a Master Formulation record (MFR).
2. Define the characteristics associated with compounding records (CRs).
3. Discuss the physical inspection, handling, storing, transporting, and documentation of compounded sterile preparations (CSPs).

Terms & Definitions

Compounding record (CR) A document created by the compounder to describe the compounding process for a specific CSP

Master Formulation record (MFR or FR) Document to record the general processes used in compounding CSPs and which can be used as a basis for the CR

SDS (Safety Data Sheet) Product safety information sheet that records chemical, physical, and health-related hazards

INTRODUCTION

Every compounding facility that prepares compounded sterile preparations (CSPs) must adhere to proper documentation and labeling requirements per the United States Pharmacopoeia (USP<797>) general guidelines. Standards operating procedures (SOPs) should include the facility's guidelines and templates for the forms to be used and kept on record. Pharmacy technicians who compound must complete all required information legibly as required and follow storage guidelines.

MASTER FORMULATION RECORD

The Master Formulation record (MFR or FR) must be completed for every CSP prepared in batches for multiple patients or any CSPs that use nonsterile ingredients in the preparation. This is compared to a baking recipe that would include ingredients, preparation or mixing instructions, storage or cooking time. Most facilities assign a designation, such as a number to these for future reference. The following information is required for the MFR per the USP<797> guidelines:

Name, strength, dosage form
A physical description of the compound
All quantities and ingredients needed

Proper container
Complete instructions with steps, supplies, and equipment needed
Beyond-use dates (BUD) and storage requirements
Quality assurance (QA) processes for release testing (sterility testing, visual inspection, etc.)

This record can be used to compound the CSPs, as long as there are no changes. If there any changes to the MFR identified, an authorized facility person must document them as part of the standing SOPs for the facility. The SOPs should be reviewed and changes made, with all compounding personnel being made aware of these changes (Fig. 11.1).

COMPOUNDING RECORD

A Compounding Record or CR is created by the compounder for each particular CSP prepared. The information on the MFR can be referenced to for the preparation process that is used. If there are any deviations from the MFR for the CSP being compounded, these must be identified on the CR. The following is required for the CR per USP chapter guidelines:

Prescription or other assigned identification number given and preparer name
Name, strength, and dosage form

Master Formula Record
(for training purposes only)

Simulated Testosterone 5% Gel 60 g

INGREDIENT/ DRUG	AMOUNT (GM)
DD Testosterone powder	5 g
DD SIMBASE gel 500 G	45 mL

Equipment and Supplies needed

Scale
Spatulas—(2) 6–8in.
Syringe adapter
Weighing boat LG
Alcohol and wipes

Gloves
60 mL syringes (2)
Syringe tip cap
Weighing papers (2 each)

NOTE: It is recommended that you follow USP<795> recommendations for potency testing, which states "each preparation shall contain no less than 90.0% and no more than 110.0% of the theoretically calculated and labeled quantity of active ingredient". In order to provide some guidance in this area, use the "percentage of error" formula to calculate potency, if required by Instructor.

This is for simulation training purposes only and has not been tested in a PCCA lab, and all required steps in process should be verified by Instructor.

Suggested Compounding Procedures

1. Perform calculations and measure each ingredient separately with a 10% excess (Testosterone on paper) and (SIMBASE in boat).

   NOTE: Some material may be lost due to sticking to sides or container. Making 10% more will provide enough to measure the full 30g needed.

2. Have your Instructor check the weights of each.
3. Using the spatula, place the SIMBASE gel and Testosterone in a glass mortar.
4. Using geometric dilution, gradually add powder to base and mix thoroughly. Combine the two ingredients completely.
5. Once mixed, draw up all the preparation into the 60ml syringe.
6. Connect the other syringe to the end by using the syringe connector and transfer contents back and forth, continuing to mix.
7. Once mixed, add the syringe tip securely.
8. Assign a BUD after compounding following USP<795> guidelines and complete compounding record/log. Estimated to be 30 days or less.

Warning: Safety precautions should be taken when compounding and using equipment. Follow all laboratory and product safety guidelines and wear appropriate personal protective equipment.

Fig. 11.1 Example of a Master Formulation record (MFR). (From DAA Enterprises, Inc.: *Pharmacy management software for pharmacy technicians: A worktext*, ed 3, St Louis, 2018, Elsevier.)

MFR reference (number) if used, or compounding preparation process details

Date and time of preparation with total prepared quantity compounded

Name of manufacturer, lot number, and expiration of each ingredient and container used

Weight or measurement of each ingredient

Calculations used to create quantities needed

Assigned BUD for CSP

QA procedures performed, such as visual inspection

Additional label for container if a batch is prepared

When preparing CSPs, the process should include a review of the MFR and CR information required and should be completed as part of preparing for aseptic technique (Fig. 11.2).

 Tech Note!

The documentation, preparation of records, and gathering of supplies and medications needed should be completed outside of the ISO Class 5 or 7 environment.

Compounding Record   Drug _____   Date _____

Prescription Number or ID Assigned	Master FR Record # Used	Name and Strength of Compound	Quantity	Actual Net Measurements	Expiration Date	MFG Lot Number	MFG Expiration Date	BUD Assigned	Date Packaged	Tech Initials	RPh Initials

Attach a prescription/patient label if applicable.

ID, Identification; *FR,* formula record; *MFG,* manufacturer; *BUD,* beyond use date; *RPh,* registered pharmacist.

Fig. 11.2 Example of a compounding record (CR). (From DAA Enterprises, Inc.: *Pharmacy management software for pharmacy technicians: A worktext*, ed 3, St Louis, 2018, Elsevier.)

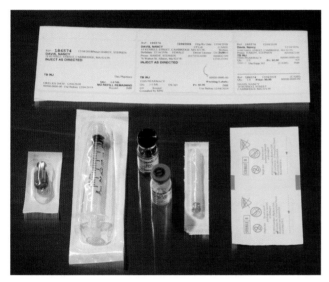

Fig. 11.3 Staged items ready for compounding.

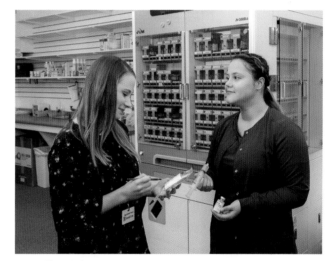

Fig. 11.4 The pharmacist checks the sterile compound.

The integrity and expiration dates of all ingredients should be checked, along with a review of the steps and process (MFR) that will take place before performing garbing and handwashing (Fig. 11.3). Once the CSP is prepared, a final review against the CR and calculations should be performed to ensure that all steps were completed and the CSP is correct. After compounding is completed, and before dispensing or transport, the CSP must be inspected to confirm integrity and a labeling match.

PHYSICAL INSPECTION

Once the sterile compound is prepared, the compounder can perform a visual inspection before the final pharmacist (RPh) check by using a black/white box test on the container. This should include visually checking for foreign matter, discoloration, cloudiness, or particulate matter. The container should be free of leaks or cracks and syringes should have sterile caps in place of needles.

The BUD should be assigned, and all reviewed documentation is signed and "staged" with the CSP and required supplies for a Pharmacist check (Fig. 11.4). Syringes used in the removal of fluids from vials should be pulled back to the correct amount added and placed with their respective medication vial. If a powder vial was used, the diluent and syringe used should also be placed together. If there was an ampule used; leave the filter straw or needle for review with the syringe used.

HANDLING AND STORING

Proper storage of prepared CSPs is very important and BUD limitations must be followed. If the CSP requires refrigeration, the temperature of the facility refrigerator must be verified at least daily and recorded on a log. If the CSP has been exposed to temperatures outside an assigned BUD range, it must be discarded (see Chapter 8) (Fig. 11.5).

Sample Pharmacy
TEMPERATURE AND HUMIDITY MONITORING LOG

Month: _____ July _____   Year: _____ 20xx

Day	1	2	3	4	5	6	7	8	9	10	11	12	13	14	15	16	17	18	19	20	21	22	23	24	25	26	27	28	29	30	31
Refrigerator Temperature: 2° to 8° Celsius (36° to 46° Fahrenheit)																															
Refrigerator #1	37°	36°	37°																												
Refrigerator #2	41°	42°	40°																												
Freezer: -25° to -10° Celsius (–13° to 14° Fahrenheit)																															
Freezer #1	–10°	–11°	–9°																												
Freezer #2	–3°	–4°	–4°																												
Incubators: High: 30° to 35° Celsius (85° to 95° Fahrenheit) and Low: 20 to 25° Celsius (68° to 72° Fahrenheit)																															
Incubator High	87°	88°	90°																												
Incubator Low	70°	70°	70°																												
Controlled Room Temperature: 20° to 25° Celsius (68° to 77° Fahrenheit) allowing excursions from 15° to 30° Celsius (59° to 86° Fahrenheit)																															
Storage #1	73°	75°	74°																												
Storage #2	72°	71°	70°																												
Buffer Room Temperature: Less than 20° Celsius (68° Fahrenheit)																															
Buffer Room #1	65°	66°	63°																												
Buffer Room #2	67	67°	66°																												
Buffer Room: Less than 60% Relative Humidity																															
Buffer Room #1	57%	59%	56%																												
Buffer Room #2	59%	56%	58%																												
Initials of Recorder	KS	KD	KW																												

Signature of Pharmacy Manager after review   _____ Date

F-210.a: 06/01/2017

Fig. 11.5 Sample temperature log, completed for the first 3 days of the month. (©1997-2019 CriticalPoint, LLC All rights reserved. Portions of this information and these forms are proprietary to and subject to copyright ownership of, CriticalPoint, LLC and have been modified by [Sample Pharmacy] under license and for limited use.)

Handling is also important. The integrity of bags or syringes must not allow for additional exposure to the outside. For example: Intravenous (IV) push syringes or prepared prefilled syringes should have a sterile cap in place of a syringe for transport. This will prevent a plunger expelling a measured dose, as well as a possible needle stick for other personnel in the delivery or administration process. In addition, tamper proof seals can be used to ensure an uncompromised CSP.

TRANSPORTING OF CSPs

The BUD requirements for the CSP must be kept throughout the transport and delivery of the prepared CSP. If the compound requires storage at refrigerator temperature, a cooler with sufficient ice to maintain this temperature must be used. If the CSP is light sensitive, then special packaging should be used. Personnel in delivery operations should have clear instructions and protect the quality of the CSP at all times. These special circumstances should be recorded on the MFR and identified in SOPs. Any persons involved in the handling and storage of the compounded CSP should be informed and know where to find this information.

 Tech Note!

If the compounded CSP is considered hazardous, USP<800> chapter guidelines must be followed.

STORAGE OF RECORDS

All records related to compounding a particular CSP, such as the MFR, the CR, and any testing results must be kept at least 3 years after the BUD of the CSP. If the state laws require longer, then those laws will be followed, as the strictest law always applies. This can be done electronically, either at the same facility or another one that is accessible within a reasonable time period. Most facilities will keep a notebook for the MFRs with easy access to compounding personnel.

To ensure patient safety and integrity of a CSP, proper documentation, handling, storage, and handling must be aligned with proper aseptic technique and environmental controls. A compounder must be aware that best practices in technique that are carried out without proper handling, labeling, and documentation compromise the system's quality.

REVIEW QUESTIONS

1. Which of the following best describes the document created by the compounder that records a patient's prepared compound?
   A. MFR
   B. CR
   C. SDS
   D. FR

2. Which of the following types of communication must be completed for CSPs prepared in batches for multiple patients or any CSPs that use nonsterile ingredients in the preparation?
   A. MFR
   B. CR
   C. SDS
   D. SOP

3. All of the following information is required on the compounding record EXCEPT:
   A. Assigned BUD
   B. Name and strength of compound
   C. Name of patient
   D. Calculations used

4. Which of the following would be appropriate for performing calculations and preparing the MFR?
   A. ISO Class 7
   B. ISO Class 5 area
   C. PEC
   D. Pharmacy counter

5. When performing a visual inspection of a completed IV preparation, which of the following should be observed?
   A. Cloudiness, particulate matter, or color change
   B. Expiration date, particulate matter, cloudiness
   C. Foreign matter, cloudiness, BUD
   D. Leaks, cracks, expiration date

6. The temperature of the facility refrigerator must be recorded at least _____ per USP<797> guidelines?
   A. Weekly
   B. Monthly
   C. Daily
   D. After every shift change

7. When dispensing an IV push medication, which of the following best describes required packaging for delivery?
   A. Add a tamper seal to the syringe and needle and place in a sealed bag
   B. Remove the needle and use a sterile cap for the syringe
   C. Use a thick bag to protect the prepared IV Push
   D. Remove the used needle and replace with a clean one and sterile seal

8. All records related to compounding, including the MFR and CR, must be kept a minimum of _____ year(s) per USP guidelines.
   A. 1
   B. 2
   C. 3
   D. 5

9. If a compound requires special storage, which of the following documents would this be recorded on?
   A. MFR
   B. CR
   C. SDS
   D. PO

10. If a CSP has been exposed to temperatures outside the BUD range, which of the following should occur?
    A. Assign a new, shorter BUD based on the manufacturer recommendations for room temperature storage
    B. Refrigerate for at least 24 hours and then dispense
    C. Discard immediately
    D. Ask the Pharmacist

CRITICAL THINKING

1. You are a compounding technician at an infusion center and receive a call from a nurse at a long-term care facility. She states that when she went to check on the delivery from you, the ice in the cooler were thawed and the IV containers seemed wet. She is questioning if she should return them, since the cooler and contents were not very cold. What would you say?
2. You are getting ready to prepare a CSP and are reviewing the MFR, when you notice a change had been made since the last time it was used. According to USP<797> guidelines, what are the steps required?

BIBLIOGRAPHY

1. General Chapter 797 Pharmaceutical Compounding—Sterile Preparations. Retrieved January 29, 2019 http://www.usp.org/compounding/general-chapter-797.

Total Parenteral Nutrition

12

Learning Objectives

1. Discuss conditions in which total parenteral nutrition (TPN) would be appropriate and list five goals of parenteral nutrition.
2. List the solution components of TPN and special considerations when preparing admixtures.
3. Discuss the preparation of total parenteral nutrition, special considerations related to forming a TPN solution, and laboratory and other additional testing requirements.

Terms & Definitions

Additives Drugs commonly added to an intravenous solution

Anorexia Extreme loss of appetite

Hypermetabolic states Condition in which an abnormal rate of metabolism occurs, such as in trauma, fever, or severe burns

Hypoglycemia Abnormally low level of glucose in the blood

Kilocalorie (kcal) A unit of measurement in nutrition

Macronutrients A source of carbohydrates, protein, and fat

Malnutrition Any disease-promoting condition that results from either inadequate or excessive exposure to nutrients

Micronutrients Additives in a total parenteral nutrition (TPN), such as vitamins, electrolytes, and trace elements

Pancreatitis Inflammation of the pancreas

Peritonitis Inflammation of the lining of the abdominal cavity

Specific gravity Weight of a substance measured in grams per milliliters as compared to an equal volume of water

Total parenteral nutrition (TPN) Nutritional support in an intravenous preparation for patients who cannot consume sufficient calories because of trauma or certain diseases

INTRODUCTION

In this chapter, we will discuss *total parenteral nutrition (TPN)*, as well as the various components, preparation techniques, and calculation and storage information related to it. There are many employment opportunities for technicians in the area of nutritional support. It is essential to understand the proper techniques, as well as the goals of TPN therapy, to prevent patient harm and provide the proper amount of calories required for a specific patient.

PATIENT CONSIDERATIONS AND RATIONAL FOR USING PARENTERAL NUTRITION SOLUTIONS

Nutritional imbalance occurs in patients who are not able to take in adequate amounts of nutrients through the gastrointestinal (GI) tract because of diseases or conditions, surgery, or trauma. Nutritional requirements for a patient can vary but commonly range from 2500 to 3000 calories per day, while on TPN therapy, which is supplied in 2 to 3 L of fluid daily. TPN solutions are intravenous admixtures that can be individually designed to meet a patient's nutritional requirements, based on their disease or condition. These must be prepared using the highest quality of aseptic technique to

prevent the spread of any bacteria that may be passed to the already critically ill or susceptible patient. They also can be very complex and require many calculations and manipulations.

The basic goals of parenteral nutrition are as follows:
- Replace nutritional deficits
- Promote wound healing
- Increase weight or diminish the rate of weight loss
- Prevent protein or caloric **malnutrition**
- Sustain nutritional balance during periods when oral or enteral feedings are not possible or sufficient.

TPN should be administered to patients who are malnourished or have the potential of becoming malnourished. Often, a good candidate has multiple problems, and TPN often follows a surgery or procedure where food intake is inhibited. Conditions can include:
- Chronic weight loss, such as from **anorexia** or chronic vomiting and diarrhea
- Conditions requiring the bowels to rest, such as massive bowel surgery, **pancreatitis**, or **peritonitis**
- Multiple trauma, coma, or critical illness (known as **hypermetabolic states**)
- Severe burns.

Hypermetabolic states, like some of those listed previously, require additional energy for the body to heal. A balance of nitrogen in the blood is essential to keep a balance of protein. A negative nitrogen balance is an indicator that lean body mass is being broken down faster than it is being replaced. When this occurs in malnourished patients, the body converts the protein to glucose (sugar) for energy. Conditions such as fever, surgery, starvation, burns, and critical illness can cause metabolism to increase in an effort to speed up the healing process.

 Tech Note!

For each gram of nitrogen loss over the amount the body requires for intake, 6.25 g of protein or 25 g of muscle tissue is lost.

SOLUTION COMPONENTS AND SPECIAL CONSIDERATIONS WHEN PREPARING ADMIXTURES

COMPONENTS

The components of TPN consist of an energy source, such as a carbohydrate, protein, or fat. These three components are known as the *base*, or **macronutrients**. Sterile water for injection is also used to adjust the volume of the final solution.

 Tech Note!

Hypertonic fluids cause the water from the cell to move outward, which causes the cell to shrink. *Hypotonic fluids* cause water to move into the cell and therefore to swell and possibly burst. *Isotonic fluids* are similar in solute concentration to body fluids and have no effect on the volume of fluid inside the cell. See Chapter 6 for additional information.

Carbohydrates

The major function of carbohydrates is to provide energy. The most common intravenous source for carbohydrates is glucose. When glucose in the form of dextrose is provided in a parenteral solution, it is completely bioavailable for the body, without any effects of malabsorption. The highest concentration that should be given through a peripheral vein is 10% dextrose in water (D10W), and it should not be given for more than 7 to 10 days (Fig. 12.1). This is considered peripheral parenteral nutrition (PPN) and is only used for short-term therapy in those whose normal GI functions will resume in 3 to 4 weeks. For TPN, a 20% to 70% solution of dextrose may be used. These solutions are administered through the central vein that leads directly to the heart because of their hypertonic qualities.

This provides calories that are essential to the patient for long-term therapy. If 20% to 70% solution of dextrose is stopped abruptly, **hypoglycemia** may occur because of an imbalance of glucose and insulin in the body resulting from the high concentration used in the solution. For this reason, TPN is started gradually and tapered off. A 10% dextrose solution may be required in some patients to allow for the dextrose load to level out.

 Did You Know?

1 g of carbohydrate = 4 kcals.
3000 mL of dextrose provides 1000 calories.

For TPN orders, the physician will order the proper amount of calories he wants the patient to have daily, and each macronutrient provides a certain amount. The amount of total fluid is important as well, so the best combination of volume and calories provided is determined.

Fats or Lipids

Intravenous fats are primarily made up of safflower or soybean oil, egg yolks, and some glycerol to provide tonicity. Fat emulsions are available in 1.1 kcal/mL, which is a 10% solution and a 2.0 kcal/mL in a 20% solution. These solutions are known as the trade name, *Liposyn*, and they are a milky, white solutions (Fig. 12.2).

Fat is a primary source of energy and heat. It provides twice as much energy calories per gram as either carbohydrates or proteins. It is essential for all

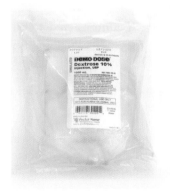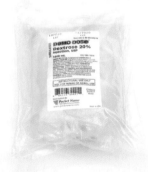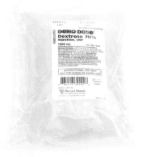

Fig. 12.1 Carbohydrate solution.

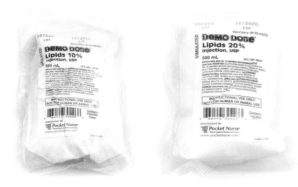

Fig. 12.2 Lipids solution.

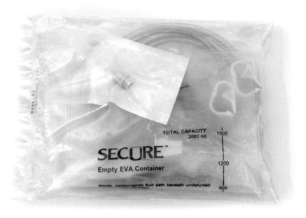

Fig. 12.4 Two-liters empty container.

structural cell membrane integrity. A condition known as *essential fatty acid deficiency (EFAD)* can occur, which causes complications, such as impaired wound healing and an increased susceptibility to infections.

> ### Did You Know?
>
> 1 g of fat (Liposyn) = 9 kcal.
> 500 mL of 20% Liposyn provides 1000 calories per day.

It is very important to carefully, visually inspect the fat emulsions for separation of the emulsion, and to not use them if there is a visible yellowish streaking.

Proteins

Proteins are body-building nutrients that promote the replacement of cells, as well as tissue growth and repair. Protein can be found in scar tissue, antibodies, and even clots. Amino acids are the basic units of proteins and are used in the TPN solution (Fig. 12.3). Some typical manufacturers' names are Aminosyn, Travasol, FreAmine, and Clinimix. These come in 3% to 15% solutions, and they are available with or without electrolytes.

The three components are added into an empty container that is usually 2 or 3 L capacity (Fig. 12.4).

Once this base is made, the next step is to add electrolytes and other ingredients based on the order.

> ### Did You Know?
>
> Protein requirements: Healthy adult = 0.8 g/kg/day.
> Protein requirements: Adult with critical illness = 1.2 to 2.5 g/kg/day.

Electrolytes

Long-term TPN requires basic electrolytes, such as potassium, sodium chloride, calcium, magnesium, and phosphorus (Fig. 12.5). Approximately 30 to 40 mEq of potassium is needed for each 1000 calories provided parenterally.

It is necessary for the transport of glucose and amino acids across the cell membranes. It may be given in the following ways:

- Potassium phosphate
- Potassium acetate
- Potassium chloride.
  Other electrolyte amounts needed are:
- Calcium gluconate or chloride: 10 to 15 mEq in 24 hours
- Sodium chloride or acetate: 60 to 100 mEq in 24 hours (maintains acid-base balance)
- Magnesium sulfate: 10 to 20 mEq every 24 hours.

These are compounded and calculated specifically for each TPN according to blood levels, acid-base balances, and disease states.

> ### Tech Note!
>
> Patients who have a decrease in renal function may require decreased amounts of potassium.

Vitamins

Certain diseases or other conditions can alter the amount of vitamins available in the body, and this

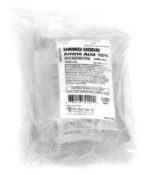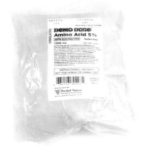

Fig. 12.3 Protein solution.

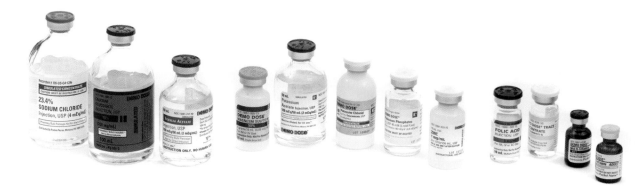

Fig. 12.5 Electrolytes.

deficiency can cause death in a critically ill patient. Vitamins, such as K1 (phytonadione), are found in lipids and therefore do not require additional injections to the patient if the patient receives this in the total parenteral admixture.

Trace Elements

These elements or microelements are found in the body in minute amounts and are beneficial in many ways. Each element is a single chemical and has its own deficiency state. Zinc aids in wound healing, copper reduces iron absorption, and iron is needed for hemoglobin production, the main component of red blood cells. Other elements, such as selenium, are important in the production of antioxidants, while fluorine and nickel are necessary for proper bone and teeth formation. Trace elements are available from the manufacturer in a single vial and are added to the TPN with the other macronutrients.

Other Additives

In addition to combining components of the base (carbohydrate, fat, and protein) and the **micronutrients** (electrolytes and vitamins) to form the TPN, other medications specific to each patient may be necessary. These may include insulin, heparin for blood thinning, and histamine-2 receptor blockers, such as famotidine (Pepcid), to prevent GI problems, such as stress ulcers.

> **Tech Note!**
>
> Always check the manufacturer's package inserts for information about any incompatibilities with the TPN solution when adding additional medications.

PREPARATION OF TOTAL PARENTERAL NUTRITION

Perform all calculations or research required to prepare the medication ordered. Once the order has been interpreted and the ingredients gathered, the TPN solution should be prepared using proper procedures and sterile aseptic technique in a certain order and in the correct environment (Procedure 12.1).

Procedure 12.1 Preparing a Total Parenteral Nutrition (TPN)

EQUIPMENT AND SUPPLIES

Medication order
Pen
Calculator
Compounded sterile preparation (CSP) label (prepared) and order
Bases (Amino Acid, Lipids, and Dextrose)
Micronutrient additives (vials of various electrolytes)
One regular needle each additive vial
3 way gravity TPN bag with leads
Sterile seal (for bag)
Personal protective equipment (PPE)

Waste container
Sharps container
Sharpie marker

STEPS: PERFORM OUTSIDE OF ISO CLASS 7 OR 8 ENVIRONMENT

1. Complete any calculations needed and prepare label before entering the ISO class 8 ante area.
   PURPOSE: The ante area is considered a controlled environment and loose papers or excessive movement or equipment introduced can create dust or the introduction of unwanted microbes.

Procedure 12.1 Preparing a Total Parenteral Nutrition (TPN)—cont'd

STEPS: PERFORM IN ANTE AREA (ISO CLASS 8)

1. Perform handwashing and garbing per USP<797> guidelines.
   Purpose: To ensure there is no contamination or transfer of infection from the compounder to the final compound

2. Ensure the laminar airflow workbench (LAFW) has been cleaned and turned on for at least 30 minutes.
   PURPOSE: The LAFW air flow must have time to circulate through the high-efficiency particulate air (HEPA) filter.

STEPS: PERFORM THE FOLLOWING IN BUFFER AREA (ISO CLASS 7)

1. Stage the bases and additives, TPN bag, label, and supplies needed on a (work surface) stainless-steel cart beside the LAFW.
   Purpose: Staging ensures there can be a review to verify that every item needed is there at arm's length; this allows less interruption once work starts inside the LAFW. Every time the compounder comes out of the primary engineering controls (PEC), there is a chance of introduction of contaminants that can be brought in from the ISO class 7 (buffer area) to the ISO Class 5 environment (PEC).

2. Mark each base with amount needed and place base items (Amino acid, Dextrose, and Lipids) and TPN empty container with leads in the LAFW one a time, hanging the bags and maintaining correct spacing of at least 6 inches. Spray each port with sterile isopropyl alcohol (IPA) 70%, after removing outer packaging at the edge of the hood.
   PURPOSE: Each item is sprayed and unwrapped before entering the ISO Class environment (PEC) to allow for less contaminants from outer wrappings or excess paper. ONLY what is needed should be in the ISO Class 5 area.

3. Attach the leads to each one of the base solutions without touching the critical site area, port tops and hang up.
   PURPOSE: The bases should be marked with a sharpie on the line where the fluid is stopped per the amount needed in the order.

4. Undue the roller clamp on the lead to each base hanging up. Stop by rolling the clamp down when the marked line is reached.
   PURPOSE: The marked line is the amount calculated for each base and all are added to an empty TPN bag for the base solution.

5. Lay the base aside for checking by Pharmacist. Once completed, discard the remaining bags of base fluid and put the TPN base to the side.
   PURPOSE: The base should be verified before adding the additives, which ensures it is correct before adding more ingredients to it.

6. Add each additive vial to the LAFW by spraying as in step 4.
   Purpose: After adding the medication to the bag per the ordered amount, the seal protects the port, which has been entered and also indicates to any person handling it that the bag has added contents in it.

7. Add a syringe and needle beside each additive withdrawn to the amount required to be withdrawn. Allow this to be checked before proceeding.
   Purpose: A check at this point ensures that validation of medications and correct calculations have been made before adding to the base. This is also a cost saving measure.

8. Withdraw each amount from each vial needed and keep the syringe and medication vials separated by laying the syringe/needle, with medication in it, next to its respective vial.
   PURPOSE: Another check by the Pharmacist may be required at this point before the additives are added to the base bag.

9. Once verified, add each additive to the port of the base bag. Do not discard syringes, just needles at this point. Affix a seal to any Multiple dose vials (MDVs) and the port of the finished TPN bag.
   PURPOSE: Once the bag is prepared and labeled, it will be checked by a Pharmacist. Each additive may also require an additional check, so stage the vials with their respective syringes for another check if needed, because of the numerous components and complicated calculations. *Remember: For any MDVs used, the time and date opened along with tech initials should be written on them.*

10. Recheck calculations.
    PURPOSE: Always recheck calculations to ensure that the correct compound was prepared. Never rely on the Pharmacist to find an error. When you are finished, consider it ready and correct and consider the Pharmacist to be a validation or second check in the system.

11. Allow the Pharmacist to check with the syringe, medication, and labeled bag "staged".
    PURPOSE: Create a "staged" layout so the Pharmacist can easily see how much you added per the syringe pulled back and the medication (ampule) you used, and can verify that the container is labeled correctly. *In some cases, they will want to see the filter straw or needle laid out to ensure it was used, so do not discard until you know.*

ANTE AREA

- Only bring outside items needed for the preparation of the TPN into the area.
- Perform proper hand hygiene, garbing, and gowning procedure.
- Put on sterile gloves.

BUFFER AREA

- Spray gloved hands with 70% alcohol or disinfectant and allow to dry.
- All supplies used in the PEC should be gathered and then decontaminated by spraying or wiping the outer surface with sterile 70% isopropyl alcohol (IPA) or removing the outer packaging at the edge of the primary engineering controls (PEC), as it is entered into the aseptic workspace. This will aid in removing dust particles and any other contaminates.
- Attach syringes to needles inside the PEC, without contact contamination or interruption of first air.
- Disinfect all critical sites using sterile 70% IPA wipes and wait to dry before use.

First, the base is made. This consists of the macronutrients, which are the amino acids, the dextrose, and the fat or lipid for the three-in-one solution. Some TPNs will call for the lipid to be infused separately; in that case, just the amino acid and dextrose will be together in the bag. The order of mixing is very important because the dextrose and the fat should not be directly combined.

GRAVITY METHOD

Each component is spiked (there is a sharp point at the end of the tubing designed to puncture the rubber port of a bag or vial) and a special empty bag that holds either 2 or 3 L is used. There are three leads attached to this bag that allow the fluid of each source to enter the empty bag by gravity. The empty bag will hold the components once they are added together, and then it will become the TPN. The fluids are transferred into the bag by hanging them up and allowing the calculated amounts to flow into the empty bag. Drawing a line with a Sharpie marker on the correct measurement before starting the flow indicates the amounts. The flow of each component is controlled by clamping off the lead of each piece of tubing.

AUTOMATED COMPOUNDER MACHINES

Automated compounder machines (also known as *compounders*) can be used to make the base as well. These automated machines allow the fluids to be measured by specific gravity, and they are programmable. **Specific gravity,** or the weight of each substance measured in grams per milliliters as compared to an equal volume of water, is programmed in the machine along with the desired volume, and the exact amount for each solution is pumped into the empty bag. For example, the specific gravity of sterile water is 1.00 g/mL

and dextrose is 1.24 g/mL because the sugar solution is heavier than water. There are many advantages to using the compounder machines; they are faster than the gravity method, there is less touch contamination, and they have better accuracy than the gravity method. Once the order is calculated, the pharmacist can input it into the system and generate a label automatically. Each bag is given a number, and the technician programs the compounder that sits directly inside the laminar airflow workbench (LAFW) and monitors the process. If there is a need to program the amounts of each source to be added, the technician can manually enter the volume to be added and the specific gravity of that source at the machine.

MICRONUTRIENTS

Once the base is prepared, it can be placed on the side of the PEC, out of the way, and the other ingredients or micronutrients can be introduced into the PEC. Each one should be drawn up individually. The amount of micronutrients that can be added vary from one or two up to as many as 14. If the gravity method is used, these will be gathered and staged in the LAFW in proper order, as described in the previous sections, "Ante Area" and "Buffer Area." Refer to the steps for drawing up a vial in Chapter 10 if needed.

The technician should always refer to the printed information from the manufacturer regarding incompatibilities and order of mixing throughout this process. For example, potassium phosphate and calcium gluconate can precipitate if they are added too closely together. These individual vials should be drawn up and then verified by a pharmacist before adding them to the bag of base solution preparation, which was made earlier.

If there is an automated compounder machine available for adding the micronutrients, this procedure is slightly different; it can be programmed to add these components similar to the way the base is made.

 Tech Alert!

Automated compounder machines are kept in the LAFW, and all aseptic technique procedures are necessary during use. Follow manufacturers' guidelines when cleaning the equipment, as well as while performing calibration to maintain the highest accuracy.

Even though TPN is most often administered in a hospital setting, a patient may receive this therapy at home. For patients who require TPN because of postoperative or preoperative procedures that prolong nutritional needs, as well as for those patients who will not ingest adequate nutrients and those who are unable to be fed by a feeding tube, a technician will prepare the TPN at a home infusion facility, where they will be delivered, and a home health nurse will administer the solution using an infusion pump.

SPECIAL CONSIDERATIONS

The U.S. Food and Drug Administration (FDA) has special steps to decrease the risk of precipitation forming in a TPN solution. Storage is extremely important because of the increased risk of microbial growth caused by the high dextrose content. Once prepared, the TPN should be refrigerated or used immediately. After they are hung, they should be infused or discarded within 24 hours. All parenteral nutrition should be filtered with a 0.2-micron filter. TPN solutions are administered through an infusion pump so that the rate can be controlled and gradually increased. Before infusion, TPN should be warmed to room temperature for approximately 1 hour. Patient care should include daily weight, vital signs, and various laboratory values every 4 to 6 hours. If TPN is stopped abruptly, a bag of D10W should be administered at the same rate that the TPN was being given, until the patient's status can be evaluated. Labeling is necessary and includes all ingredients and amounts added to the bag along with the expiration, rate to be infused, and the proper signatures of the preparer and a pharmacist.

Because of the complexity of TPN orders and the amounts of **additives** that must be combined, it is even more important to follow the strictest aseptic technique to avoid potential infections to critically ill patients (Fig. 12.6). The more manipulations that need to be involved in the preparation, the higher the risk of contamination of the parenteral admixture. Technicians should be extremely cautious when calculating the amounts of the additives, as well as when observing proper technique and storage requirements.

LABORATORY AND OTHER ADDITIONAL TESTING REQUIREMENTS

The patient on TPN must be monitored closely by a pharmacist and nutritional specialists to ensure the amount of carbohydrates, protein, and vitamins and minerals, such as trace elements, are appropriate. Since the patient on TPN is dependent on it for their only source of nutrients, slight changes in the blood levels can indicate that changes to the components are required. This has to be monitored through weekly and sometimes daily blood tests to check for levels in the blood. For instance, if the glucose level becomes too high because of too much dextrose in the TPN, this can cause the patient to become hypoglycemic, which can lead to death. The TPN order would need to be adjusted by a physician and a new bag prepared by the pharmacy, according to the new order presented. If a particular micronutrient level, such as potassium chloride, is too high, the amount in the TPN can be decreased to the next bag. Pharmacy technicians must be aware of the constant monitoring and possible order changes with TPN in order to provide the patient with the proper nutrients at all times.

REVIEW QUESTIONS

1. Which of the following is NOT a macronutrient used in a TPN?
   A. Electrolytes
   B. Protein
   C. Carbohydrate
   D. Fat
2. Which of the following would be considered a micronutrient component of a TPN?
   A. Dextrose 10%
   B. Liposyn 5%
   C. Potassium Phosphate
   D. Amino acid
3. A balance of _____ in the blood is essential to keep a balance of protein.
   A. potassium
   B. nitrogen
   C. sodium chloride
   D. magnesium
4. The highest concentration that should be given through a peripheral vein is _____ dextrose in water.
   A. 20%
   B. 10%
   C. 50%
   D. 70%
5. This condition may cause an abnormally low amount of glucose in the blood because of an imbalance of glucose and insulin in the body.
   A. Hyperglycemia
   B. Hypoglycemia
   C. Anorexia
   D. Malnutrition
6. Which subsequent condition describes what can occur to a patient because of trauma, fever, or severe burns?
   A. Hyperglycemia
   B. Hypoglycemia
   C. Hypermetabolic state
   D. Peritonitis
7. Nutritional requirements for a patient through a TPN usually occur in what range of calories?
   A. 1000–1500
   B. 1500–2000
   C. 2000–2500
   D. 2500–3000
8. Which trace elements add to wound healing in the body?
   A. Selenium
   B. Zinc
   C. Fluorine
   D. Nickel
9. The order of mixing is very important, so which of these components should not be directly combined?
   A. Dextrose and lipids
   B. Amino acid and dextrose
   C. Amino acid and lipids
   D. Dextrose and sterile water

TPN ORDER SHEET

HOME HEALTH		DATE
PATIENT	ADDRESS	

TPN FORMULA:

	mL
AMINO ACIDS: ☐ 5.5% ☐ 8.5% ☑ 10%	
☐ WITH STANDARD ELECTROLYTES	*425*
DEXTROSE: ☐ 10% ☐ 20% ☐ 40% ☐ 50% ☑ 70%	mL
(check one)	*357*
LIPIDS: ☐ 10% ☑ 20%	mL
FOR ALL-IN-ONE FORMULA	*125*

FINAL VOLUME		mL
qsad STERILE WATER FOR INJECTION *400 mL*	*1248*	

Calcium Gluconate	0.465 mEq/mL	*5*	mEq
Magnesium Sulfate	4 mEq/mL	*5*	mEq
Potassium Acetate	2 mEq/mL		mEq
Potassium Chloride	2 mEq/mL		mEq
Potassium Phosphate	3 mM/mL	*15*	mM
Sodium Acetate	2 mEq/mL		mEq
Sodium Chloride	4 mEq/mL	*35*	mEq
Sodium Phosphate	3 mM/mL		mM
TRACE ELEMENTS CONCENTRATE	☐ 4 ☐ 5 ☐ 6		mL

Patient Additives:

☐ MVC 9 + 3 10 mL Daily

☐ HUMULIN-R *10* units DAILY

☐ FOLIC ACID _____ mg
_____ times weekly

☐ VITAMIN K _____ mg
_____ times weekly

☐ OTHER: *MVI 10 mL/daily*

☐ OTHER: _____

Directions:

INFUSE: ☐ DAILY

☐ _____ TIMES WEEKLY

OTHER DIRECTIONS:

_____

_____

_____

_____

Rate: ☐ CYCLIC INFUSION:	"	☐ CONTINUOUS INFUSION:	"	☑ STANDARD RATE:
OVER _____ HOURS	"	AT _____ mL PER HOUR	"	AT *104* mL PER HOUR
(TAPER UP AND DOWN)	"		"	FOR *12* HOURS

LAB ORDERS:

☐ STANDARD LAB ORDERS
SMAC-20, CO2, Mg+2 TWICE WEEKLY
CBC WITH AUTO DIFF WEEKLY
UNTIL STABLE, THEN:
SMAC-20, CO2, Mg+2 WEEKLY
CBC WITH AUTO DIFF MONTHLY

☐ OTHER: _____
_____
_____

VALIDATION:

_____
DOCTOR'S SIGNATURE

Print Name: _____

Office Address: _____

_____

Phone: _____

WHITE: Home Health   CANARY: Physician

Fig. 12.6 Sample total parenteral nutrition (TPN) order. (From Brown M, Mulholland JL: *Drug calculations: process and problems for clinical practice*, ed 8, St Louis, 2007, Mosby.)

TPN ORDER SHEET

HOME HEALTH		DATE
PATIENT	ADDRESS	

TPN FORMULA:

	mL
AMINO ACIDS: ☑ 5.5% ☐ 8.5% ☐ 10%	*400*
☐ WITH STANDARD ELECTROLYTES	
DEXTROSE: ☑ 10% ☐ 20% ☐ 40% ☐ 50% ☐ 70% (check one)	*350* mL
LIPIDS: ☑ 10% ☐ 20% FOR ALL-IN-ONE FORMULA	*200* mL

FINAL VOLUME qsad STERILE WATER FOR INJECTION *400 mL*	*1350* mL

Calcium Gluconate	0.465 mEq/mL	*5* mEq
Magnesium Sulfate	4 mEq/mL	*10* mEq
Potassium Acetate	2 mEq/mL	mEq
Potassium Chloride	2 mEq/mL	*20* mEq
Potassium Phosphate	3 mM/mL	mM
Sodium Acetate	2 mEq/mL	mEq
Sodium Chloride	4 mEq/mL	*30* mEq
Sodium Phosphate	3 mM/mL	mM
TRACE ELEMENTS CONCENTRATE	☐ 4 ☐ 5 ☐ 6	mL

Patient Additives:

☐ MVC 9 + 3 10 mL Daily

☐ HUMULIN-R _____ units DAILY

☐ FOLIC ACID _____ mg
_____ times weekly

☐ VITAMIN K _____ mg
_____ times weekly

☐ OTHER: _____

☐ OTHER: _____

Directions:

INFUSE: ☐ DAILY

☐ _____ TIMES WEEKLY

OTHER DIRECTIONS:

_____

_____

_____

_____

Rate:	☐ CYCLIC INFUSION: OVER _____ HOURS (TAPER UP AND DOWN)	" " "	☐ CONTINUOUS INFUSION: AT _____ mL PER HOUR	" " "	☑ STANDARD RATE: AT _____ mL PER HOUR FOR *12* HOURS

LAB ORDERS:

☐ STANDARD LAB ORDERS
SMAC-20, CO2, Mg+2 TWICE WEEKLY
CBC WITH AUTO DIFF WEEKLY
UNTIL STABLE, THEN:
SMAC-20, CO2, Mg+2 WEEKLY
CBC WITH AUTO DIFF MONTHLY

☐ OTHER: _____
_____
_____

VALIDATION:

_____
DOCTOR'S SIGNATURE

Print Name: _____

Office Address: _____

_____

Phone: _____

WHITE: Home Health   CANARY: Physician

Fig. 12.6, cont'd

10. What method is used to measure fluids when using an automated compounder?
    A. Weight of each component in g/mL
    B. Weight of each component in grams
    C. Volume of each component in ounces
    D. Volume of each component in milliliters

CRITICAL THINKING

1. Would a patient who refuses to eat be a viable candidate for long-term TPN, and if so, why?
2. Why is periodic laboratory work important when administering TPN? Discuss the type of laboratory tests that are being done and why.

BIBLIOGRAPHY

1. Pharmaceutical compounding-sterile preparations (general information chapter 797). In: *The United States Pharmacopeia, 27th rev. and The National Formulary*, ed 22, pp. 2350–70, Rockville, MD, 2004, The United States Pharmacopeial Convention.
2. Gahart BL, Nazareno AR: *2007 Intravenous medications*, ed 23, St Louis, 2007, Mosby.
3. Phillips LD: *Manual of I.V. therapeutics*, ed 4, Philadelphia, 2005, F.A. Davis Company.
4. *Taber's cyclopedic medical dictionary*, ed 22, Philadelphia, 2013, F.A. Davis Company.
5. Trissel LA: *Handbook on injectable drugs*, ed 15, Bethesda, MD, 2016, American Society of Health-System Pharmacists.

United States Pharmacopeia<800> Hazardous Pharmaceuticals

13

Learning Objectives

1. List examples of ways that exposure to hazardous drugs (HDs) can occur.
2. Discuss inventory management considerations related to HDs.
3. Describe the environment necessary when HDs are being handled.
4. Discuss compounding personnel requirements related to HDs.
5. Describe the labeling, transport, and disposal of HDs.

Terms & Definitions

Active Pharmaceutical ingredient (API) Any substance or mixture of substances used in the compounding process

C-PEC Controlled primary engineering control, such as the class II BSC (biologic safety cabinet)

C-SEC containment secondary engineering control Room with fixed walls with airflow and pressure requirements where the C-PEC is placed

Deactivation Changing an HD to a less hazardous substance on surfaces by use of heat, sterilization, light

Decontamination Using chemicals to remove, deactivate, or neutralize an HD substance

Hazardous Drugs (HD) Antineoplastic and other drugs considered hazardous, as identified by the NIOSH organization

NIOSH National Institute for Occupational Safety and Health

Spill kit A special kit used to clean a spill for HDs

Supplemental engineering control An additional control used along with a primary or secondary engineering control, such as a BSC (biologic safety cabinet), which is used to enhance protection from an HD

INTRODUCTION

Before July 2018, the guidelines for handling a hazardous drug or HD was listed under chapters USP<795> or <797>. Following a revision process by USP, chapter 800 Hazardous Drugs—Handling in Healthcare Settings, has now been created and is in effect. This chapter is specific to HDs, either when performing nonsterile or sterile compounding, and the quality standards for handling, as well as storage, receipt, compounding, dispensing, administration, and disposal. All facilities that have potential exposure to these drugs are required to follow the guidelines.

The list of HDs can be found at the National Institute for Occupational Safety and Health (NIOSH), as discussed earlier, and this should be reviewed periodically to ensure a knowledge of current medications. There are over 200 drugs on the list, which are categorized in the following order:
- Any active pharmaceutical ingredient or API that is considered hazardous
- Any antineoplastic (chemotherapy agent) (Fig. 13.1).

EXPOSURE TYPES

Some drugs may pose a threat because of their direct exposure when compounding through skin or inhalation contact alone. Confining these drugs is a must to protect the compounder, as well as the patient care activities, with nursing personnel. Exposure could also occur during receipt, packaging, or disposal. Performing a risk assessment allows the facility to identify the various ways exposure can occur and what occupational actions should be taken.

Each activity used when handling HDs should be reviewed for each HD drug, and actions should be taken to protect the worker as well as any personnel who may be exposed to the drug.

Examples of ways that exposure can occur include:

Inventory processes	when receiving inventory, there may be residue on packaging
Dispensing	this may include counting an HD tablet/pill or administering IV therapy
Compounding	during the process, handling of powders or solutions can allow for skin or inhalation contact

Cleaning/ deactivation	during the cleaning process, residue exposure may occur through inhalation or contact
Administration	priming an IV line and administering medication to a patient may allow for undue exposure to the healthcare worker and patient. Can also include exposure from waste or body fluids of the patient receiving the medication
Spills	inhalation and possible skin contact while cleaning
Transport	moving these medications within the healthcare setting can allow for exposure through contact or inhalation
Waste	discarding supplies used in compounding as well as any items used in administration or waste can allow for exposure

IV, Intravenous.

INVENTORY MANAGEMENT CONSIDERATIONS

Facilities that prepare IV hazardous medications must follow the USP<800> and <797> guidelines for the environment. Engineering controls are specialized for HDs and certain areas must have negative pressure to protect the surrounding areas. There should be a back-up system to maintain the negative pressure atmosphere in the case of a power loss.

Storage of HDs is also critical. HDs should not be stored on the floor nor in areas that are high risk for flooding or high traffic. All inventory processes, such as unpacking, should occur in a neutral or negative pressure area to prevent particles from being transferred into the air where compounding takes place. There should be a dedicated refrigerator for the storage of HDs, separate from all other stock.

If a shipment appears to be damaged and the container does not require opening, label it as "hazardous" and return it to the wholesaler or manufacturer. If the container is broken or opened, open it in the controlled primary engineering control (C-PEC) on a plastic backed mat. Wipe the outside and placed it in a plastic bag. Either return it or dispose of it after deactivating or decontaminating, following the USP<800> guidelines.

ENVIRONMENT

The space/device where sterile compounding takes place must be in an ISO class 5 or better air quality. The PEC laminar airflow workbench (LAFW) should not be used. The acceptable C-PECs for compounding of HDs are as follows:

- Class II biologic safety cabinet—BSC
- Compounding aseptic containment isolator—CACI.

These "hoods" must be placed in a containment secondary engineering control room (C-SEC), which is of ISO class buffer room and ante room quality (Fig. 13.2).

The air quality in the C-SEC (room) where the hoods are placed must have air exchanges of at least 12 air changes per hour and be externally vented. There should be fixed walls in the ISO class 7 room and monitoring of air exchanges, temperature, and humidity is required. A sink must be placed at least 1 meter from the entrance to the negative pressure buffer room.

CONTAINMENT SUPPLEMENTAL ENGINEERING CONTROLS

The most common piece of additional equipment used to protect the compounder from exposure to aerosols, from the medication being withdrawn from a vial, is a closed-system drug transfer device or CSTD (Fig. 13.3). This device allows for a closed filter

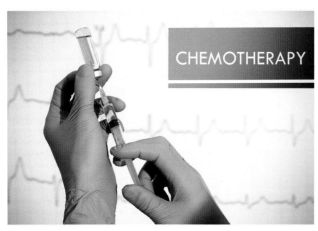

Fig. 13.1 Antineoplastics is a category on the National Institute for Occupational Safety and Health (NIOSH) list. (Copyright © iStock.com/GreenApple78.)

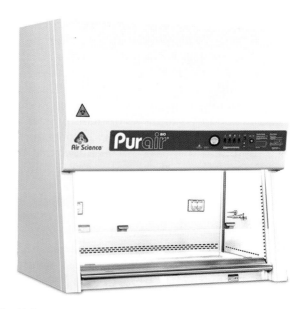

Fig. 13.2 Class II BSC (biologic safety cabinet). (Courtesy Air Science, Fort Myers, Florida.)

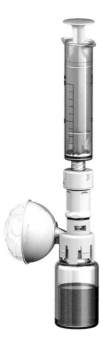

Fig. 13.3 CSTD (closed-system drug transfer device). (Courtesy and © Becton, Dickinson and Company.)

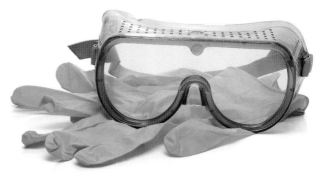

Fig. 13.4 Proper personal protective equipment (PPE) includes goggles and gloves. (Copyright © robeo/iStock/Thinkstock.com.)

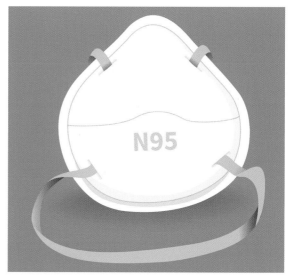

Fig. 13.5 N95 mask. (Copyright © aekgasit mabobut/iStock/Thinkstock.com.)

that captures aerosols that can escape from the vial as well as a needle-less puncture system to avoid a stick from an HD contaminated needle.

See Chapter 15 for more information.

COMPOUNDING PERSONNEL REQUIREMENTS

All personnel who handle HDs must be trained based on their job functions and reassessed every year. The training must include the following:

- Overview of HDs and their risks
- Proper use of personal protective equipment (PPE) and performance of handwashing
- Proper use of equipment to include cleaning (deactivation, decontamination)
- Spill management
- Review of the facilities standard operating procedures (SOPs)
- Proper disposal requirements.

Proper PPE must be worn during handling, which includes compounding, receipt of inventory, storage, transport, administration, cleaning, spills, and disposal. Handwashing must take place following the USP<797> guidelines and HD PPE is required. The gloves are different, however, in that they are chemotherapy gloves, which are thicker and must meet the American Society for Testing and Materials (ASTM) requirements. There are two pairs used, the outer pair being sterile. They should be changed every 30 minutes and discarded if pin holes or tears are found.

The gown is disposable and should be resistant to permeability of HDs. They must not have seams or closures where HDs can penetrate, and cloth gowns are not permissible. If there is no permeation, change them every 2 to 3 hours.

Head, hair, shoe, and sleeve covers are also required. In addition to these, goggles must be worn. Face shields and goggles are required, even if glasses are worn (Fig. 13.4).

When handling HDs, the risk of respiratory exposure is great. The compounder must protect themselves from inhalation of these drugs and wear a surgical type mask, such as those worn with non-HD compounding, is not sufficient. The use of an N-95 fitted mask is required. These should be worn during the deactivation, decontamination, compounding, or unpacking of HDs (Fig. 13.5).

Disposing of the worn PPE should take place before leaving the C-SEC area and should be performed into an approved hazardous containment device or sealable bag. Gloves and sleeves should be discarded in a sealed bag inside the C-PEC (Fig. 13.6).

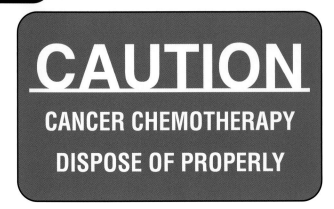

Fig. 13.6 Warning label. (Courtesy Healthcare Logistics, Circleville, Ohio.)

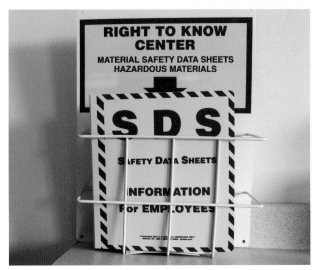

Fig. 13.8 Certificate of analysis (COA) and safety data sheet (SDS) information should be kept and reviewed as part of the facility's documentation. (Copyright © iStock.com/ROAProductions.)

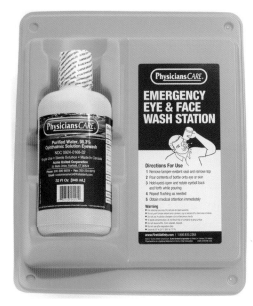

Fig. 13.7 The facility is required to have an eye wash station in case of eye exposure.

In case of eye exposure, an eye wash station is required for the facility (Fig. 13.7).

ENVIRONMENTAL CLEANING GUIDELINES

ALL areas where the handling of hazardous takes place and where any reusable equipment or supplies must be deactivated, decontaminated, disinfected, and cleaned.

The differences between these terms are important and each compounder or personnel handling HDs must know the process and common agents used.

PROCESS	PURPOSE	EXAMPLE OF AGENTS USED
Deactivation	Used to make a compound inert or inactive	Hypochlorite, hydrogen peroxide
Decontamination	Removes HD residue	Alcohol, water, hydrogen peroxide, sodium hypochlorite

PROCESS	PURPOSE	EXAMPLE OF AGENTS USED
cleaning	Removes inorganic or organic material	Germicidal agent
Disinfecting	Destroys microorganisms	Sterile alcohol or other EPA approved disinfectant

EPA, Environmental Protection Agency.

Materials and surfaces should be compatible with each chemical agent, so manufacturer information, such as the certificate of analysis (COA) and the safety data sheet (SDS) information, should be kept and reviewed as part of the facility's documentation (Fig. 13.8). Compounding personnel performing any of the cleaning activities listed previously must be garbed and wear appropriate respiratory gear.

Applying the agents with wetted wipes and discarding in hazardous waste containers are necessary. Decontaminating surfaces, such as carts, shelving, or the work tray in the C-PEC, should be performed by applying the agent to a disposable wipe or towel while wearing a respiratory mask.

Cleaning is used to remove contaminates, such as soil, dust, or residue. Before performing the disinfecting process with sterile alcohol (isopropyl alcohol [IPA] 70%), the surface or object should be cleaned with alcohol, water, or a germicidal agent. See Procedure 13.1 for instructions on cleaning a Biologic Safety Cabinet.

LABELING, TRANSPORTING, AND DISPOSAL

The facility must have SOPs for HDs, just as in USP<797>, for nonhazardous sterile compounds. These SOPs will describe the designation of HD areas, training requirements for compounders, receipt and

Procedure 13.1   Cleaning a Biological Safety Cabinet

Goal: To learn to properly clean a biologic safety cabinet.

EQUIPMENT AND SUPPLIES

- Biologic safety cabinet
- Lint-free cloths
- Manufacturer's recommended product for cleaning agent followed by isopropyl alcohol (IPA) 70% for disinfecting
- Sealable chemo-waste container small enough to sit inside the biologic safety cabinet (BSC)
- Chemo mat

PROCEDURAL STEPS

1. Perform hazardous garbing and handwashing in the Ante room before entering the buffer area.
   PURPOSE: When entering the SCA or segregated compounding area, personnel must avoid the introduction of pathogens. Because patients receiving intravenous medications have compromised immune systems and may be more susceptible to infection from contamination or transfer of germs from the compounding person to the product.

2. Place the chemo-waste container inside the BSC on the mat.
   PURPOSE: Hazardous waste (wipes used and outer gloves) should be discarded in hazardous container inside the BSC, sealed, and then placed in the proper trash to prevent transferring material to the outside. By not placing items on the direct work surface it will keep them from being contaminated with any material on the work surface.

3. Spray cleaning agent or alcohol on the front lip (tray area near edge of BSC) and wipe with cloth. Discard in the container inside the BSC.
   PURPOSE: Cleaning the tray first will help eliminate the sleeves from getting contaminated while performing the rest of the procedure.

4. Next, clean the intravenous (IV) pole and sides. Wipe with overlapping strokes, from top to bottom, downward toward the work surface. Discard in the container inside the BSC when done.
   PURPOSE: Cleaning should start at the top and work downward because a BSC is a vertical airflow hood.

5. Clean the work surface wfrom back to front, around the mat, moving outward with overlapping strokes.
   PURPOSE: Cleaning the work surface last will ensure any loose material has been caught from previous areas and moving from back to front will bring all contaminates out without pushing material into the hood.

6. Clean the inner view screen (glass front) of the BSC. Discard the cloth in waste container.
   PURPOSE: The inner glass view screen may have contaminants and should be cleaned with other surfaces.

7. Pinch the mat and place in the waste container.
   PURPOSE: The mat can be removed and discarded now to be able to get to the area of the work surface where it was sitting.

8. Remove the outer pair of gloves and discard them in the waste container.
   PURPOSE: The outer pair of gloves has been used to clean entire BSC and now coming outside with them on would containment the environment (air) of the buffer area.

9. Clean the outside of the view screen. Discard cloth in the waste container.

10. Remove the container and place it in the outer trash container marked Hazardous. Degown and place all personal protective equipment (PPE) in the same trash.
    PURPOSE: The cleaning items and PPE were all exposed to Hazardous material and must be placed in designated trach containers for proper disposal.

storage procedures, hand hygiene and garbing requirements, transport and administration, disposal, and environmental sampling and monitoring guidelines. Any persons transporting HDs must be trained in Occupational Safety and Health Administration (OSHA) standards for hazardous waste operations.

The risk factor of exposure for HDs to a person's health is greater, since these medications are often chemotherapy treatments for cancer or other hazardous medications. Transporting these medications must include clear labeling to identify them as HAZARDOUS, and personnel who deliver them must be trained in the risk of exposure.

The final product should be labeled and then placed in a hazardous labeled sealed bag, in case of a leak or spill (Fig. 13.9). Syringes that are prefilled

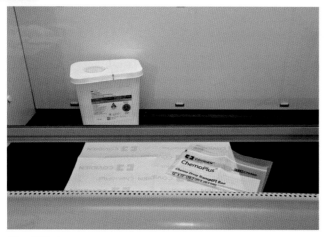

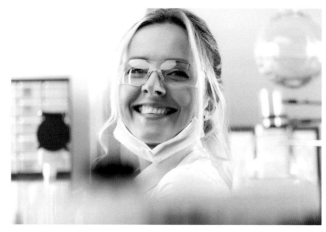

Fig. 13.9 Transport bag for final product. (From Davis K, Guerra A: *Mosby's pharmacy technician*, ed 5, St Louis, 2019, Elsevier.)

Fig. 13.11 Worker protection is essential when handling hazardous drugs. (Copyright © iStock.com/scanrail.)

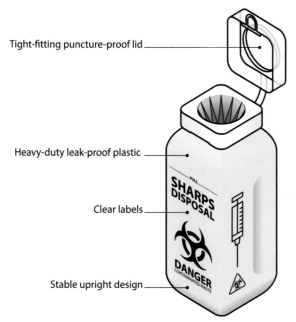

Tight-fitting puncture-proof lid

Heavy-duty leak-proof plastic

SHARPS DISPOSAL

Clear labels

DANGER CONTAMINATED WASTE

Stable upright design

Fig. 13.10 Hazardous sharps container. (Copyright © ZemLiew/iStock/Thinkstock.com.)

should be capped and should not be delivered with a needle attached.

Any persons or companies involved in disposal of HDs must also be trained in the proper trash containers and disposal guidelines per state, local, and federal requirements (Fig. 13.10).

MEDICAL SURVEILLANCE

The new USP<800> guidelines also include a comprehensive exposure plan, which reviews the protection provided by environmental controls, practices, and education. Workers are also monitored for future health changes due to exposure to HDs. This is accomplished by continuous monitoring and reporting of the worker's hours spent handling HDs, urine and blood

tests, and exit examinations for employees who leave. If any symptoms or physical changes are noted, the facility should take measures to review the data and make changes to protect the worker (Fig. 13.11).

Handling hazardous drugs can be intimidating to some technicians, but the key is to be aware and properly trained. Staying current with the facility's SOPs and following the practices to protect yourself, such as wearing proper garb, ensures the risk of exposure is minimal. Following the USP<800> guidelines that are designed to protect workers, patients, and administering personnel will provide a safe environment and enable technicians to provide the highest quality HD therapy available.

REVIEW QUESTIONS

1. Which of the following equipment is required to be used when withdrawing hazardous medication from a vial to capture aerosol contaminates?
   A. Compounding aseptic containment isolator
   B. C-SEC
   C. CSTD
   D. CACI
2. Decontamination is best described by which of the following?
   A. Using chemicals to neutralize an HD substance
   B. Using heat to change an HD to a less hazardous substance
   C. Using light to change an HD to a less hazardous substance
   D. Using sterilization to change an HD to a less hazardous substance
3. Which of the following best describes equipment required when compounding hazardous medications?
   A. Double gloves and safety mat
   B. Sterile gloves and use of CSTD
   C. Safety glasses and vented needle
   D. Regular needle and CSTD

4. Which of the following types of mask is required when preparing hazardous medications?
   A. Mask with eye shield
   B. Mask without eye shield and goggles
   C. N95 respirator mask
   D. Surgical type face mask
5. Which of the following types of C-PEC's are approved for the preparation of HDs?
   A. CACI and BSC
   B. LAFW and BSC
   C. CAI and LAFW
   D. Restricted Access Barrier system
6. Sterile alcohol is used for which of the following processes?
   A. Disinfection
   B. Decontamination
   C. Deactivation
   D. Both A and B
7. Which of the following organizations maintains a list of antineoplastic and other hazardous drugs?
   A. USP
   B. NIOSH
   C. ASHP
   D. NVVLP
8. In which of the following environmental conditions should inventory tasks, such as unpacking a shipment of hazardous medications, occur?
   A. Negative pressure room
   B. Positive pressure room
   C. Segregated area
   D. ISO class 5 area
9. How often should personnel who handle HDs be reassessed for their job functions?
   A. Monthly
   B. Yearly
   C. Every 3 months
   D. Every 6 months

10. Wearing PPE is required for all of the following functions EXCEPT:
    A. Decontamination
    B. Compounding HD medications
    C. Unpacking HD medications
    D. Ordering HD medications

CRITICAL THINKING

1. As a hazardous compounding technician, why is it important to have a set of baseline data and be observed under the medical surveillance program required by USP<800>?
2. Name at least three components covered in a facility's SOPs for HDs? Why is each important?

BIBLIOGRAPHY

1. Beans BE: (2017). USP <800> adds significant safety standards: facility upgrades needed to protect employees from hazardous drugs. *P & T: A Peer-Reviewed Journal for Formulary Management*, 42(5), 336-339, 2017.
2. Reed M: Key Points to Consider From USP<800>. Retrieved October 2, 21, 2018 from https://www.pharmacytimes.com/publications/health-system-edition/2018/january2018/key-points-to-consider-from-usp-800.
3. USP General Chapter <800> Hazardous Drugs-Handling in Healthcare Settings. Retrieved July 2, 2019 from http://www.usp.org/compounding/general-chapter-hazardous-drugs-handling-healthcare.

Hazardous Drug Preparation

14

Learning Objectives

1. Define the set criteria to identify drugs as being hazardous.
2. Discuss cancer and common chemotherapy medications used in cancer treatment.
3. Describe preparation of chemotherapy agents.
4. Discuss special considerations, techniques, equipment, and precautions related to hazardous intravenous (IV) drugs.
5. Describe how to clean up a spill and discuss the specific education and training requirements related to handling hazardous drugs.

Terms & Definitions

Antineoplastic agent An agent that prevents the development or growth of malignant cells

Chemotherapy Treatment of disease with chemicals that destroy disease-causing cells

Chronic anemia Condition in which there is a prolonged loss of red blood cells

Cytotoxic agents Antineoplastic agents that kill dividing cells

Hazardous Drugs (HD) Antineoplastic and other drugs considered hazardous, as identified by the NIOSH organization

Malignant Tending to or threatening to produce death; a neoplasm that is cancerous as opposed to benign

Metastasize Spreading of cancer cells to other organs or tissues

NIOSH National Institute for Occupational Safety and Health

INTRODUCTION

Once a drug has been identified as a hazardous drug or HD per National Institute for Occupational Safety and Health (NIOSH) listings, any personnel compounding HDs, either sterile or nonsterile, must adhere to compounding techniques/preparation under chapters USP<795> or <797>. The USP<800> guidelines, Hazardous Drug—Handling in Healthcare Settings, require outlining the specific techniques, equipment, and training to ensure minimal exposure for the preparer and the patient receiving the medication.

HAZARDOUS DRUG CRITERIA

The NIOSH organization has set criteria to identify HDs. Some drugs may be considered HDs for direct exposure by skin or inhalation. This can also be caused by containment, packaging, the dosage form, or most commonly, can include any antineoplastic (chemotherapy drug).

Antineoplastic agents or "cancer drugs" are designed to kill cancerous cells, but in the process, they also cause damage to healthy cells. All personnel who handle these medications must be aware of the risks and adhere to strict guidelines related to handling these products. With the ever-growing elderly population, there are more patients requiring this therapy, and there is a growing demand for **chemotherapy** clinics that have technicians preparing these medications for hospitals, outpatient clinics, and home administration. In this chapter, we will discuss the most common types of medications being used in cancer therapy, proper techniques and equipment, and training guidelines to ensure that technicians and patients will be protected.

 Tech Note!

Proper garbing is always required when handling HDs in any way.

CANCER AND CYTOTOXIC AGENTS USED IN ITS TREATMENT

Cancer, or neoplastic diseases, involves abnormal tissues (neoplasm) that grow excessively through uncontrolled cell division (Fig. 14.1). They can **metastasize** or invade the surrounding healthy tissues and cells, interfering with their function. Antineoplastic drugs, also referred to as *chemotherapy agents*, are used to either destroy these cells or control their growth.

Chemotherapy drugs are designed to affect cells that divide and grow rapidly. Since the **malignant** cells have these fast-growing properties and a high

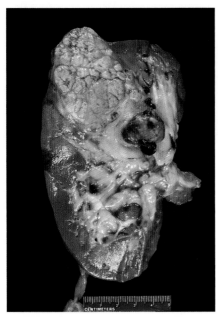

Fig. 14.1 A cancerous tumor in an adult kidney. (From Leonard PC: *Building a medical vocabulary with Spanish translations*, ed 8, St Louis, 2012, Elsevier Saunders.)

metabolic rate, the chemotherapy drugs affect them more. However, cells of the oral mucosa, gastrointestinal tract, bone marrow, and lymph tissues also grow rapidly and are affected by these drugs as well. This is the main disadvantage of using these agents; they destroy normal cells as well as cancer cells. If too much damage is done to normal cells before the cancer is brought under control, treatment must sometimes be withdrawn.

There are also many side effects and complications associated with these drugs, such as severe pain, nausea and vomiting, hair loss, and a compromised immune system. Patients often have to receive additional supportive agents, such as epoetin alfa (Epogen, Procrit), to prevent **chronic anemia** that occurs because of the use of chemotherapy agents. These supportive agents are hormones that help to rebuild red blood cells that have been destroyed because of the medication. Since the chemotherapy medications are considered toxic or hazardous, special considerations must be observed when preparing them aseptically.

COMMON CHEMOTHERAPY MEDICATIONS USED IN CANCER TREATMENT

There are several classes of chemotherapeutic agents used in intravenous (IV) therapy. They are classified as the following:
- Alkylating
- Antitumor antibiotics
- Antimetabolites
- Hormones
- Enzyme inhibitors
- Immunomodulating agents
- Miscellaneous agents.

Alkylating

These attach "alkyl groups," or side chains, to the proteins within the cancer cell and interfere with their function. Common drugs include:
- carboplatin
- cisplatin
- cyclophosphamide
- mechlorethamine oxide Mustargen, also known as *nitrogen mustard N-oxide hydrochloride.*

 Did You Know?

Nitrogen mustard was discovered as a result of experiments with poisonous gas during World War I.

Antitumor Antibiotics

These antibiotics interfere with the deoxyribonucleic acid (DNA) or ribonucleic acid (RNA) synthesis. Common drugs include:
- bleomycin
- doxorubicin (Adriamycin)
- mitomycin
- dactinomycin (Cosmegen).

Antimetabolites

These substances replace, compete with, or antagonize a metabolic or body function by interfering with a specific phase of cell metabolism. Common drugs include:
- methotrexate (Rheumatrex Dose Pack, Trexall)
- fluorouracil (Adrucil)
- cytarabine
- gemcitabine (Gemzar).

Hormones

Hormones antagonize certain reproductive tumors and accessory tract organs by altering hormonal balance. Common drugs include:
- fulvestrant (Faslodex)
- leuprolide (Eligard, Lupron)
- triptorelin pamoate (Trelstar).

Enzyme Inhibitors

Enzyme inhibitors interfere with tumor enzymes. Common drugs include:
- asparaginase (Elspar)
- irinotecan (Camptosar)
- pegaspargase (Oncaspar).

Immunomodulating Agents

Immunomodulating agents inhibit growth of the cells. Common drugs include:
- aldesleukin (Proleukin).

Miscellaneous Agents

Miscellaneous agents are mitotic inhibitors, which means they interfere with cellular division.

Chemotherapy treatment can be administered in a hospital or inpatient setting, as well as in an outpatient setting. It can also be accomplished by intermittent therapy, where high doses are given weekly or monthly, with a "rest period" in between. This allows the patient to gain strength and recover from some of the side effects that occur. Doses may be prepared in IV bags or as IV push in syringes. Common drugs include:

- vincristine (Vincasar)
- vinblastine (Toposar).

For a complete listing of hazardous drugs, refer to the NIOSH website at https://www.cdc.gov/niosh/index.htm.

PREPARATION OF CHEMOTHERAPY AGENTS

Aseptic technique should be followed when preparing any IV admixture, but when handling HD or **cytotoxic agents**, there are additional precautions. American Society of Health-System Pharmacists (ASHP) and USP<800> have specific guidelines concerning hazardous drugs and include special procedures, disposal, storage, and delivery of the medication to prevent unnecessary exposure. Occupational exposure can result in skin rashes, adverse reproductive effects, and even cancer. See Procedure 14.1.

Procedure 14.1 Preparing a Hazardous (Chemotherapy) Preparation

EQUIPMENT AND SUPPLIES

Medication order
Pen
Calculator
Compounded sterile preparation (CSP) label (prepared)
Closed system vial-transfer device (CSTD)
Regular needle
Intravenous (IV) container (fluid)
Syringe
IV tubing
Chemo mat
Spill kit
Transport bag and CHEMO labels
Sterile seal (for bag)
Personal protective equipment (PPE)
Waste container
Red sharps container
Yellow sharps container
Hazardous waste container

STEPS: PERFORM OUTSIDE OF ISO CLASS 7 OR 8 ENVIRONMENT

1. Complete any calculations needed and prepare label before entering the ISO class 8 ante area.
   PURPOSE: The ante area is considered a controlled environment and loose papers or excessive movement or equipment introduced can create dust or the introduction of unwanted microbes.

STEPS: PERFORM IN ANTE AREA (ISO CLASS 8)

1. Perform handwashing and garbing per USP<800> guidelines.
   PURPOSE: To ensure there is no contamination or transfer of infection from the compounder to the final compound
2. Ensure the biologic safety cabinet (BSC) has been cleaned and is on.

PURPOSE: The BSC air flow must have time to circulate through the high efficiency particulate air (HEPA) filter.

STEPS: PERFORM THE FOLLOWING IN BUFFER AREA (ISO CLASS 7)

1. Stage the medication, bag, label, and supplies needed on a (work surface) stainless-steel cart beside the BSC.
   PURPOSE: Staging ensures there can be a review to verify that every item needed is there at arm's length; this allows less interruption once work starts inside the LAFW. Every time the compounder comes out of the primary engineering control (PEC), there is a chance of introduction of contaminants that can brought in from the ISO class 7 (buffer area) to the ISO Class 5 environment (PEC).
2. Lay out the mat in the BSC and items needed for priming the bag.
   PURPOSE: The mat is used to capture any spills or droplets that occur during the compounding process. Priming the IV bag first without opening the hazardous drug (HD) ensures less exposure time or possible contamination for both the operator and the other items being used.
3. Prime the IV bag with clean fluid by attaching the spike end of the tubing to the bag. Allow fluid to reach the end of the tubing and then clamp the line off.
   PURPOSE: Priming the bag before adding the HD will ensure that the administration personnel or patient is not exposed to an HD or chemotherapy medication while inserting the IV line. Any drainage during this process will be HD-free.
4. Place primed bag with its tubing to the side and add other items in the BSC, one at a time, maintaining correct spacing of at least 6 inches,

Continued

Procedure 14.1   Preparing a Hazardous (Chemotherapy) Preparation—cont'd

spraying each item with sterile isopropyl alcohol (IPA)70%, and removing outer packaging at the edge of the hood.

   PURPOSE: Each item is sprayed and unwrapped before entering the ISO Class environment (PEC) to allow for less contaminants from outer wrappings or excess paper. ONLY what is needed should be in the ISO Class 5 area.

5. Before spiking the vial of HD medication, discard all trash possible (before exposure to the chemo drug) in regular trash or sharps if needed.

   PURPOSE: Discarding now helps with waste management costs, and any items not exposed can be placed in regular trash. Once the CSTD is attached, all trash is hazardous and must be placed in YELLOW marked containers.

6. Attach the CTSD to the medication vial without touching the critical site areas (spike end).

   PURPOSE: The CSTD spike end is considered a critical site, just as is the hub of a needle.

7. Withdraw the contents using just a syringe attached via luer lock to the CSTD. There will be no need for using the seesaw method or removing air bubbles, since the CSTD is a vented, closed transfer system.

   PURPOSE: The CTSD has a top that attaches directly to the syringe and a built-in filter with no needle. This allows for containment of aerosols and requires no needle.

8. Add a needle to the filled syringe and inject the medication into the IV bag and affix a seal on the port of the bag.

   PURPOSE: After adding the medication to the bag per the ordered amount, the seal protects the port, which has been entered and also indicates to any person handling it that the bag has added contents in it.

9. Inspect the bag for leaks, cloudiness, or particulate matter. Place the labeled bag in a labeled or marked as HAZARDOUS/CHEMO delivery bag. Wipe the bag with an alcohol wipe.

   PURPOSE: A visual inspection can find incompatibilities or leaks before patient administration. Wiping the bag down will ensure any contaminants that may have gotten on the bag do not come outside the BSC. Staging items will allow the Pharmacist to validate the compound without reaching in the BSC and risking exposure.

10. Discard unneeded items except vial, mat, and prepared compound. Lay out both the syringe drawn back to amount added and the drug inside the BSC and ask for a Pharmacist check.

    PURPOSE Discarding excess items in the marked HD containers inside the BSC and leaving out what should be checked allows for an easy visual check without the clutter.

11. Once the bag is checked, it can be removed. While still sitting at the BSC, discard trash and medication in the appropriate containers (yellow sharps for the syringe, needle, medication) and yellow container for the mat, only the OUTER pair of gloves, supplies, and any other items left in BSC.

    PURPOSE: Discarding items that have been exposed to HDs while still inside the BSC will ensure fewer exposure possibilities and proper disposal in HD marked containers. Keeping the INNER pair of gloves on protects from removing additional PPE outside the BSC.

12. Remove PPE (HD) including the INNER (second) set of gloves outside BSC and place in larger hazardous waste container in the ISO Class 7 area.

13. Wash hands again in the ante area before leaving the sterile compounding area.

    PURPOSE: Washing hands again after working with HDs will ensure more personnel and coworker protection upon leaving the sterile environment.

There are special supplies used in preparing sterile HDs (Fig. 14.2). Some are similar to those used in sterile preparation of nonhazardous compounds, but differences include:

- Yellow disposal containers (verses red)
- Special spill kits
- Chemo gloves
- Use of a preparation mat
- Gowns that close in the back with closed cuffs of elastic or knit.

PRIMARY ENGINEERING CONTROLS FOR HD PREPARATION

The ISO Class 5 environment primary engineering control (PEC), which is used in preparing HDs, requires a controlled (C)-PEC, such as a Class I or II biologic safety cabinet (BSC), a containment ventilated enclosure (CVE), or a compounding aseptic containment isolator (CACI). These C-PECs are externally ventilated cabinets that move air downward through a high-efficiency particulate air (HEPA) filter to avoid a flow of air across the work surface into the operator's face. They should be placed away from air currents and out of personnel traffic, inside a Class 7 environment or better (Fig. 14.3).

The downward air does not expose the operator to the air, as does the outward flow of air in a horizontal laminar airflow workbench (LAFW) hood. The BSC should also be placed away from the other preparation areas and allowed to remain running 24 hours a day.

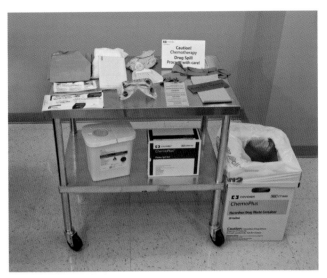

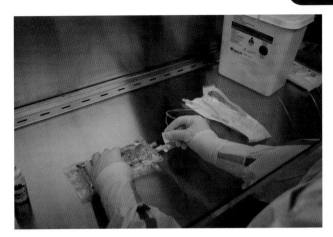

Fig. 14.4 A sharps container for hazardous waste may be placed in the biologic safety cabinet. (Courtesy CriticalPoint, LLC, Totowa, New Jersey.)

Fig. 14.2 Special chemotherapy supplies and equipment used in the preparation of a hazardous medication. (From Davis K, Guerra A: *Mosby's pharmacy technician*, ed 5, St Louis, 2019, Elsevier.)

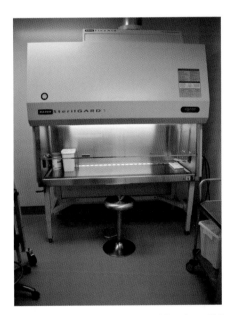

Fig. 14.3 Biologic safety cabinet, a type of Laminar Airflow System (LAFS). (Courtesy CriticalPoint, LLC, Totowa, New Jersey.)

Often a large hospital will have a separate department for chemotherapy infusion where this may be accomplished. Gowns, face masks, eye protectors, hair covers, shoe covers, and double gloving with special sterile chemo-type gloves are required during the preparation of all hazardous materials. A special sharps container, marked with "CAUTION: BIOHAZARDOUS WASTE" or "CHEMOTHERAPY WASTE", should be placed in the BSC and used as well (Fig. 14.4). Yellow (marked chemo or HD) bags and red disposal bags or biohazard bags for trash should be used instead of the regular trash bags. Place all waste generated in the BSC in a small sealed plastic bag before removing it from the BSC. A special

leak-proof absorbent pad should be placed on the work surface of the BSC to catch any small spills that may occur during manipulations. Only necessary items used in the preparation of the admixture should be placed in the BSC, because any items exposed to open vials or ampules must be disposed of in the hazardous waste bags.

Tech Alert!

Never hang bags above the work surface in a BSC because they obstruct the air from above.

SPECIAL CONSIDERATIONS, TECHNIQUES, EQUIPMENT, AND PRECAUTIONS

Placement of items should allow for the air above each item to be unobstructed during any manipulations. As trash is accumulated, discard it to the side of the work space (inside the BSC) in a puncture-proof container marked as *hazardous*. Any opened liquids should also be discarded in this container. Other materials used, such as wrappers and alcohol swabs, which have had minimal exposure, can be placed in a sealed plastic bag and transferred to a container outside the hood.

If possible, open packaging, such as syringes, tubing, and plastic bags, *before* opening the HD itself. This will allow much of the trash to be thrown away in the regular bag and avoid additional costs for special hazardous waste disposal.

Did You Know?

Hazardous waste, including sharps containers and any red bags marked "hazardous," must be incinerated, which costs enormous amounts of money.

To avoid unnecessary exposure to the nursing staff and the patient, tubing should be primed before adding the cytotoxic agent to the IV bag. This is accomplished by allowing "clean" fluid from the bag to run through the IV tubing and by attaching a Luer-Lok fitting device at the end before adding the cytotoxic agent to the bag.

> **! Tech Alert!**
>
> Always prime tubing and perform any manipulations that can be done before opening any HD. This will avoid unnecessary exposure to the caregiver and the technician preparing the medication.

Since spray often occurs with withdrawal of the contents from a vial, a closed system vial transfer device (CSTD) must be used when the dosage form allows. These devices are needleless and contain a 0.2-micron hydrophobic filter that allows the air to escape through the closed system rather than in the air. The spike end is inserted into the vial, a syringe is attached on the device by Luer-Lok, and the contents are withdrawn. If a CSTD is not available, there are some special considerations to observe when using a syringe and needle in the preparation and delivery of chemotherapy medications (Fig. 14.5).

- Use caution to avoid pressure build-up inside the vial that may result in spray or leakage.
- When adding diluent to a vial, inject slightly less air into the vial than required to maintain "negative" pressure.
- Keep the access pin or needle in the vial when measuring the dose.
- Use syringes that are large enough that the solution drawn up does not take up more than three-fourths of the space to avoid the plunger from coming out.

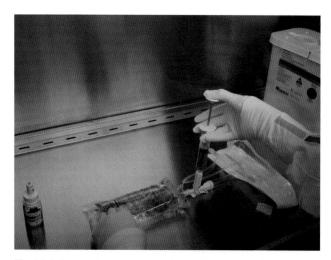

Fig. 14.5 If not using a closed system vial-transfer device, there are special considerations when using a syringe and needle in the preparation and delivery of chemotherapy medications. (Courtesy Critical-Point, LLC, Totowa, New Jersey.)

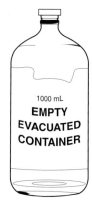

Fig. 14.6 Empty evacuated container (EEC)

- When removing the syringe from the vial, use a steady, slow motion while holding back on the plunger to avoid leakage or spray.
- When removing air bubbles from a syringe, clear any solution from the hub of the needle by drawing additional air into the syringe. Any excess drug should be expelled into a closed container, known as an *empty evacuated container (EEC)* (Fig. 14.6), rather than expelling it into the air.
- In the case of an IV push order, *never* transport drug-filled syringes with needles attached. Replace the needle with a push-on or twist-on cap, being careful to not contaminate the surface of the cap or the syringe tip.

  If an ampule is used, follow these guidelines:
- Tap down any drug from the top of the ampule and put gauze around the neck when you break it.
- Change the standard needle to a filter device or filter needle before adding the solution to the IV solution container.
- Dispose of any remains of the ampule in the puncture-proof container that is marked *hazardous*.

  Once the admixture is completed, the bag should be checked for leakage and wiped down with moist gauze. Wipe the entry port and place it in a zipped-lock bag. It should be labeled with an additional warning label that reads *"Caution: Hazardous Drug. Handle with Gloves. Dispose of Properly"* on the drug container itself, as well as on the outside of the bag used for transport.

> **Tech Note!**
>
> Never transport cytotoxic drugs through a pneumatic system.

HDs should be stored separately from other inventory to prevent contamination and unnecessary exposure and misadventures or errors, such as pulling the wrong drug. Wearing appropriate chemotherapy gloves and other required personal protectice equipment (PPE, see Ch. 14) is required when handling, stocking, distributing, preparing, and performing inventory control. Access should also be limited to only those personnel who are involved in HD preparation. When wearing double gloves, tuck the cuff of the inner glove under the gown sleeve, and tuck the cuff of the outer glove over the gown sleeve. If the outer gloves become contaminated, change them immediately. If the outer glove is punctured or torn, change both gloves.

 Tech Note!

Follow these steps in this order for removal of gloves and gown once manipulations are complete:
1. Remove the outer pair of gloves in the BSC and place them in a sealed bag.
2. Remove the gown.
3. Remove the inner pair of gloves, and discard all of the aforementioned items in the hazardous waste container.

CLEAN UP

Trained personnel must clean up spills immediately. Garb should include an outer pair of utility gloves and an inner pair of chemo gloves, gown, eye protection, and a respirator if aerosol droplets or powder is present. If a large spill occurs, the area should be restricted and an absorbent pad should be used. There are standard chemotherapy spill kits available that include all of the necessary items needed to contain a spill, including protective gear and disposal bags. Spills on the skin should be washed with soap and water immediately, and contact with the eyes should be followed by a 3- to 5-minute rinse. All technicians involved in the preparation of HD products should be familiar with site-specific procedures and protocols.

EDUCATION AND TRAINING REQUIREMENTS

The ASHP and USP<797> have specific guidelines for handling HDs that include training and education guidelines. According to USP<800>, "Personnel who compound hazardous drugs should be fully trained in the storage, handling, and disposal of these drugs" (USP). Training should occur before preparing or handling, and testing of specific techniques should be included at least annually. This should include didactic overview of drugs and ongoing training for new drugs, as well as safe manipulation practices, negative pressure techniques, correct use of CSTD devices, containment and clean up of spills, and exposure treatment.

Disinfecting and deactivating the environment, including sampling of surface areas such as the BSC and counter tops for HD environment, adhere to the same scheduling as USP<797> guidelines. Compounding personnel with reproductive capability should confirm in writing their understanding of the

risks. The ASHP Technical Assistance Bulletin on Handling Cytotoxic and Hazardous Agents is also a comprehensive source of current information. It states, "Conduct regular training reviews with all potentially exposed workers in workplaces where hazardous drugs are used" (NIOSH). Disposal of all contaminated waste should follow federal and state regulations.

Always use proper aseptic technique when preparing any IV admixture. Extra precautions should be observed when handling HDs. All required PPE (e.g., gowns, gloves, and masks) are always used, and disposal of contaminated waste should follow procedures. Cleaning of the BSC should occur daily or when a spill occurs. All PPE should be worn to avoid contact with any HD residue. Patients with cancer have many additional complications and are very susceptible to infections caused by compromised immune systems and general weakness. It is extremely important to remember to follow guidelines to safeguard yourself as well as your patient and other healthcare workers who are associated with HDs.

REVIEW QUESTIONS

1. Which of the following supply items must be used when compounding hazardous medications?
   A. Vented needle
   B. Regular needle
   C. Filter needle
   D. Chemo dispensing pin
2. All of the following cells are most affected by chemotherapy medications EXCEPT?
   A. Mouth area cells
   B. Cells in the gastrointestinal tract
   C. Cells in bone marrow
   D. Cells in the lung area
3. Which of the following is a common medication used to rebuild red blood cells destroyed by chemotherapy medication?
   A. Procrit
   B. Hematocrit
   C. Adrucil
   D. Mitomycin
4. Which of the following medications is an example of an antibiotic chemotherapy drug used to treat tumors?
   A. Adriamycin
   B. Adrucil
   C. Elagard
   D. Elspar
5. All of the following are special supplies required when compounding hazardous sterile medications EXCEPT?
   A. Yellow disposal containers
   B. Spill kits
   C. Sterile gloves
   D. Preparation mat

6. Which terms best describe the process of filling the IV tubing with clean fluid from the IV bag (before the hazardous medication is added)?
   A. Preparing the tubing
   B. Priming the tubing
   C. Pinching the tubing
   D. Placing the tubing

7. What is the primary function of the absorbent mat used when preparing sterile hazardous compounds?
   A. To absorb spills outside the PEC
   B. To absorb spills inside the PEC
   C. To clean up spills outside the PEC
   D. To clean up spills inside the PEC

8. Which of the following hazardous medications works by interfering with tumor enzymes?
   A. Trelstar
   B. Gemzar
   C. Elspar
   D. Cosmegan

9. With regard to the BSC, which of the following describes the airflow direction?
   A. HEPA filtered air flows vertically and is vented externally
   B. HEPA filtered air flows horizontally and is vented internally
   C. HEPA filtered air flows vertically and is vented internally
   D. HEPA filtered air flows horizontally and is vented externally

10. Which of the following terms describes a neoplasm that has become cancerous?
    A. Metastasize
    B. Malignant
    C. Cytotoxic
    D. Chronic

CRITICAL THINKING

1. You are the chemotherapy technician for the day at the hospital. It is time to put on your garb and prepare for the batch due this afternoon. When you start to put on your garb, you notice the gloves in the bin are not chemo gloves—but rather sterile gloves from the IV room. Can you double glove and use these instead? Explain your answer.

2. You must prepare a replacement chemo IV preparation for a patient whose line infiltrated and will need another one as quickly as possible. The nurse says she will wait, and you start. You are in a hurry and forget to take all of the necessary steps. You add air to the vial, which causes spray all over the bag, as well as your gloves and sleeves. Explain what you would do in detail.

BIBLIOGRAPHY

1. Pharmaceutical compounding-sterile preparations (general information chapter 797). In: *The United States Pharmacopeia, 27th rev. and The National Formulary*, ed 22, pp. 2350–70, Rockville, MD, 2004, The United States Pharmacopeial Convention.
2. Gahart BL, Nazareno AR: *2007 Intravenous medications*, ed 23, St Louis, 2007, Mosby.
3. Phillips LD: *Manual of I.V. therapeutics*, ed 4, Philadelphia, 2005, F.A. Davis Company.
4. *Taber's cyclopedic medical dictionary*, ed 22, Philadelphia, 2013, F.A. Davis Company.
5. Department of Health and Human Services, Centers of Disease Control and Prevention, National Institute for Occupational Safety and Health: *NIOSH alert: preventing occupational exposures to antineoplastic and other hazardous drugs in health care settings.* www.microcln.com/PDF/2004_165.pdf. Accessed March 1, 2013.

United States Pharmacopeia<825> Radiopharmaceutical—Preparation, Compounding, Dispensing, and Repackaging

15

Learning Objectives

1. Describe practice and quality standards for handling radiopharmaceuticals, including radiation detection and measuring devices.
2. Discuss personnel training and qualifications necessary for personnel who work with radioactive material. Also,

discuss handwashing, garbing order, and the necessary environment.

3. Describe remote aseptic processing, quality controls and testing, additional considerations, and transporting guidelines related to radiopharmaceuticals.

Terms & Definitions

ALARA represents "as low as (is) reasonably achievable". The effort of maintaining exposures to ionizing radiation as low as possible

Dynamic operation condition existing conditions in the segregated radiopharmaceuticals compounding processing area (SRPA) or classified area, where compounding activity is taking place

Hot-cell a device made of lead that is used to shield or contain radioactive materials

Hot lab a nonclassified radiopharmaceutical processing area without a primary engineering control (PEC)

Kit A commercially available kit that contains everything to compound a radiopharmaceutical EXCEPT the radionuclide

Kit-splitting (fractionation) dividing a kit's vial contents to transfer aliquots into other containers

Radioactive materials (RAM) license document that is issued by the United States or an agreement state that allows for various activities involving radioactive materials, such as compounding, distribution, medical use, and possession

Radio assay measurement with a special device for amount of radioactivity present in a container

Radiopharmaceutical a finished dosage form that contains a radioactive substance. Term is interchangeable with "radioactive drug"

Segregated radiopharmaceutical processing area (SRPA) the designated area that contains the PEC, where radiopharmaceutical compounding takes place

INTRODUCTION

Many of the techniques and required practices for handling radiopharmaceuticals are the same as USP<797>, with some additional requirements. There is the additional need to protect the compounding personnel, as well as the public, from exposure to radiation. In some cases, this may cause deviations to some of the sterile practices and adherence to Chapter 825 provides those guidelines. Additional supplies, such as vial shields, are used for contamination control. Environment controls, training, techniques, and documentation will be discussed here.

REGULATORY ORGANIZATIONS

Radiopharmaceuticals are considered a set inside radioactive materials and fall under the control of the US government Nuclear Regulatory Commission (NRC), as well as the US Food and Drug Administration (FDA). The regulations are designed for safe preparing, dispensing, and delivery of human and animal radioactive medications. Federal and state

organizations limit radiation exposure to all personnel who handle radiopharmaceuticals and require detection and measuring devices to be used.

Time, distance, and shielding are all part of the efforts to protect anyone near radioactive medications.

 Tech Note!

USP<825> includes the further processing or manipulation even after release.

TIME

When handling radiopharmaceuticals, the time that aseptic preparation is performed must be balanced with the exposure time to the medication. The ALARA or as "low as reasonably achievable" practice is used to ensure safety and the least time of exposure possible. Measuring devices must be used to allow the compounder to know the exposure readings. The goal is to handle the medication and perform

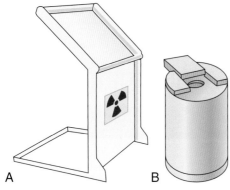

Fig. 15.1 (A) L-block. (B) Shield.

compounding as quickly as possible and to limit the time and hand movements in and out of the ISO Class 5 environment (primary engineering control [PEC]).

DISTANCE

The distance from the handler and the radiopharmaceutical should be limited. The closer to the radioactive material the person is, the more exposure there will be. There are remote special tools that can be used to allow more space between the compounder and the material.

SHIELDING

Shielding refers to special equipment, such as vial and syringe shields made of lead or tungsten, that are used to protect the radiopharmaceutical exposure to the compounder. There are also torso vests and L-blocks, which are mini walls that the compounder works around when performing aseptic technique (Fig. 15.1).

EXAMPLES OF STERILE RADIOPHARMACEUTICALS

All injectables, including intravenous, subcutaneous, intraperitoneal, inhalations, ophthalmics, intradermal, and intrathecal, are considered sterile radiopharmaceuticals. These medications are usually packaged in vials, and using aseptic techniques found in USP<797>, such as disinfecting the vial septum with a 70% isopropyl alcohol (IPA) sterile wipe, is still performed. In addition, the shields discussed earlier are used to decrease exposure from the radioactive medications being drawn up.

Radioisotopes are often used for diagnostic procedures, such as imaging tests or diagnoses. Some common examples include gallium, technetium Tc99m lidofenin, or technetium Tc99m mebrofenin. Certain cancers of the bone, thyroid, or prostate use radioactive drugs. Iodine can be injected with a prepared syringe for thyroid cancer. They are commonly given by injection and give off radiation to kill the cancer cells. Examples include: radioactive iodine, strontium, samarium, and radium.

RADIATION DETECTION AND MEASURING DEVICES

Personnel who are handling radiopharmaceuticals must wear extremity dosimeters, which are devices used to measure long-term radiation exposure. This is usually worn on the ring finger and under the gloves. A body dosimeter is also used and worn under the gown. Additional measuring devices may be placed inside the ISO Class 5 PEC.

PERSONNEL TRAINING AND QUALIFICATIONS

In addition to following the USP<797> guidelines for aseptic compounding, the personnel who work with radioactive material must have additional training and knowledge of exposure risks to this special group of drugs. Competencies that include aseptic technique, garbing, PEC cleaning, media fill testing, and gloved fingertip sampling must be reviewed every 12 months. Anyone who has rashes, sunburn, recent tattoos, or respiratory infections should be carefully reviewed, as these conditions may allow for an increased risk to exposure. If a person fails any of the evaluations, they must pass reevaluations before resuming processing of sterile radiopharmaceuticals.

HANDWASHING AND GARBING ORDER

Before entering the segregated radiopharmaceuticals compounding processing area (SRPA), also referred to as the buffer room, personnel must perform handwashing (hands and arms up to elbows) and remove all outer clothing and jewelry. Once in the SRPA, don shoe covers, head/hair covers, and face mask, then use an alcohol-based hand sanitizer. Next, don a low-lint disposable gown with cuffs that fit snuggly to wrists. Last, don sterile, powder-free gloves that cover the cuffs and leave no skin exposed. When leaving the SRPA, the garb must be discarded, and new garb must be put on for each reentry.

ENVIRONMENT

The PEC, such as the laminar airflow workbench (LAFW) or biologic safety cabinet (BSC), should be placed in a classified area, following the USP<797> guidelines for ISO Class 7 or better buffer room and ISO Class 8 or better ante room with fixed doors and walls. If using an LAFW, the airflow is vertical unidirectional high-efficiency particulate air (HEPA) filtered air. The BSC has an open front and inward and downward airflow that is HEPA filtered exhaust.

Temperature and humidity control, as well as cleaning of surfaces to include walls, floors, ceilings, and surfaces should follow the USP<797> guidelines.

REMOTE ASEPTIC PROCESSING

A **hot-cell** may be used to provide a physically segregated ISO Class 5 processing area. This is a device that allows the operator to work remotely and outside of the PEC, which limits exposure distance. This may be integrated with the HEPA filtration system and should be checked with smoke pattern tests periodically.

QUALITY CONTROLS AND TESTING

Surface sampling, media fill testing of personnel, and daily monitoring of temperature and humidity are required.

AGENT	PURPOSE
Cleaning agent	Removes residue like dirt, debris, and residual drugs/chemicals from surfaces
Disinfecting agent	Destroys fungi, viruses, bacteria
Sporicidal agent	Destroys bacterial and fungal spores

Cleaning and disinfecting are performed daily for the PEC and torso shield, surfaces, such as sink, hot-cells interior, if used, and equipment within the PEC. Absorbent contamination pads are used to apply chemicals.

Walls, ceiling, and storage shelving should be cleaned and disinfected monthly, and sporicidal should be used.

 Tech Note!

A complete list of chemicals to use is provided in USP<1072> Disinfectants and Antiseptics.

ADDITIONAL CONSIDERATIONS

Any radiation shielding equipment used in the SRPA or PEC that is also exposed to patient care areas, must be cleaned and disinfected before returned to the classified areas. Syringes used in patient administration should never be brought back into PEC or SRPA areas.

BUD ASSIGNMENT

When assigning a beyond-use date (BUD) for a radio-pharmaceutical, the time starts with the first puncture into the vial septum. There are **kits** made from the manufacturer, which may include suggested times in the packaging information. Several other considerations must be included:

- radiochemical stability—may be affected by packaging type, stabilizing agents used, or storage temperature
- radionuclidic purity—radioactive materials decay over time and must be considered in assigning a BUD
- age of generator—this refers to chemical changes to the atoms and nuclides of the material, which naturally occur
- others include specific activity and number of particles.

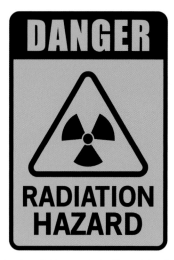

Fig. 15.2 Standard radiation symbol. (Copyright © duleloncar_ns/iStock/Thinkstock.com.)

DOCUMENTATION AND LABELING

Documentation should include the facility maintaining Master Formula Records (MFR) if compounding a radioactive preparation with minor deviations. This would be specific processes or methods outside of FDA-approved labeling. Labeling requirements are governed by several agencies including State Boards of Pharmacy and Federal agencies.

Some special requirements for the INNER label include:
- Standard radiation symbol (Fig. 15.2)
- The words "caution-Radioactive Material"
- Radionuclide and chemical name
- Radioactivity (units at time of calibration). The OUTER shield or label must include:
- Standard radioactive symbol
- The words "caution-Radioactive Material"
- Radionuclide and chemical name
- Radioactivity (units at time of calibration)
- Volume dispensed
- Number of dosages
- BUD.

TRANSPORTING GUIDELINES

The ports or generator needle must be capped with sterile protectors within the ISO Class 8 environment or better. Special leaded containers are used to deliver the doses.

The basic guidelines for preparation, environment, and documentation, under USP<797> for sterile, and USP<795> for nonsterile compounding, is used; and in addition, special consideration for radiopharmaceuticals are included. These radioactive materials present an additional risk to compounders and patients and should be followed per the USP<800> chapter guidelines. All personnel handling radioactive materials should be aware of all three guidelines and protect themselves from exposure, whenever possible. Using proper equipment and measurement devices are additional protective supplies that will enhance the safety of all workers.

REVIEW QUESTIONS

1. Which of the following substances is a hot cell made of?
   A. Stainless steel
   B. Lead
   C. Copper
   D. Steel
2. What term describes the existing conditions in the SRPA, where radiopharmaceutical compounding occurs?
   A. Radioactive compounding
   B. Dynamic operations
   C. Radioactive operations
   D. Hazardous compounding
3. The term ALARA can be defined as which of the following?
   A. As low as is reasonably achievable
   B. As low as radioactivity is allowed
   C. All radioactivity allowed
   D. Always aware of radioactivity
4. A radio assay is a measurement of which of the following?
   A. Radioactivity of a drug
   B. Radioactivity reading for the compounder
   C. Radioactivity of the container
   D. Radioactivity of completed compound
5. Which of the following organization(s) does Radio-pharmaceuticals fall under the control of?
   A. NRC and FDA
   B. USP and FDA
   C. USP and NRC
   D. NRC and NABP
6. Which of the following describes the mini walls that the compounder works around when preparing radiopharmaceuticals?
   A. L block
   B. H block
   C. Glass block
   D. R block
7. All of the following are common injections used to give off radiation to kill cancer cells in bones EXCEPT:
   A. Gallium
   B. Radioactive iodine
   C. Strontium
   D. Radium

8. Compounding personnel handling radiopharmaceuticals must be evaluated at least every _____ for proper aseptic technique.
   A. Year
   B. 6 months
   C. 30 days
   D. 90 days
9. When assigning a BUD for a radiopharmaceutical, which of the following describes when the time starts?
   A. With the first puncture into the vial
   B. With the first entry into the container
   C. With the first contact of the packaging
   D. With the first contact with syringe being used
10. Which of the following is a requirement for the OUTER label of a compounded radiopharmaceutical that is not required for the INNER label?
    A. Standard radiation symbol
    B. The words "caution-Radioactive Material"
    C. Radionuclide and chemical name
    D. BUD

CRITICAL THINKING

1. You are the compounding technician today and receive a phone call from a facility that administers radiation therapy for cancer patients. The nurse states she has a patient with some adverse drug effects and wants to know to whom she should report this. What would you tell her? And why?
2. You are compounding a radioactive injection of Iodine for a local clinic. What would this typically be used for? How would you package this?

BIBLIOGRAPHY

1. American Cancer Society: Systemic Radiation Therapy. Retrieved February 28, 2019 from https://www.cancer.org/treatment/treatments-and-side-effects/treatment-types/radiation/systemic-radiation-therapy.html.
2. APhA: Nuclear Pharmacy Resources. Retrieved March 20, 2019 from https://www.pharmacist.com/nuclear-pharmacy-resourcesUSP<825>.
3. Ponto J: USP<797> and <825> Current and future standards for preparation and compounding of radiopharmaceuticals. Retrieved March 12, 2019 from https://apha2018.pharmacist.com/sites/default/files/slides/Radiopharm_Reg_Pharmlaw_Update_3-17-18_105A_HO.pdf.
4. USP General Chapter <825> Radiopharmaceuticals—Preparation, Compounding, Dispensing, and Repackaging. Retrieved January 11, 2019 from http://www.usp.org/chemical-medicines/general-chapter-825.

Quality Management, Safety, and Patient Compliance

16

Learning Objectives

1. Identify training and reevaluation programs for personnel who are compounding sterile preparations per USP guidelines.
2. Describe several types of errors that can occur in preparation of compounded sterile preparations (CSPs).
3. Describe media fill testing, as well as when it is necessary to reevaluate and retrain personnel.
4. List possible sources of medication errors, as well as ways to prevent these errors from occurring.
5. List the patient rights of administration.
6. Define quality assurance and quality control and list the major components of a quality assurance program.
7. Discuss adverse event reporting and the responsibility of compounding personnel.

Terms & Definitions

Media fill test A test designed to access the quality of compounding processes or aseptic technique of personnel by using a microbiologic growth medium

Quality assurance (QA) A system of procedures, activities, and management to ensure a set of predetermined standards are met

Quality control (QC) The actual sampling, testing, and documentation of quality assurance results or evidence to ensure a quality product

Release testing Process to ensure that a compounded sterile preparation (CSP) meets a predetermined set of requirements or characteristics

Responsible person An individual who is held accountable for an activity

Standard operating procedures (SOPs) Set of procedures, including environmental controls, personnel training, and validation of technique, to ensure the sterility of all CSPs

INTRODUCTION

The roles of pharmacy technicians have changed greatly over the years. In addition to performing aseptic technique and routine prescription processing, the roles have expanded to include more innovative responsibilities, such as administration, in some states. Participating in medication error prevention and quality assurance (QA) programs has expanded the level of education and training, as well as opened up specialty areas. In this chapter, we will discuss the components of a QA plan and the compounder's role in preventing and reporting adverse events per Unites States Pharmacopoeia (USP<797>) guidelines.

USP<797> GUIDELINES

Compounding sterile preparations requires proper techniques, equipment, training, and standards to ensure a high quality compounded sterile preparation (CSP). The USP compounding chapters, as well as the American Society of Health-System Pharmacists (ASHP) technical assistance bulletin, describes conditions and practices that will prevent harm, and even death, to a patient. Patient safety, accuracy, and the prevention of errors should be priorities in every aspect of the aseptic preparation of CSPs. There should be **standard operating procedures (SOPs)** in place, as well as a QA program to ensure that personnel involved in the preparation of CSPs are trained and that the environment and processes meet established criteria for accuracy. USP<797> states, "every facility must have a formal, written QA and quality control (QC) program to establish a system of adherence to procedures, prevention detection of errors and other quality problems along with the corrective actions needed".

It is not enough to be trained and adhere to the processes required for aseptic compounding. There must be a plan in place to review, test, and record any errors and ensure the requirements for sending a prepared CSP out to the public are met.

ADVERSE EVENTS AND REPORTING

During preparation of CSPs, there are several types of errors that may occur. The most common error is microbacterial contamination, or nonsterility. This may be because of microbial, physical, or chemical contamination, such as improper handwashing, improper compounding environment, or incorrect manipulations or procedures. For instance, if handwashing is

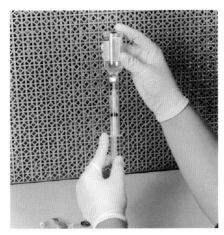

Fig. 16.1 A syringe being held properly in the hood. (From Hopper T: *Mosby's pharmacy technician principles & practice*, ed 3, St Louis, 2012, Elsevier Saunders.)

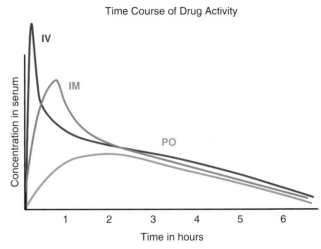

Time Course of Drug Activity

Fig. 16.2 Timing of routes of administration through the bloodstream. (From McKenry LM, Tessier E, Hogan MA: *Mosby's pharmacology in nursing*, ed 22, St Louis, 2005, Mosby.)

not done properly, contamination may occur because of physical contact.

If critical areas are compromised through either touch or interruption of first air in the laminar airflow workbench (LAFW), contamination may occur. If the LAFW is not cleaned properly or is not turned on for the required 30 minutes before manipulations, contamination may occur.

Any direct or physical contact with critical site areas poses the greatest risk to the patient, and compounding personnel must always be conscientious of this fact. A technician *must* have a responsible attitude when performing aseptic compounding. Some errors may occur that would not be recognized by a pharmacist checking a final intravenous (IV) solution, such as the occurrence of a touch contamination (without being seen by the pharmacist), a wrong strength of an ingredient, or a syringe pulled back to the correct amount but not actually added to the admixture (Fig. 16.1). Preparation of CSP must occur in the primary engineering control (PEC) located in the ISO Class 5 environment. Final check of a retail prescription can easily include verification of the amount of tablets found in the bottle. How does a pharmacist measure the amount of additive in the admixture? The **staging** of a completed CSP with the syringe drawn back and the container labeled properly is essential to the Pharmacist's verification process.

Environmental conditions where compounding takes place must also meet certain standards to ensure sterility. Proper cleaning, placement, and environmental sampling should be incorporated to provide the cleanest environment for aseptic compounding. This is why the USP<797> provides environmental quality specifications and monitoring standards. Tasks, such as proper garbing and handwashing, air quality, and equipment calibrations, should be incorporated as standard procedures to prevent contamination and subsequent harm to the patient. USP<797> guidelines provide a sampling plan for air and surface compounding areas. These include areas within the ISO Class 5 area and surrounding surfaces, as well as the ISO Class 7 and 8 areas, which should be collected and reviewed on a periodic basis. Equipment should be kept in operating condition according to manufacturers' specifications. Accuracy of automated compounding devices, such as that used in total parenteral nutrition (TPN) preparation, and balances should also be tested to prevent errors in measurements. Proper storage instructions and **beyond use dates (BUDs)** should also be included.

Incorrect dosages and strength and quality of correct ingredients are also types of errors. Labels for CSPs should include correct amounts and names of all ingredients, total volume, appropriate route of administration, and storage conditions. Patient names should be double-checked, as well as all calculations, additives, and fluids used. All finished CSPs should undergo **release testing**, either visual or sterility depending on the assigned BUD.

> ### 💬 Tech Note!
>
> *Remember:* CSPs are potentially the most hazardous to patients because they bypass the digestive tract (oral route of administration) and are administered parenterally (into the bloodstream), which is one of the fastest routes of administration (Fig. 16.2).

> ### 💬 Tech Note!
>
> Use reference guides (e.g., Trissel's *Handbook on Injectable Drugs, Drug Facts & Comparisons,* and package inserts) for compatibility, dilution, preparation, and storage information.

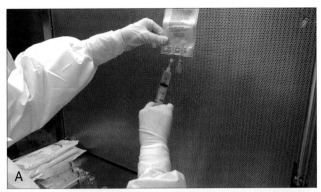

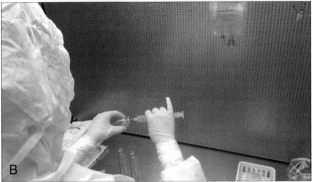

Fig. 16.3 Example of a media fill test. Transfer the compound out of the bag (A) and into the vial (B). (Courtesy CriticalPoint, LLC, Totowa, New Jersey.)

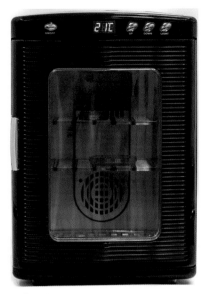

Fig. 16.4 Incubator for media fill tests.

MEDIA FILL TESTING (VALIDATION OF ASEPTIC TECHNIQUE)

After successfully completing hand hygiene and garbing, compounding personnel should have their techniques tested per USP guidelines. This is accomplished by performing media fill tests. This is recorded in the personnel's record and repeated quarterly.

The basic procedure is as follows:

- Perform test during the most challenging compound during a normal work shift
- Do not interrupt the test once started
- If all components are sterile, transfer a sterile soybean-case in digest into a similar container to simulate the process. There are kits available for this process (Fig. 16.3)
- Incubate the media-filled vials at 20 to 35 °C, for a minimum of 14 days, or one lower and one higher temperature for 7 days each, depending on media growth used (Fig. 16.4)
- Review the results with personnel and if needed, repeat the test.

Tech Note!

Always check storage and expiration dates on media fill tests components before using in tests to avoid an error in results

REEVALUATION AND RETRAINING SCHEDULING

Every compounder must undertake refresher training annually in the core competencies, such as visual observations, sampling, media fill, cleaning and disinfecting, and after any pause of 3 months or more in compounding. A person who fails any written tests, observations, or sampling and media fill, must undergo repeat training and requalifications before compounding again. Once retrained, personnel must pass a series of three successive tests before resuming compounding.

MEDICATION ERROR PREVENTION

Medication errors can occur because of poor handwriting that is difficult to read, confusion about drugs with similar names, or a lack of training and knowledge of sterile technique and best practices. In the institutional setting, there are several ways to prevent medication errors. Some of them include:

- Rechecking calculations and interpretations of orders. This may be accomplished by simply allowing another technician or pharmacist to read the same order
- Reconfirming confusing or specialty orders. This may be done by reviewing websites (such as the Institute for Safe Medical Practices [ISMP] at http://ismp.org/) for high-risk drug information and sound-alike/look-alike drugs, or printed pharmacy references, such as *Drug Facts and Comparisons* or *Mosby's Drug Guide for Nursing Students*
- *Always* check reference materials for unusual doses and consult the pharmacist—especially for TPN or chemotherapy orders—before preparing the compounded product

- Check for drug incompatibilities. Use reference sources, such as the *Handbook on Injectable Drugs* by Trissel or *2018 Intravenous Medications* by Gahart and Nazareno, to verify proper diluents, stability, and any special storage or preparation information
- Do not store sound-alike drugs or look-alike drugs on the same shelf. Follow standards of practice and procedures to verify these drugs and ask someone to check with you. For a complete listing of sound-alike/look-alike drugs, see the ISMP website (http://ismp.org/)
- Always work as a team to ensure the best patient care and continue to gain knowledge in the field. The IV technician is part of a team that should continuously look for ways to improve and expand knowledge about the quality of sterile preparations
- Always continue to gain knowledge about new medications through continuing education and by staying current in the practice to ensure that the most up-to-date information and practices are used.

 Tech Note!

When in doubt, check it out. If the order seems unusual or the interpretation is not clear, ask a colleague to read it, or discuss it with them.

PATIENT RIGHT OF ADMINISTRATION

Patient safety should always be the most important aspect of any healthcare worker's job, and patients are guaranteed certain rights when it comes to medication, including infusion therapy. They are as follows:

- *Right patient*: Be certain that names, birth dates, and any other identifying information specific to the patient is checked, when interpreting the order and preparing the IV therapy
- *Right medication*: Check the order for accuracy and completeness. Use references, such as Trissel's *Handbook on Injectable Drugs*, and package inserts for dilution, storage, and mixing instructions
- *Right strength*: Check the order for the correct dosage or strength, and label it accurately
- *Right route*: Check references for the appropriate route, such as IV push, piggyback, or intramuscular (IM) injection
- *Right time*: Verify the directions for the proper intervals for infusion, for labeling, and for the storage requirements.

QUALITY ASSURANCE PRACTICES AND QUALITY CONTROL ELEMENTS

A QA program consists of a way to monitor, evaluate, correct, and then improve all of the aspects of compounding sterile preparations. Anyone who is involved in the delivery of medication should be included in this QA process, including, but not limited to, technicians, pharmacists, physicians, nurses, and others in supportive roles. A QA program ensures that the quality of products and services meet a set of standards defined by the organization. This QA plan, or program, should include several components to ensure that the highest possible standards for high quality CSPs are met. The QA plan should include a formalized, written plan, which is provided to all of the appropriate personnel involved in compounding of CSPs.

The plan should include SOPs to describe processes and **responsible persons** associated with each. They should be detailed and include step-by-step instructions to guide a compounder through each procedure, along with dates of implementation, changes, and authorizing persons. The program should address, at a minimum, the following per USP guidelines.

- Personnel qualifications and required training

  This includes periodic review of files for basic qualifications and completion with dates for required training and qualifications. Sampling results, such as glove fingertip/thumb and media-fill testing. Results of observations of performance competencies that include handwashing, proper garbing techniques, cleaning and disinfecting procedures, and aseptic manipulation skills (*process validation*, a term used to describe the checking of the preparer's aseptic technique for sterility).

- Design and maintenance of environment (facilities and equipment)

  This is to ensure the environment and facilities are being assessed periodically through cleaning and disinfection and step-by-step SOPs to describe timelines and steps involved (Fig. 16.5). Any out of normal records of air or humidity, storage temperatures, and results from outside certifications or testing of equipment must be kept and reviewed.

- Component selection and handling

  Ensure quality of components from US Food and Drug Administration (FDA) qualified vendors and proper inventory and disposal.

- Actual compounding processes

  This includes SOPs and reviews of processes used in compounding, such as final labeling and documentation, to include compounding records and master formulas. In addition, there should be processes for investigations of any deviations or errors found.

- Final release of CSPs procedures

  This should include the types of inspections are required, and a description for each type of testing for compliance.

SOP No. 102

Title of SOP: Facility and Personnel Specifications

Original: Yes _____ No _____   Revision: Yes _____ No _____   Revision No.: _____

Responsibility:
The pharmacist-in-charge is responsible for this procedure.

Purpose:
The purpose of this standard operating procedure (SOP) is to ensure that the personnel and facilities meet all requirements per USP<797>. Facilities in which compounding takes place must be maintained to prevent airborne contaminants of CSP's. Personnel must demonstrate a theoretical and hands on proficiency in required practices, and all required documentation must be maintained.

Equipment/Supplies Required:
• Current USP<797> guidelines and facility prepared logs

Procedure:
1. All personnel performing compounding must demonstrate proficiency through initial and refresher training and testing in the required core competencies.

2. All personnel must be able to demonstrate proficiency in the theoretical principles of sterile manipulations.

3. Each employee active in this SOP must review, understand, and document this understanding by signing the appropriate log.

4. Each employee reviews the requirements on an annual basis. This review is documented and signed by both the employee and appropriate supervisor.

5. Documentation of personnel qualifications is placed in both the employee's employment folder and reviewed accordingly.

6. Documentation of facilities compliance is maintained in the SOP master book and reviewed for accuracy and timely information.

Approved by _____   Date _____

Implemented by _____   Date _____

Page 1 of 1

Fig. 16.5 Sample standard operating procedure (SOP).

• Documentation
  This should include the SOP creation and review or change procedure, complaint handling, and management procedures the facility adheres to.
  The QA program should evaluate the overall compliance regarding compounding sterile preparations SOPs, identify and analyze problems, and provide solutions or improvements to prevent medication errors or harm to patients.

COMPLAINT HANDLING AND REPORTING OF ADVERSE EVENTS

Compounding facilities must have a formal plan for receiving and reviewing complaints. They must keep written records of questions with responses and identify the facility's personnel who are qualified for review. If that person determines that complaint indicates a potential problem or need for assessment, there must be an investigation, with documentation, performed. If corrective action is required, the related SOPs should be reviewed and any identified problems must be corrected.

A written record of each complaint must be kept by the facility and include the following:

- Name of complainant
- Date received
- Nature of complaint
- Any identifying information, such as name and strength of CSP, lot number, prescription number
- Any findings and follow up.

These reports should be reviewed periodically as part of the QA program in an effort to prevent future occurrences. If there are problems with manipulation or aseptic technique skills, printed materials (e.g., checklists or instructions provided during or after training) may be helpful. If deficiencies in procedures or technique are found, reinstruction and reevaluation of the compounding personnel must occur. The quality of a product is determined at the time it is compounded by the person who is compounding it. Proper technique, environmental controls and barriers, along with monitoring, is essential to ensure that patients receive the proper medication.

 Tech Note!

All of the procedures to prevent medication prevention errors do no good without a follow-up evaluation of why they happened and a solution to prevent them from occurring again.

Successful QA programs and medication error prevention is a team effort. Each and every person, especially those who are compounding, is responsible for ensuring the integrity of the final preparation. The process should include SOPs that outline tasks, environmental controls, validation methods, and provide education and training.

Reporting of adverse events of CSP must be reviewed promptly, and if serious or unexpected adverse events are evident, they must be reported to FDA through MedWatch (Fig. 16.6). If it is animal-related, the Form FDA 1932a should be used.

A good QA program can provide the foundation for a clear understanding of the aseptic technique and facility policies and procedures that are essential to quality patient care. The five rights of the patient should always be a consideration when preparing any medication. Performance improvement programs allow healthcare team members to review and identify problems or errors, evaluate causes, develop solutions, and monitor the results. This, along with patient education and proper compounding personnel training, can greatly decrease medication errors.

 Did You Know?

According to an article published by ASHP on CSPs, "The essence of quality assurance is proving that you are really doing what you say you are doing."

As the roles of pharmacy technicians continue to expand, the specialty areas and administration opportunities will also increase. Technicians should always strive to gain knowledge in the field through participating in organizations, obtaining certification, and enrolling in advancing education. The more knowledgeable the technician is, the better equipped he or she is at performing the correct practice. Continuing education for technicians is often free and can be found through a variety of sources. Organizations offering continuing education include:

- ASHP
- The Society for the Education of Pharmacy Technicians (SEPhT)
- American Association of Pharmacy Technicians (AAPT)
- National Pharmacy Technician Association (NPTA)
- POWER-PAK C.E.
- RxSchool
- Pharmacy Technician Certification Board (PTCB).

Your facility is also a great resource for education, as well as some state boards of pharmacy.

Patient safety is every healthcare worker's responsibility, and technicians should take an active role in QA programs and error prevention. This is the only way to ensure the safest and highest quality care for all patients.

 Tech Note!

Technicians should be aware of their state's requirements for practice. For a complete listing of the state Boards of Pharmacy, go to the National Association of Boards of Pharmacy (NABP) at http://www.nabp.net.

REVIEW QUESTIONS

1. List three requirements for records of complaints that must be kept by the facility.
2. Define *QA*, and list four elements that should be included.
3. Name at least three common practices associated with CSPs that should be evaluated on a periodic basis.
4. List the five rights of a patient.
5. List three ways used to avoid medication errors.

CRITICAL THINKING

1. Discuss how you, as a technician, can participate in a QA program. Working at the technician level in a hospital system, name specific ways that you can improve patient safety, and give an example of a problem and a solution.
2. Explain the following statement in your own words, "All personnel who prepare CSPs are responsible for understanding these fundamental practices and precautions, developing and implementing appropriate procedures, and continually evaluating these procedures and the quality of final CSPs to prevent harm."

DEPARTMENT OF HEALTH AND HUMAN SERVICES
Food and Drug Administration

Form Approved: OMB No. 0910-0291
Expiration Date: 6/30/2015
(See PRA Statement on preceding
general information page)

MEDWATCH Consumer Voluntary Reporting
(FORM FDA 3500B)

Section A – About the Problem

What kind of problem was it? *(Check all that apply)*

☐ Were hurt or had a bad side effect *(including new or worsening symptoms)*

☐ Used a product incorrectly which could have or led to a problem

☐ Noticed a problem with the quality of the product

☐ Had problems after switching from one product maker to another maker

Did any of the following happen? *(Check all that apply)*

☐ Hospitalization – admitted or stayed longer

☐ Required help to prevent permanent harm *(for medical devices only)*

☐ Disability or health problem

☐ Birth defect

☐ Life-threatening

☐ Death *(Include date):* _____

☐ Other serious/important medical incident *(Please describe below)*

_____

_____

_____

Date the problem occurred *(mm/dd/yyyy)*

Tell us what happened and how it happened. *(Include as many details as possible)*

_____
_____
_____ | Continue Page |

List any relevant tests or laboratory data if you know them. *(Include dates)*

_____
_____
_____ | Continue Page |

For a problem with a product, including

- prescription or over-the-counter medicine
- biologics, such as human cells and tissues used for transplantation (for example, tendons, ligaments, and bone) and gene therapies
- nutrition products, such as vitamins and minerals, herbal remedies, infant formulas, and medical foods
- cosmetics or make-up products
- foods (including beverages and ingredients added to foods)

⇨ **Go to Section B**

For a problem with a medical device, including

- any health-related test, tool, or piece of equipment
- health-related kits, such as glucose monitoring kits or blood pressure cuffs
- implants, such as breast implants, pacemakers, or catheters
- other consumer health products, such as contact lenses, hearing aids, and breast pumps

⇨ **Go to Section C (Skip Section B)**

For more information, visit *http://www.fda.gov/MedWatch*

Submission of a report does not constitute an admission that medical personnel or the product caused or contributed to the event.

Fig. 16.6 US Food and Drug Administration MedWatch form. (Courtesy Drug Enforcement Administration, Washington, DC.)
Continued

Section B – About the Products

Name of the product as it appears on the box, bottle, or package *(Include as many names as you see)*

Name of the company that makes the product

Expiration date *(mm/dd/yyyy)*	Lot number	NDC number

Strength *(for example, 250 mg per 500 mL or 1 g)*	Quantity *(for example, 2 pills, 2 puffs, or 1 teaspoon, etc.)*	Frequency *(for example, twice daily or at bedtime)*	How was it taken or used *(for example, by mouth, by injection, or on the skin)?*

Date the person first started taking or using the product *(mm/dd/yyyy)*: _____

Date the person stopped taking or using the product *(mm/dd/yyyy)*: _____

Why was the person using the product *(such as, what condition was it supposed to treat?)*
_____
_____
_____

Did the problem stop after the person reduced the dose or stopped taking or using the product? ☐ Yes ☐ No

Did the problem return if the person started taking or using the product again? ☐ Yes ☐ No ☐ Didn't restart

Do you still have the product in case we need to evaluate it? *(Do not send the product to FDA. We will contact you directly if we need it.)* ☐ Yes ☐ No

⇨ *Go to Section D (Skip Section C)*

Section C – About the Medical Device

Name of medical device

Name of the company that makes the medical device

Other identifying information *(The model, catalog, lot, serial, or UDI number, and the expiration date, if you can locate them)*
_____
_____
_____

Was someone operating the medical device when the problem occurred? ☐ Yes ☐ No

If yes, who was using it?
☐ The person who had the problem
☐ A health professional *(such as a doctor, nurse, or aide)*
☐ Someone else *(Please explain who)*
_____

For implanted medical devices ONLY *(such as pacemakers, breast implants, etc.)*

Date the implant was put in *(mm/dd/yyyy)*	Date the implant was taken out *(If relevant) (mm/dd/yyyy)*

⇨ *Go to Section D*

For more information, visit *http://www.fda.gov/MedWatch*

Submission of a report does not constitute an admission that medical personnel or the product caused or contributed to the event.

Fig. 16.6, cont'd

Section D – About the Person Who Had the Problem

Person's Initials	Sex	Age *(at time the problem occurred)* or Birth Date	Weight *(Specify lbs or kg)*	Race
	☐ Female ☐ Male			

List known medical conditions *(such as diabetes, high blood pressure, cancer, heart disease, or others)*

_____

_____

Please list all allergies *(such as to drugs, foods, pollen, or others)*.

List any other important information about the person *(such as smoking, pregnancy, alcohol use, etc.)*

List all current prescription medications and medical devices being used.

_____

_____

| Continue Page |

List all over-the-counter medications and any vitamins, minerals, supplements, and herbal remedies being used.

| Continue Page |

⇨ **Go to Section E**

Section E – About the Person Filling Out This Form

We will contact you only if we need additional information. Your name will not be given out to the public.

Last name	First name
Number/Street	City and State/Province
Country	ZIP or Postal code
Telephone number	Email address	Today's date *(mm/dd/yyyy)*

Did you report this problem to the company that makes the product (the manufacturer)? ☐ Yes ☐ No	May we give your name and contact information to the company that makes the product (manufacturer) to help them evaluate the product? ☐ Yes ☐ No

Send This Report by Mail or Fax

Keep the product in case the FDA wants to contact you for more information. Please do not send products to the FDA. Mail or fax the form to:

Mail:	**Fax:**
MedWatch Food and Drug Administration 5600 Fishers Lane Rockville, MD 20857	1-800-332-0178 (toll-free)

Thank you for helping us protect the public health.

For more information, visit *http://www.fda.gov/MedWatch*	Submission of a report does not constitute an admission that medical personnel or the product caused or contributed to the event.

Fig. 16.6, cont'd

COMPETENCIES

QUALITY ASSURANCE AND MEDICATION ERROR PREVENTION

Evaluation Key: S = Satisfactory   NI = Needs Improvement

Name: _____   Quarter: _____   Date: _____

COMPETENCIES	STUDENT			INSTRUCTOR		
Student will be able to:	S	NI	Comments	S	NI	Comments
Discuss the USP<797> guidelines regarding compounding personnel and their responsibilities.						
Discuss common types of errors that may occur when compounding CSPs.						
Identify several examples of errors that may not be noticed by pharmacist checking.						
Discuss USP's sampling plan for air and surfaces.						
List the items found on an IV label.						
List two references that may be used when compounding CSPs and the type of information found in them.						
List several ways to prevent medication errors.						
Given a scenario, describe a QA program and its elements.						
Describe a media fill test.						
Discuss low risk level CSPs, including some examples, storage, and QA procedures.						
Discuss medium risk level CSPs, including some examples, storage, and QA procedures.						
Discuss high risk level CSPs, including some examples, storage, and QA procedure.						

Review each concept to ensure that the learning objectives for the chapter have been met. Your instructor or supervisor will evaluate this as well.

LAB ACTIVITY

You have been working as a technician student in a hospital pharmacy accredited by The Joint Commission (TJC) for about 2 weeks. One day, while you are replenishing the operating room (OR) trays, you decide to look at a drug that you are not familiar with. When reviewing the package insert, you discover that the expiration date that is being marked on the labels on the vials in the tray is wrong. A homemade chart on the refrigerator that the technicians follow indicates the drug is good at room temperature for 30 days, but the insert says the drug is good at room temperature for *14 days*. In addition, the drug becomes toxic after the 14-day time period, and more than 20 trays of this drug are currently on the OR floor.

Answer the following:
1. Why do you think this happened?
2. Could it have been avoided?

3. What were the correct steps that you, as the technician student, took?
4. Thinking about the components of a good QA plan, who should you tell first, and what should you do with the drugs in the trays on the OR floor?
5. What actions should follow this discovery to prevent it from happening again in the future?
6. Use the previous scenario to create your own QA program to prevent this from happening again. *Remember*: A good plan must have a way to monitor a process, evaluate what happened, correct it, and then improve the results or prevent the incident from happening again. Include all of the elements of a good QA plan, including a summary of what happened, any patient consequences that could have occurred, a detailed description of the correct storage and expiration of this drug, and any processes that you would put in place, along with the required reporting elements for USP. Your plan will be graded using the following chart:

BIBLIOGRAPHY

1. Pharmaceutical compounding-sterile preparations (general information chapter 797).

Third-Party Billing, Reimbursement, and Inventory Management

17

Learning Objectives

1. Identify common aspects of billing for infusion therapy, including additional supplies and drugs that could be billed in addition to the infusion therapy itself.
2. Identify best practices for inventory control.
3. Discuss purchasing processes, management of shortages, pharmacy and therapeutics (P&T) committees, and drug use reviews (DUR) or evaluations (DUE).
4. Describe continuous quality improvement (CQI).

Terms & Definitions

Current Procedural Technology (CPT) codes A set of codes used to identify surgical, diagnostic, and medical procedures, used for billing services

DUR/DUE (Drug use review, drug use evaluation) a review of the drugs within an organization to determine where improvements in the process can occur

Electronic health record (EHR) Computer-based record that records patients information to include demographic information and overall medical and medication information

HCPCS Health Care Financing Administration (HCFA) Common Procedures Coding System Uniform language using codes to describe procedures, services, and diagnoses for billing purposes for Medicare and third-party providers

INTRODUCTION

Infusion billing is complicated and is often the reason facilities will opt for working through an outside agency for their intravenous (IV) therapy. As a pharmacy technician working in infusion services, it is important to understand the billing aspect of compounding. If a facility does not bill correctly and receives payment for the medications that are being sent out, the compensation will be incorrect and can cause rebilling and audits, as well as confusion. Hand in hand with billing and reimbursement is inventory management. Knowing a drug's level, when to reorder, and handling shortages are a basic part of every compounding pharmacy. Maintaining the most efficient inventory levels allows for the greatest profit margin, as well as on-time patient care, and provides a team approach to the patient's care while allowing all the caregivers to share information (Fig. 17.1).

COMMON ASPECTS OF BILLING

There are specific codes set each year by the Health Care Financing Administration known as *Health Care Financing Administration Common Procedures Coding System* (HCPCS) codes and Current Procedural Technology (CPT) codes provided by the American Medical Association (AMA). In general, the codes are used as the same identifiers, but when billing Medicare, the HCPCS codes are used. This coding system allows for a universal system to use for billing IV compounds and supplies or equipment used in their administration.

Infusions are based on three categories: IV, intravenous push (IVP), or injections, which can be subcutaneous or intramuscular (IM).

In addition to the categories, these routes of administration define the method of administration the medication is to be given.

There are medication levels or types of service. These include:
- Chemotherapy/biologic
- Therapeutic or diagnostic medication
- Hydration (Fig. 17.2).

When a medication is being administered, the time of service, which can be billed, is only the time the medication is going into the patient (being infused). This does not include the time the patient is physically at the office visit, the time it takes to prepare the medication, or the consultation, if applicable.

Time is also a critical factor to billing. If the time it takes for the medication to be infused is less than 15 minutes, it is considered an IVP and must be billed as such. If the time goes 16 minutes or over, it can be billed for an hour of infusion.

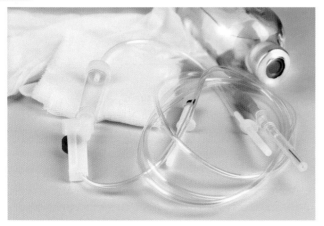

Fig. 17.1 Infusion billing can be complex. (Copyright © iStock.com/belchonock.)

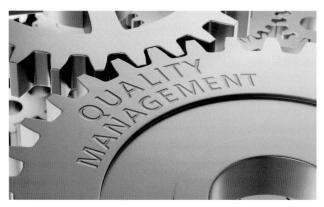

Fig. 17.2 The many aspects of billing contribute to quality management as a whole. (Copyright © iStock.com/Zerbor.)

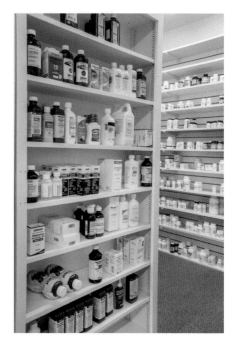

Fig. 17.3 Additional supplies are billed in home health settings.

ADDITIONAL SUPPLIES

In addition to the medications being billed, in home health settings, the supplies and equipment used for administering is also billed using the same coding system. Typical additional supplies will include:

- Syringes and needles for flushing the peripherally inserted central catheter (infusion line)
- IV pole (if stationary pump is used)
- IV pump (if applicable)
- Gloves
- Alcohol swabs
- Heparin and saline vials for flushing the IV line between administration
- Sharps container
- Batteries (back up for electrical outages) (Fig. 17.3).

MECHANICS OF INVENTORY CONTROL

Inventory for any pharmacy is the single largest investment that can be made. There should be enough medications to prepare IV compounds, but not an excess that will expire or take up profits while sitting on a shelf. Ordering the right amount and in the right package size is important as well. For instance: if you receive an order to prepare the following sterile compound, which

would be the most appropriate size vial to use, based on the information provided subsequently?

Tech Note!

Furosemide is a very commonly prescribed IV, IM, and IVP medication.

1. Furosemide 40 mg in Dextrose 5% 50 mL x 7 bags.
2. Furosemide (40 mg/4 mL) vial cost $7.00.
3. Furosemide (100 mg/10 mL) multidose vial (MDV) cost $16.00.
4. Furosemide (20 mg/2 mL) vial cost $2.25.

Each vial has a 10 mg/mL concentration, but if you need x7 bags with 40 mg in each, that will be 280 mg total. Here are the choices:

- Purchase of x3 of the MDV would be 300 mg total, which would leave 2 mL or a 20 mg dose of waste. The cost would be $16.00 x 3 or $48.00
- Purchase of x7 40 mg/4 mL to get 280 mg in vials would be $7.00 x 7 or $49
- Purchase of x14 of the 20 mg/mL vials to get 80 mg would be $2.25 x 14.00 or $31.50.

The best choice is the MDV. Even though there will be some waste, the cost is less and the remainder from an MDV can be stored for some time. This may allow the left over dose to be used up, but even if that does not occur, it is more economic to purchase it for the seven bags needed (Fig. 17.4).

The inventory may include all three of the aforementioned package sizes, but as the compounding pharmacy technician, you will need to choose the most appropriate vial, based on costs, time to prepare, and beyond use date. In some cases, it may be feasible to use single dose vials, but this will depend on the setting, order instructions, and circumstances for administration. In the outpatient setting, where delivery to a patient occurs weekly, compounding the seven bags at once will be needed. In a hospital (in-patient setting), the order may call for a dose made every 24 hours, so as to not have unused medications, if they are discharged.

Even though the concentration (mg/mL) is the same for all the vial choices, using the stock that saves compounding time is also important. To withdraw the contents of 14 vials, as listed earlier, to make the seven bags, would take a total of 14 each syringe, needle, and alcohol wipes (per each vial). This is costly and time consuming. In addition, it entails more manipulations and a much higher possibility of touch contamination. Using the MDV, or even the seven in the other choices, would be quicker and take less supplies, as a single larger syringe could be used to withdraw the contents of the entire vial and inject required amounts into the seven containers. All these considerations are part of the technician's role in compounding.

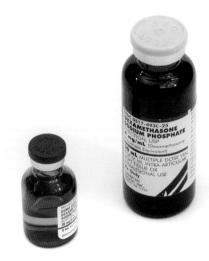

Fig. 17.4 The remainder from an multidose vial (MDV) can be stored for some time.

PURCHASING AND SHORTAGES MANAGEMENT

Sources for inventory can vary from one facility to another, but can work either direct from manufacturer or, as is the case for most, are indirectly purchased through agreements with wholesalers (Fig. 17.5).

There are also group purchasing organizations or GPOs, which is where organizations negotiate contracts with drug manufacturers on the members' benefit. This

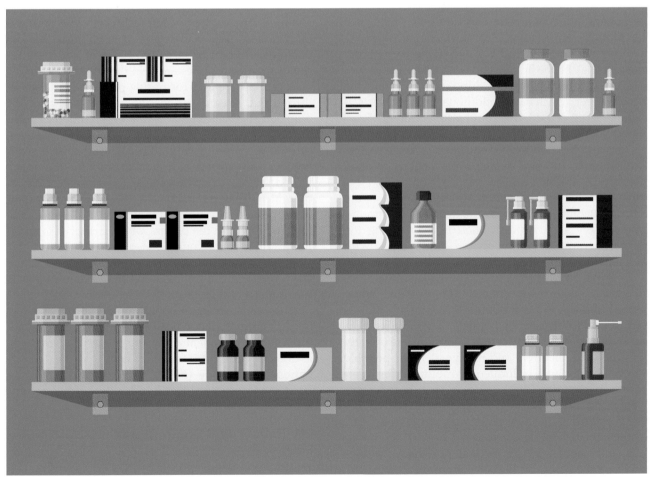

Fig. 17.5 Inventory can come directly from the manufacturer or through an agreement with wholesalers. (Copyright © iStock.com/drogatnev.)

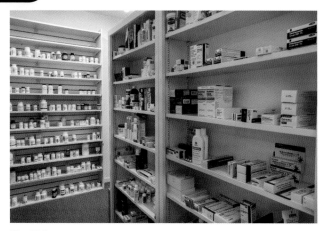

Fig. 17.6 Most inventory is ordered through a Just-in-Time approach, so that a minimum inventory amount can be kept.

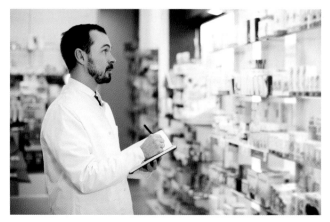

Fig. 17.7 The best way to control inventory is visually—looking at what is on the shelf and maintaining a periodic automatic replenishment (PAR) level. (Copyright © iStock.com/JackF.)

could be a hospital system, a chain drugs store system, or outpatient facility, with several clinics across the country. A purchase order (PO) is a document used to order and track items. Most items are ordered through a Just-in-Time approach. This allows for a minimum inventory amount to be kept, which reduces the amount of the business's capital tied up in medications (Fig. 17.6).

Shortages can cause extra attention in the form of disrupting normal ordering procedures and a delay in compounded medications to the patient. This can affect the patient's treatment and cost additional money, if substitutions are required. For instance; if a generic medication is ordered and is shorted, the only option available may be the brand. This is usually more expensive and can require special shipping direct from the manufacturer, which incurs additional time and costs. If a similar drug is used, this could also require the Practitioner and pharmacist to have to calculate equivalent dosages and provide further education of the alternate medication to the patient and other healthcare team members. A shortage can last days or months, and it is imperative that the compounding technician be aware of the availability when reviewing the order. Communication is key and any disruption in maintaining the normal medication supply should be discussed with the Pharmacist and inventory personnel.

Working proactively should be a systemwide approach to ensure medications are available when needed to prepare a compound. If the organization is part of a GPO or uses a wholesaler for supplies, provide additional benefits, as they communicate directly with the manufacturers and receive alerts or possible upcoming shortages or limited distribution. This is effective in ensuring the supply is distributed more evenly and allows for time to discuss alternatives before the shortage occurs. If the hospital is in a GPO, keeping the pricing lower is also a benefit. Buying in bulk and negotiating for several pharmacies allows pricing to be based on higher volumes. Knowing the contracts and relationships for your organizations will create an efficient process for ordering and maintaining a proper stock level.

Controlling inventory through use of a GPO or wholesaler is just one part of inventory management. In addition, the best way to control inventory is visually. This is basically, looking at what is on the shelf and maintaining a periodic automatic replenishment (PAR) level. This is the least amount that should be on the shelf at any given time (Fig. 17.7).

If it is known that a shortage alert has been discussed, it may be time to order extra (above the PAR level). As the compounding technician is working in the IV room on a daily basis, it is obvious that that person will know what is on the shelf and how fast medication or supplies are being used up. The time of year can also be a factor in this process. For instance, during FLU season, vaccines are in high demand. This may be a medication that is rendered limited distribution from the onset. It may require additional delivery time and ordering from the manufacturer directly. Being aware of this and stocking up for the season would be the best approach, if possible. Staying current with alerts, media flyers, and any correspondence related to a specific medication and sharing that information with the buyers and Pharmacist is an important part of the compounder's responsibility.

In a hospital, the IV department may be separated and order their supplies individually or provide the list of items and medications needed through a single inventory technician or department. This may be done by listing items electronically, throughout the day, and them submitting them at the end of each day. Ordering is done by using a tracking system that involves the national drug code (NDC) numbers and bar codes. Each medication is identified by its labeler, product and package size (Fig. 17.8).

PHARMACY AND THERAPEUTICS COMMITTEE (P&T)

Most hospitals and managed care organizations rely on a team approach to deliver optimal patient care. Often a representative from the IV department is part of this group and provides valuable information based

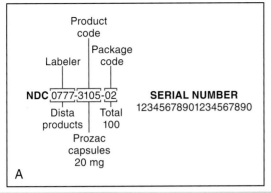

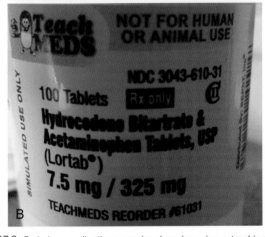

Fig. 17.8 Ordering medications can be done by using a tracking system that involves national drug code (NDC) numbers and bar codes. (A) Example of an NDC, broken down by section. (B) Bar code sample. (C) Label sample. (A, From Davis K, Guerra A: *Mosby's pharmacy technician*, ed 5, St Louis, 2019, Elsevier.)

on routine compounding processes. This is a team effort and includes a review of the formulary on a regular basis. As part of good inventory management practices, this oversight group is comprised of Practitioners, pharmacy personnel, dieticians, and other healthcare team members who participate in the medication delivery process. The primary focus is divided in three parts:

- Maintain a medication list
- Develop policies for adding and deleting medications to the list

- Maintaining medication information, such as dosing, effectiveness, and availability.

Providing useful background and medication inventory practices, both good and bad, are used for quality control and the group's development of best practices (Fig. 17.9).

DRUG USE EVALUATION (DUE) OR DRUG USE REVIEW (DUR)

Organizations, such as The Joint Commission and the National Committee for quality Assurance (NCQA) provides guidance for performing an evaluation of drug use. It is designed to improve use within the organization.

> **Tech Note!**
>
> DUE is a term for the process used by The Joint Commission. DUR is the same process mandated by OBRA-90 (Omnibus Budget Reconciliation Act-1990).

STEPS IN THE JOINT COMMISSION'S DUE PROCESS

The steps in the DUE process include the following:
1. Assign responsibility and obtain administrative approval to conduct DU—performed by the P&T committee
2. Delineate scope of drug usage within the organization—review of drug literature and clinical practice guidelines
3. Identify specific drugs that should be monitored and evaluated—identify high risk, high usage, or high cost drugs
4. Identify indicators—develop criteria for a drug to be used
5. Establish thresholds—establish the limits for optimal use of a drug
6. Collect and organize data
7. Evaluate drug use
8. Performs actions from information gathered to improve drug usage
9. Communicate the findings and improvements to the appropriate responsible parties.

CONTINUOUS QUALITY IMPROVEMENT (CQI)

An organization should be continuously reviewing and improving services to deliver medications on time and safely to patients. Each employee works in an individual capacity, as well as with the team. As a compounding technician, there is an opportunity to share the best elements of the inventory processes in the department and allow for feedback for improvements. This may be turnaround time for orders, a better process for checking for outdates or expired drugs, or even the process of placing an order.

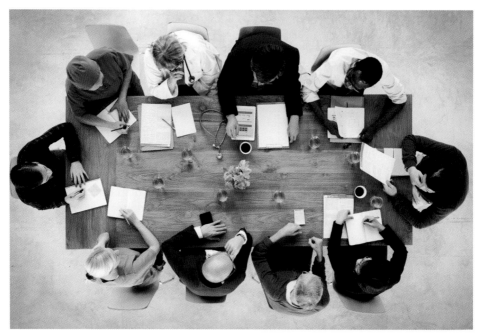

Fig. 17.9 A pharmacy and therapeutics committee is a part of good inventory management practice. (Copyright © iStock.com/Rawpixel Ltd.)

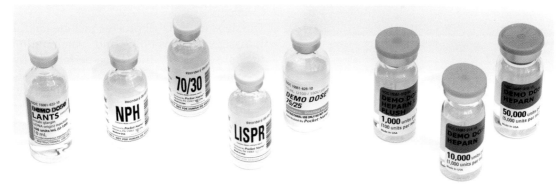

Fig. 17.10 High alert medications, such as insulin or heparin, should be double-checked for accuracy.

The medication use system is the most common method to organize errors:
- Errors involving selecting medications
- Errors involving ordering medications
- Errors involving dispensing medications
- Errors involving administering medications
- Errors involving monitoring medications.

As part of the inventory management process, selecting and ordering are important. Selecting medications is probably the easiest way to cause an error. There can be several ways this can occur. There should be a process established for all personnel who must perform selection. In the IV department, something as simple as shelf placement can be a cause of a selection error. Medications with similar names (look-alike and sound-alike) should have special marking or possibly special placement. When

compounding medications and choosing the medications, it is easy to select a drug that may be confused with another.

For instance:
- Dopamine and Dobutamine
- Morphine and Hydromorphone
- Lantus or Lente insulin

The Institute for Safe Medication Practices (ISMP) provides Practitioner's with several listings of common mistaken drugs at www. https://www.ismp.org/. These include: Look-alike, sound-alike, High alert, confused names, and Tall man lettering. High alert medications, such as insulins or heparin, should be double-checked (Fig. 17.10).

One universal industry standard way to identify confusing drugs is using the Tall man lettering font. This alerts the person dispensing to a name alert.

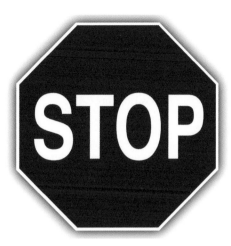

Fig. 17.11 Special stickers can be used on bins to prevent dangerous mistakes. (Copyright © iStock.com/aydinynr.)

Examples include:
- diphenhydrAMINE and dimenhryDRINATE
- DOPamine and DOBUTamine

For a complete listing, see www. https://www. ismp.org/recommendations/tall-man-letters-list.

There are also special stickers that can be used on the bins to indicate an alert for the drugs (Fig. 17.11).

As part of inventory management, the compounding technician must be aware of the dangers of selection and ordering wrong IV medications. If there are best practices, such as using special stickers or placement on the shelves, this should be implemented and shared with all compounding personnel.

Using a continuous evaluation and monitoring process in inventory management is critical to the organization's ability to provide cost-effective mediations safely and timely to patients. As a compounding technician, identifying best practice and ways to improve medication dispensing tasks, should go hand in hand with adhering to aseptic technique practices. Knowing the possible pitfalls of selection and ordering errors and participating in the organization's efforts to bill and prepare medications properly, are key to the safest and most cost-effective delivery of medication.

REVIEW QUESTIONS

1. Based on the HCPCS coding system, infusions are based on all the following categories EXCEPT:
   A. IV
   B. IM
   C. IVP
   D. Intradermal (ID)
2. Based on HCPCS, which of the following is a type of service used in billing infusion therapy?
   A. Hydration
   B. Pain management
   C. Antibiotic therapy
   D. Cardiac therapy

3. If a medication is administered in 15 minutes or less, what type of infusion service must be billed for?
   A. 10 minutes
   B. 15 minutes of less
   C. 30 minutes of less
   D. One hour or less
4. Which type of organization negotiates contracts with drug manufacturers on the members benefit?
   A. GPO
   B. PO
   C. GMP
   D. CPT
5. Which of the following best describes the least amount of inventory that should be maintained on the shelf at any given time?
   A. PRE
   B. PAR
   C. POR
   D. PAT
6. The P&T committee responsibilities include all the following EXCEPT:
   A. Maintaining a medication list
   B. Developing policies for adding and deleting medications to and from the list
   C. Maintaining medication dosing information
   D. Validating Pharmacist credentials
7. Which organization publishes a list of Look-alike-Sound-alike medications?
   A. ASHP
   B. ISMP
   C. USP
   D. US Food and Drug Administration (FDA)
8. If two drugs have similar names, which of the following would be appropriate method of preventing a selection error?
   A. Change their shelf placement
   B. Add an alert sticker to the bin
   C. Notify all personnel in the department
   D. Both A and B
9. The Joint Commission identifies the program for performing an evaluation of drug use by which acronym?
   A. DUR
   B. DUE
   C. DME
   D. DMR
10. Which of the following is the component identifiers in a drug's NDC number?
    A. Labeler, product and package size
    B. Manufacturer, lot number, and package size
    C. Expiration date, labeler, and package size
    D. Manufacturer, expiration date, and date made

CRITICAL THINKING

1. As the compounding technician in a busy hospital, you notice that there are errors occurring

with two drugs that have very similar names. They are located next to each other on the shelf. What could you do to avoid a future medication error from occurring? How would you use this example when trying to train a new technician?

BIBLIOGRAPHY

1. HMSA Provider Resource Center: Intravenous Therapy—General and Billing Information. Retrieved March 28, 2019 https://hmsa.com/portal/provider/zav_pel.fh.INT.800.htm.
2. Institute for Safe Medication Practices. Retrieved April 6, 2019 from https://www.ismp.org/.

Operations and Emergency Preparedness

18

Learning Objectives

1. Identify common types of emergencies or disasters that require additional preplanning tasks related to sterile compounding.
2. Describe planning requirements for disasters, including the roles of organizations associated with emergency planning and how they relate to sterile compounding.
3. Describe special storage and delivery considerations for medications to be used in emergencies, including the Strategic National Stockpile (SNS).

4. List and explain the six sections of the National Boards of Pharmacy's (NABP"s) "Model Emergency Disaster Preparedness and Response Plan."
5. Describe the various roles of pharmacy personnel in the immediate response to an emergency.

Terms & Definitions

Disaster An emergency that requires outside assistance

Disaster Medical Assistance Team (DMAT) Team that set up temporary treatment medical sites to treat burns and mental health emergencies

Disaster Mortuary Operations Response Teams (DMORT) Made up of mortuary directors, pathologists, dental assistants, medical examiners, medical record technicians, and mental health staff, which are responsible for identification of victims and support family members in the grieving process in a disaster or emergency event

Emergency An event which affects public safety, health, or welfare

FEMA The Federal Emergency Management System

International Medical Surgical Response Team (IMSRT) This team performs as an operating room in the field and manages major traumas

National Incident Management System (NIMS) Established by the Department of Homeland Society to manage the coordination and support of needed facilities and establish

guidelines for responders to understand ways to assist before, during, and after an emergency

National Veterinary Response team (NVRT) Team responsible for treatment and care of working and victim animals in affected area

Natural Disaster Medical System (NDMS) A department of the Federal Government, which is responsible for sending out medical teams, equipment, and supplies to the disaster areas affected

Strategic National Stockpile (SNS) The United States national repository for medications and supplies needed for disasters or emergencies

The National Pharmacy Response Team (NPRT) An organization, which provides mass immunizations and is made up of pharmacy technicians and Pharmacists

U.S. Public Health Service (USPHS) A bank of trained healthcare professionals ready to act once needed in a disaster or emergency

INTRODUCTION

As a compounding technician working in the pharmacy, the impact of emergencies or disasters impacts the delivery of medical services that must be provided to the public before, during, and after an event. Miscommunication between the locally affected areas and responders can result in wrong or incomplete information and delay responses. There may be damage to healthcare facilities, that is known and unknown, which result in loss of phone lines, supplies, patient records, and staff shortages. These challenges affect coordination between emergency and healthcare providers and can result in extreme situations and a lack

of proper care for victims. Without patient histories or medication records for a surge of patients, the focus must remain on patient safety and treatment using the best sources for information available (Fig. 18.1).

As a significant part of the healthcare team, this also presents different challenges to pharmacy staff and supplies. Responses must be preplanned and include ways to provide an effective, safe, and confident approach for medication delivery. Each disaster or emergency brings their own set of challenges that requires planning, preparation and training for pharmacy personnel. If supplier facilities are damaged for instance, supplies and medications may need to be brought in

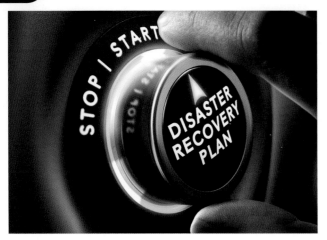

Fig. 18.1 Disaster plans must focus on patient safety and treatment. (Copyright © iStock.com/olm26250.)

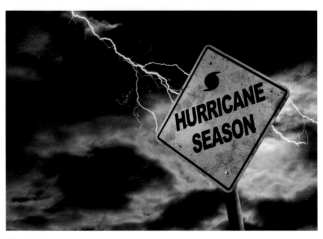

Fig. 18.3 Providing medications to communities that have become isolated because of wind- and water-related disasters, such as hurricanes can be challenging. (Copyright © iStock.com/ronniechua.)

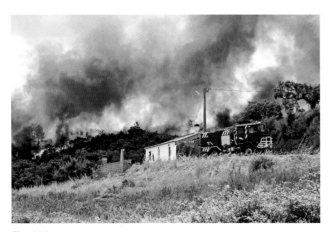

Fig. 18.2 Wildfires can cause significant respiratory events, as well as burns. (Copyright © iStock.com/Nisangha.)

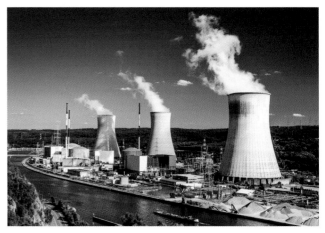

Fig. 18.4 Radiologic exposure at, for instance, a nuclear power plant, may require intravenous therapy. (Copyright © iStock.com/jotily.)

from outside sources, which may require additional security measures, such as in the case of controlled medications, and a longer delivery time.

TYPES OF EMERGENCIES OR DISASTERS

Each disaster or emergency presents its own set of challenges. The following is a list of common disaster or emergencies and some common sterile compounds associated with each.

WILDFIRES

This can cause significant respiratory events because of smoke inhalation, as well as burns. The type of medications most closely associated would include breathing treatment solutions, wound care (washes or baths), intravenous (IV) antibiotics, large volume bags for hydration, immunizations, such as tetanus, and IV or intramuscular (IM) pain medications (Fig. 18.2).

TORNADOS, HURRICANES, FLOODS (WIND OR WATER RELATED) EVENTS

These events can render a community cut off from others because of road closures, debris, or flooding. Medications, such as IV pain management, antibiotic

therapy, immunizations, and chronically ill patient's medications that must be uninterrupted, are common challenges (Fig. 18.3).

RADIOLOGIC OR CHEMICAL EXPOSURE

With these critical events, often IV therapy is the quickest way to react as fast as possible. This may include antibiotics, antidotes, burn-related therapy, such as wound washes, hydration, or sterile preparations for the eyes (Fig. 18.4).

PLANNING REQUIREMENTS FOR DISASTERS

Before an event, there must be plans in place and coordination efforts with organizations that will work together in the response (Fig. 18.5). In 2006 the National Boards of Pharmacy (NABP) developed a guide known as *"Recommendations for Preparing and Responding to an Emergency or Disaster"*. This includes responses and a planning template for events that affect the United States drug distribution system. Under this guide, the state boards of pharmacy are encouraged to develop plans more specific to their community's needs.

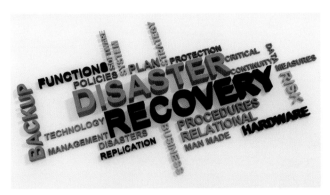

Fig. 18.5 Disaster planning is crucial. (Copyright © iStock.com/levoncigol.)

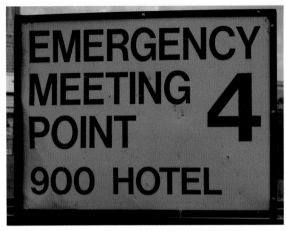

Fig. 18.6 Temporary sites must be part of disaster planning. (Copyright © iStock.com/dallaspaparazzo.)

The federal government has set up the Natural Disaster Medical System (NDMS), which coordinates with US Departments of Homeland Security, Defense, and Veterans Affairs. They are responsible for sending out medical teams, equipment, and supplies to the disaster areas affected. Under this organization, there are specialized teams, which include volunteers that are registered and trained beforehand. The personnel are required to participate in drills, attend training sessions, and stay current in their field. These teams include:

TEAM	FUNCTION
Disaster Medical Assistance Team (DMAT)	Sets up temporary treatment medical sites to treat burns and mental health emergencies
Disaster Mortuary Operations Response Teams (DMORT)	Made up of mortuary directors, pathologists, dental assistants, medical examiners, medical record technicians, and mental health staff, which are responsible for identification of victims and support family members in the grieving process in a disaster or emergency event
National Veterinary Response team (NVRT)	Responsible for treatment and care of working and victim animals in affected area
International Medical Surgical Response Team (IMSRT)	Performs as an operating room in the field and manages major traumas

Other organizations, such as The Joint Commission, include disaster planning and drills in their accreditation requirements for hospital systems and other related facilities. Larger communities may have a designated business or agency, where this takes place. Records are another challenge. Victims are confused and unable to communicate their medication histories, so maintaining these in secured locations and electronically is often required. Even simple information, such as vendor contacts, employee contact information, and master formula records must be obtainable. Often a duplicate source may be kept with these records, in case of destruction of a facility or inability to reach it.

Temporary sites must be part of the preplanning (Fig. 18.6). How do you perform sterile compounding in a temporary facility that may not meet the required USP<797> standards? This is where your expertise and understanding of the compounding processes comes into play. Handwashing is still critical and good aseptic TECHNIQUE is everything. Preparing IV medications in a less than perfect environment may be the only option during the event, so preparation and planning ahead is key. Thinking through the challenges, such as a setting up an alternate compounding environment, with or without electricity. This will have to include some type of primary engineering control (PEC), stockpiling and safe storage of supplies, and record keeping, as part of the compounding technician's role. Staying current in practices and participating in the facilities plan is essential to being prepared. These are not ideal situations for performing sterile compounding, but in a disaster, there may be no choice.

SPECIAL STORAGE AND DELIVERY CONSIDERATIONS

Per USP<797> and <800>, there are specific guidelines for assigning beyond use dates (BUDs) and storage conditions for sterile compounds. There must be consideration made for special delivery and storage for medications in the event of loss of electricity. If the compounded medication BUD assignment requires refrigerated storage, the pharmacy may have to provide a cooler and ice or ice packs, when delivering the medication. Since many IV medications require refrigeration, there will be a need to purchase and have on hand extra coolers, ice, or other means to keep the sterile preparations cold. Delivery of extra medications may need to be coordinated days ahead of the event and assigning BUDs will be a challenge. Regardless of the circumstances, all USP<797> guidelines must be considered.

Some events, such as hurricanes, give a window of time for preplanning, such as preparation of batches or extra medications in preparation for loss of electricity or supplies. This will require additional stocking and ordering ahead of medications and supplies, as well as alternative and additional storage efforts. Items, such as syringes, needles, coolers, ice packs, personal protective equipment (PPE, alcohol-based hand sanitizer) should be stockpiled in addition to the medications.

STRATEGIC NATIONAL STOCKPILE

The US government maintains a storage of certain medications that are normally required in a disaster event. The Strategic National Stockpile (SNS) is operated by the Center for Disease Control and Prevention (CDC) and includes a collection of chemical antidotes, immunizations, antitoxins, antiviral drugs, PPE, medical/surgical items, and ventilators. The CDC keeps large amounts of these medical supplies and medications, known as *Push packs*, which are delivered within 12 hours of a federal decision. The packs can treat thousands of patients and are color coded and numbered for tracking. Once federal and local agencies agree supplies are needed, the Push Packs can be delivered to any state within 12 hours. Each state should have a plan for receiving and distributing these to the affected areas.

In addition, local pharmacies and hospitals work with the Homeland Security and local Public Health departments to house a stockpile of similar items to be available, as a first response, or until the CDC can deliver inventory to an established point of distribution (POD) for distribution. The rule is usually to stockpile at least 72-96 hours of medications and supplies (inventory). The stock is maintained separately from the facilities normal stock and inventories are conducted regularly for expiration and updating. Antibiotics, vaccines, antidotes, contraception, Insulin, medications for pain control, life support and surgical medications are commonly stored items. In addition, IV pumps and fluids, respiratory products and supplies, diabetic supplies, and additional items such as batteries, alcohol, waste containers, and personal protective equipment are also stocked in quantity. Updating or increasing the PAR levels of medications in stock- There may be a need to increase the amount on hand for specific medications ahead of a disaster. Coordinate with vendors to ensure inventory is sufficient during and for restocking after (Fig. 18.7).

Maintaining current ordering and contact information for vendors should be a routine task along with checking expiration dates, monitoring manufacturer shortages, changes in the SNS recommended list from the CDC, or rotating stock out to the main pharmacy or returning to the wholesaler to replace with longer dated medications (Table 18.1).

The stockpile will vary based on the input of local pharmacies, other community organizations and regional needs. As a compounding pharmacy technician, it is important to understand the policies and

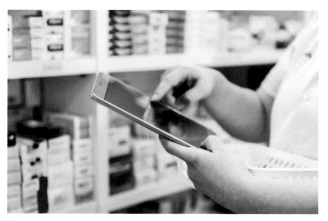

Fig. 18.7 There may be a need to increase the periodic automatic replenishment (PAR) levels of medications ahead of a disaster. (Copyright © iStock.com/MJ_Prototype.)

Table **18.1**	Commonly used Medications During Disasters.
THERAPEUTIC CLASS	**MEDICATIONS**
Analgesics	PO: hydrocodone/acetaminophen, oxycodone, acetaminophen, ibuprofen IV: morphine, fentanyl
Antibiotics, broad-spectrum with low allergy risk	PO and IV: levofloxacin PO: doxycycline, ciprofloxacin
Antibiotics, others	PO and IV: penicillin, clindamycin, metronidazole IV: vancomycin
Antidotes	Various
Antiemetics	PO and IV: ondansetron
Antipsychotics	PO and IV: haloperidol
Anxiolytics	PO and IV: lorazepam
Burn care agents	Topical: silver sulfadiazine, bacitracin
Ear, nose, and throat agents for tympanic membrane perforation	Otic: Neomycin/Polymyxin B, and hydrocortisone otic suspensions
Intubation medications	IV: etomidate, succinylcholine, and vecuronium
IV fluids	0.9% sodium chloride Dextrose 5% in water Lactated Ringer's solution
Ocular medications	Proparacaine ophthalmic ointment, erythromycin ophthalmic ointment
Respiratory	Inhalation: albuterol
Vaccines	Tetanus toxoid vaccine

IV, Intravenous; *PO*, oral.

From Bell C, Daniel S: Pharmacy leader's role in hospital emergency preparedness planning. *Hospital Pharmacy*, 49(4), 398–404, 2014. http://doi.org/10.1310/hjp4904-398.

procedures for handling a stockpile and ensuring readiness at all times. The victims will go to the POD, who will have both medical and pharmacy personnel working together to distribute and administer medications, such as immunizations, and often the National Pharmacy response Team (NPRT) sends professionals to work along-side local pharmacy employees and other volunteers. This is a team effort, but many victims will rely on their local pharmacy for knowledge of their medication history. For example, a known allergy history must be considered when administering a vaccine.

NABP'S "MODEL EMERGENCY DISASTER PREPAREDNESS AND RESPONSE PLAN"

Organizations offer templates for plans for organizations to use for readiness. The NABP's "Model Emergency Disaster Preparedness and Response Plan", is provided to state boards of pharmacy to assist them in planning for disasters in each of their states. The plan consists of six sections that can be used to develop a template.
- Section 1: Emergency planning.
- Section 2: Maintaining board of pharmacy operations.
- Section 3: Communication.
- Section 4: Evacuation planning.
- Section 5: Shelter in place planning.
- Section 6: Protecting resources.

SECTION 1: EMERGENCY PLANNING

This section comprises the following subsections:
- Contact listing for all personnel with address, phone numbers, and emergency contact information
- A risk assessment that determines what impacts different disasters may cause. This is used to determine a warning time and what efforts should be made ahead of time, such as evacuation or sheltering in place
- Emergency supply list of items and essential records that should be stored in fire and water-proof containers
- Immunization records of staff and board members
- Training records and participation in drills.

SECTION 2: MAINTAINING BOARD OF PHARMACY OPERATIONS

This section comprises the following elements:
- Listing that defines the leadership and individual roles of members and staff
- Remote access for individuals to have access to records in case of damaged facilities
- An alternate site location for operations
- A critical function listing for each member is identified
- A listing of suppliers and wholesalers for medications and supplies
- Record preservation methods for prescription and medical histories—both electronic and hard copy.

SECTION 3: COMMUNICATION

This section explains methods to communicate before, during, and after the event. This may be websites, local news stations, telephone call tree, or special passwords for entry into records.

SECTION 4: EVACUATION PLANNING

This section explains procedures to evacuate if needed. It includes communication methods, primary and secondary locations, reporting managers, and "all clear" methods.

SECTION 5: SHELTER IN PLACE PLANNING

This section provides instructions for staying in the event of a disaster, methods to identify those entering and leaving, and any special training for warnings, such as tornados.

SECTION 6: PROTECTING RESOURCES

This section explains cyber security measures, such as technology used to maintain patient histories and records, which must be protected even in a disaster. In the event computer hardware is damaged, there should be a back-up in place to replace or recoup that information.

This section also discusses ways to support staff as a valuable resource. The wellbeing of personnel is critical for proper functioning during the event, and the plan should include providing counselors for stress or burn out.

IMMEDIATE RESPONSE

The initial response should be coordinated among key agencies to provide food, water, and essentials to life first. This is "all hands-on deck" and will include all pharmacy personnel. You may be asked to work at a POD to give out the basics, such as food and water. Once this immediate need to prepare batches response phase is done, there may be the need for sterile medications ahead. Regardless of what your normal or routine activities are in the pharmacy, you may be asked to perform different tasks initially in the disaster response. Staying current in your field, participating in drills, and being a team member in planning and advanced preparation efforts, will ensure each person works together and provides a smooth workflow process. Pharmacy personnel must be aware of the dangers associated with the disaster encountered and prepare themselves to safely interact with and provide victims with appropriate assistance. Staying current with immunizations, cardiopulmonary resuscitation (CPR), and additional training related to assisting victims is important.

Tasks, such as handwashing may be reduced to handwashing without water. Using PPE, such as masks, gloves, gowns, shoe and hair covers may be required to work in the PODs or deliver medications to community areas (Fig. 18.8). In disasters that include air contaminates, which are determined by Occupational Safety and Health Administration (OSHA), respirators may be required. It is the pharmacy technician's responsibility to know these procedures and be able to comply in different disasters.

If isolation patients require medications, you must be aware of the protocols associated. You may be asked to deliver medications to a facility set aside for evacuees or those requiring isolation and you must protect yourself, as well as the patient from contamination.

In addition, knowing your department or facility's response plan is essential to being effective before, during, and after the emergency. If training, such as CPR/First AID is required of all pharmacy team members, it must be kept up to date. Waiting until an imminent disaster is on the horizon will not be the best use of your talents nor will it allow you to help your department when you are needed (Fig. 18.9).

Before medication can be distributed in cases, such as hurricanes, floods, or tornados for instance,

the victim's personal safety and control over their medication needs must come first. There may need to be sheltering-in-place or an evacuation, depending on the effects on the disaster. Determining the risks associated with a location or type of disaster must be always be determined first. There are zones to assess the locations with the contamination or risk assessment:

- Hot zone—the area where the event took place
- Warm zone—area at least 300 ft from the event
- Cold zone—area close to the warm area but away from the event.

Identifying "high risk" groups is an important part of the pharmacy's role. Creating manual lists that your pharmacy serves, such as for elderly, pediatric, and patients with chronic disease, such as diabetes, may be a task assigned to a compounding pharmacy technician. These may require special kits that are ready for distribution early on. An example would be insulin, needles and syringes for diabetic patients (Fig. 18.10).

As the compounding technician, it may be necessary to provide prefilled syringes of certain medications or batch immunizations for teams in the field to administer (Fig. 18.11). Communication is key when

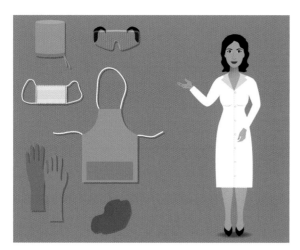

Fig. 18.8 Personal protective equipment, such as masks, gloves, gowns, shoe and hair covers, may be required to work in the point of distributions or deliver medications to community areas. (Copyright © iStock.com/S_Veresk.)

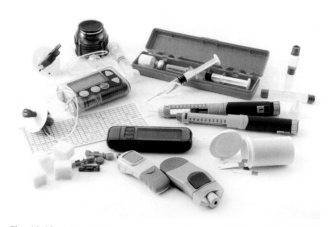

Fig. 18.10 "High risk" groups may require special kits, such as this kit for diabetic patients. (Copyright © iStock.com/MihaPater.)

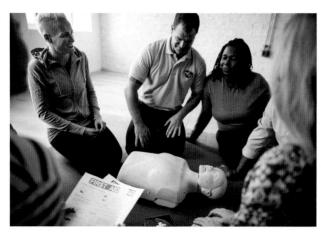

Fig. 18.9 Cardiopulmonary resuscitation (CPR) training must be kept current if it is required of all pharmacy team members. (Copyright © iStock.com/Rawpixel Ltd.)

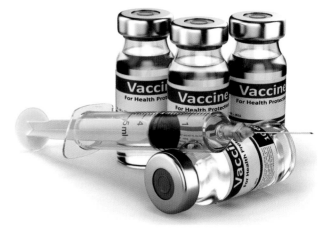

Fig. 18.11 Compounding technicians may need to provide prefilled syringes of certain medications or batch immunizations for teams in the field to administer. (Copyright © iStock.com/Bet_Noire.)

working with other facilities or agencies. Using good communication and team building skills provides a calming and effective environment for the victims, which leads to better compliance and safer practices. In every instance, always use your experience and training to perform whatever important services are needed.

The key to disaster preparedness is being ready and knowing the role you play, understanding the established plan for your facility, and the impacts or risks associated with the disaster being faced. As a compounding pharmacy technician, you have a particular set of skills that are vital in planning and participating both during and after a disaster. You will encounter patients and other community and healthcare members who require assistance for their medication needs, and serving as a response team member is rewarding and can provide victims with assurance and a sense of comfort.

REVIEW QUESTIONS

1. Which team is responsible to set up temporary medical sites to treat burns and mental health issue in times of disaster or emergency?
   A. NVRT
   B. DMORT
   C. NPRT
   D. DMAT
2. Which team is responsible for the treatment and care of working and victim animals in affected areas because of a disaster or emergency?
   A. DMORT
   B. NPRT
   C. DMAT
   D. NVRT
3. Which team is responsible for providing mass vaccinations during a disaster or emergency?
   A. NPRT
   B. NVRT
   C. NDMS
   D. National Incident Management System (NIMS)
4. Which of the following was established by the Department of Homeland Security to manage the coordination and support of facilities during a disaster or emergency?
   A. NIMS
   B. NDMS
   C. FEMA
   D. NABP
5. As a pharmacy technician, which of the following would be appropriate to be a member of as a trained professional ready to work in a disaster or emergency situation?
   A. NABP
   B. NPRT
   C. NVRT
   D. DMORT

6. In a radiation exposure type of disaster, which of the following treatments would most likely be required?
   A. Immunization
   B. Chronic disease management
   C. Pain management
   D. Sterile eye preparations
7. Which of the following organizations maintains a national stockpile of medication for use in disasters or emergencies?
   A. CDC
   B. NABP
   C. USP
   D. ASHP
8. Which of the following terms is used to describe a ready set of medications and supplies sent to a disaster area?
   A. Push boxes
   B. Push Packs
   C. Pull Packs
   D. Ready Packs
9. Which of the following organizations has prepared a document known as the "Model Emergency Disaster Preparedness and Response Plan" to be used for disaster planning?
   A. USP
   B. Department of Homeland Security
   C. NABP
   D. CDC
10. Which of the following zone identifiers is used to identify an area that is 300 feet away from the event or disaster?
    A. Hot zone
    B. Warm zone
    C. Cold zone
    D. POD

CRITICAL THINKING

1. As a compounding technician in a local pharmacy, it is your responsibility to maintain a stockpile of vaccines and common disaster related medications. What are some of the steps that would be involved in this process?
2. The news has announced that a hurricane could affect your immediate area. The Pharmacist states that everyone should make sure their department is ready and well stocked. What common sterile compounding and delivery supplies should be evaluated for your area?

BIBLIOGRAPHY

1. General Chapter <797> Pharmaceutical Compounding—Sterile Preparations. http://www.usp.org/compounding/general-chapter-797. Retrieved August 26, 2018.
2. American Society of Health-System Pharmacists: ASHP Guidelines on Quality Assurance for Pharmacy-Prepared

Sterile Products. http://www.ashp.org/s_ashp/docs/files/BP07/Prep_Gdl_QualAssurSterile.pdf. Accessed August 26, 2018.

3. Centers for Disease Control and Prevention: Guideline for hand hygiene in health-care settings: recommendations of the healthcare infection control practices advisory committee and the HICPAC/SHEA/APIC/IDSA hand hygiene task force, *MMWR* 51(RR-16:2, 29-33). October 2002: http://www.cdc.gov/mmwr/PDF/rr/rr5116.pdf. Accessed August 27, 2018.

4. *Dorland's illustrated medical dictionary*, ed 31, Philadelphia, 2007, Saunders.

5. ISMP: Sterile Compounding Tragedy is a Symptom of a Broken System on Many Levels. https://www.ismp.org/resources/sterile-compounding-tragedy-symptom-broken-system-many-levels. Retrieved September 28, 2018.

6. Sir Joseph Lister: Developer of Antiseptic Surgery. *essortment* (website): http://www.essortment.com/sir-joseph-lister-developer-antiseptic-surgery-37935.html. Accessed September 2, 2018.

7. MD: Medical Errors—Third Leading Cause of Death. https://www.mdmag.com/conference-coverage/aapa-2017/medical-errors-the-third-leading-cause-of-death-in-the-united-states. Accessed September 17, 2018.

8. Mitchell J, Haroun L: *Introduction to health care*, ed 2, Clifton Park, NY, 2007, Thomson Delmar Learning.

9. The Joint Commission: Medication—Sterile Compounding—Compounding Staff Competency Requirements. https://www.jointcommission.org/standards_information/jcfaqdetails.aspx?StandardsFaqId=1624&ProgramId=46. Accessed September 2, 2018.

10. CDC: Strategic National Stockpile (SNS) (webpage). Retrieved Mar 7, 2019 from www.cdc.gov/phpr/stockpile/stockpile.htm.

11. U.S. Department of Health and Human Services: Stockpile Products. Retrieved March 9, 2019 from https://www.phe.gov/about/sns/Pages/products.aspx.

12. WHO. International travel and health: situation as on 1 January 2010. 2010. http://www.amazon.com/International-Travel-Health-2009-Situation/dp/9241580429/ref=s r_1_17?ie=UTF8&s=books&qid=1271876707&sr=1-17# reader _9241580429.

Looking Forward

19

Learning Objectives

1. Discuss advanced training opportunities and certifications for sterile preparation through the Society for the Education for Pharmacy Technicians, CriticalPoint, and the National Pharmacy Technician Association, as well as additional training opportunities.

2. Discuss the specialty certification for Certified Sterile Processing technician (CSPT).
3. Describe patient-centered care and the future of sterile compounding.

Terms & Definitions

CSPT (Certified Sterile Processing Technician An advanced certification in sterile compounding offered by Pharmacy Technician Certification Board (PTCB)
PCCA Professional Compounding Centers of America
Pharmacy Patient Care Process (PPCP) Plan designed to assist patients in their overall wellness and disease management

Point of Care (POC) testing Immediate tests performed in Pharmacies
NPTA National Pharmacy Technician Association
SEPh The Society for the Education of Pharmacy Technicians

INTRODUCTION

As the pharmacy profession changes and healthcare advancements focus on patient-centered care, pharmacy technicians will have opportunities to advance their knowledge in specialty areas.

Informatics and digital health in the future offer an interdisciplinary approach and rely on communication with every team member associated with a patient (Fig. 19.1). Sterile compounding is just one aspect of the whole picture and will require more and more work with automation and other dispensing technology. The basics of good aseptic technique will never change, however.

ADVANCED TRAINING OPPORTUNITIES

There are several organizations and educational institutions that offer specialized or advanced training in sterile compounding. Much of this includes material to read with a hands-on or skills-based session and provide the technician with continuing education (CE) credit through Accreditation Council for Pharmacy Education (ACPE). This organization is recognized by state Boards of Pharmacy and meet requirements for maintaining Pharmacy Technician Certification (CPhT) through the Pharmacy Technician Certification Board (PTCB).

SOCIETY FOR THE EDUCATION FOR PHARMACY TECHNICIANS

The Society for the Education for Pharmacy Technicians (SEPhT; www.thesepht.org) offers ACPE skills-based certification training (boot camp) for sterile compounding. This includes a 12-hour session with information regarding USP<797>, basic handwashing and garbing, and simulated IV preparation. In this one day and a half course, the student will achieve the following:

- Participants will discuss the latest USP<797> and <800> guidelines and common practices used in aseptic technique of nonhazardous and hazardous sterile compounds
- Participants will demonstrate procedures for using vials, powder vials, ampules, bags, and preparation of batch/bulk medications and hazardous drugs containment devices
- Participants will demonstrate cleaning and disinfecting procedures, handwashing, garbing, and the safe use and cleaning techniques of equipment and common supplies used in sterile compounding
- Participants will use a database software program to create labels from physician orders and perform all calculations required
- Participants will use references for compatibilities and storage/expiration information and complete all required documentation

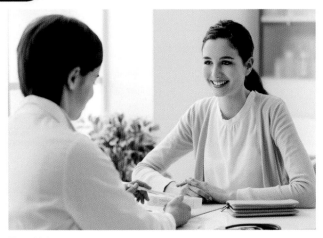

Fig. 19.1 As the pharmacy profession changes and healthcare advancements focus on patient-centered care, pharmacy technicians will have opportunities to advance their knowledge in specialty areas. (Copyright © iStock.com/demaerre.)

- Participants will discuss quality control measures, training requirements, and sampling.

CRITICALPOINT

CriticalPoint (https://www.criticalpoint.info/) offers ACPE accredited custom training and compliance tools in sterile compounding in a state-of-the-art sterile processing center. The courses are web based and include skills (hands on) sessions, as with garbing, techniques, and lecture. The 28 lessons (33 hours of ACPE-approved CE) cover all topic areas relevant to sterile compounding.
- The History of Compounding and USP<797>.
- Determining Beyond-Use Dating.
- Quality Releases and Final Checks of CSPs.
- Labeling and Packaging.
- Master Formulation and Compounding Records.
- Purpose and Effective Use of Policies and Procedure.
- General Elements of Documentation.
- Primary Engineering Controls: Function, Use, Testing and Certification (2 hours CE).
- Secondary Engineering Controls: Function, Use Testing and Certification (2 hours CE).
- Personnel Hand Hygiene, Garbing and Gloved Fingertip Sampling (2 hours CE).
- Personnel Aseptic Media Fill and Competency Evaluation.
- Volumetric Air Sampling.
- Surface Sampling.
- Overview of Cleaning and Disinfection of Pharmacy Controlled Environments.
- Cleaning and Disinfection of Primary Engineering Controls.
- Cleaning and Disinfection of Secondary Engineering Controls and Segregated Compounding Areas.
- Overview of Quality and Responsibilities of Compounding Personnel.
- Proper Material Handling.
- Use of Syringes, Needles, Vials, Ampules and Filters.
- Aseptic Technique and Conduct in Controlled Environments.

- Sterile Compounding on Patient Units (for nursing and medical staff).
- Filtration and Sterility Testing.
- Moist and Dry-Heat Sterilization.
- Bacterial Endotoxin (Pyrogen) Testing.
- Hazardous Drug Introduction and Overview.
- Engineering Controls and Personal Protective Equipment (2 hours CE).
- Hazardous Drug Work Practice Strategies (2 hours CE).

NATIONAL PHARMACY TECHNICIAN ASSOCIATION

The National Pharmacy Technician Association (NPTA; www.npta.org) offers an ACPE accredited IV certification course, with at home modules, and a session of on-site training. The course participants will work through the following concepts:
- Facilities, Garb and Equipment
- Aseptic Calculations
- Properties of Sterile Products
- Aseptic Technique
- Sterile Product Preparations
- Total Parenteral Nutrition (TPN)
- Chemotherapy
- Quality Control and Assurance.

ADDITIONAL TRAINING OPPORTUNITIES

There is also internet-based CE courses offered from several organizations, such as Power-Pak CE., PharmacyTech CE, Pharmacy Tech Topics, and many others.

American Society of Health-System Pharmacists (ASHP) has two meetings each year with CE sessions to cover a variety of pharmacy topics. As a technician, you can attend and gain ACPE credits toward state board or certification requirements. As a member, there are other opportunities to attend webinars, lectures, and state sponsored affiliate meetings. Look for content related to sterile compounding to ensure that you are staying current in your practice setting and up to date on regulations.

CSPT

The PTCB (www.ptcb.org), which provides national certification through testing known as *CPhT*, recently began offering a specialty certification for a Certified Sterile Processing technician or CSPT. The candidate who wishes to test must be a CPhT in good standing to start. They must have completed a PTCB recognized sterile compounding education course, an ASHP accredited program AND have one year of work experience in sterile compounding. Another option is to have completed 3 years of work experience in sterile compounding.

The test consists of questions broken into different sections known as *domains*. These are key areas that are covered in the test. The percentages are the weight of each domain in the test.
- Medications and Components (17%).
- Facilities and Equipment (22%).

- Sterile Compounding Procedures (53%).
- Handling, Packaging, Storage, and Disposal (8%).

MEDICATIONS AND COMPONENTS CONTENT

This domain covers the drugs, (brand and generic), dosages, characteristics, stability, storage, and safety information found in the Safety Data Sheets or SDS.

FACILITIES AND EQUIPMENT

This domain covers equipment, such as primary engineering controls, environmental monitoring, and operational standards per USP<797> guidelines.

STERILE COMPOUNDING PROCEDURES

This is over half of the test's content and relates to the actual aseptic technique procedures, calculations, procedures for cleaning and decontamination, handwashing, and garbing and gowning.

HANDLING, PACKAGING, STORAGE, AND DISPOSAL

This domain relates to supplies used, disposal of sharps and other supplies, and handling of completed compounded sterile preparations.

PATIENT-CENTERED CARE (THE FUTURE OF PRACTICE)

The term patient-centered care refers to an approach of treating the patient as a whole entity. More emphasis is on the patient's overall wellbeing and disease management, and with pharmacy being the first point of contact in many cases, pharmacy technician roles are needed for support and preparation of sterile compounds and other sterile medications for distribution. As part of the Patient Protection and Affordable Care Act, offered called the *Affordable Care Act* or *ACA*, Medicare must provide coverage for wellness and preventive services. These services may be conducted either by a physician or another licensed healthcare professional who is acting under the physician's direction, the latter of which has opened the door for pharmacists in many states to become much more involved in direct patient care, along with providing medications. As the role of the pharmacist expands, so does the role of the pharmacy technician. The day-to-day operations, including management initiatives and dispensing tasks, make up just a few of the responsibilities that technicians are taking on, as the pharmacists become more involved in a clinical role.

Additional training is available in many areas to allow trained pharmacy technicians in support roles to participate in some of the following:
- Anticoagulation or blood draws
- Immunizations
- Compliance and patient safety
- Medication reconciliation
- Preadmission histories

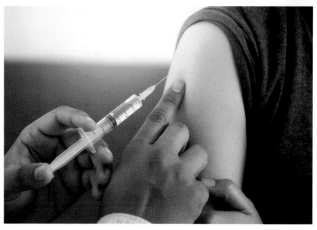

Fig. 19.2 Immunizations are being done in the pharmacy as part of the Pharmacy Patient Care Process. (Copyright © iStock.com/juststock.)

- Education regarding smoking, alcohol, diet, and exercise.

Technicians are already involved in community outreach programs for smoking cessation, diabetes management, or support personnel for "in house" pharmacy clinic settings. As part of the Pharmacy Patient Care Process or PPCP program, immunizations and other "point of care" (POC) tests, such as hemoccult, strep tests, human immunodeficiency virus (HIV), and blood pressure readings, are being done in the pharmacy (Fig. 19.2).

A pharmacy technician can assist the administration of vaccinations, although the actual administration must be performed by the pharmacist. The medications often require refrigeration, and ordering can be seasonal, as in flu vaccines for flu season. Pharmacy technicians often ensure proper documentation and billing through third-party insurance providers. The recommended schedules for adults and children can be found through the Centers for Disease Control and Prevention (CDC) website and are updated annually. These tasks can be performed by trained pharmacy technicians to allow pharmacists more time to spend with each patient (Fig. 19.3).

Pharmacy and wellness visits are a perfect pair, as more than 90% of Americans live less than a mile or two from a pharmacy. With today's fast-paced world and changes in third-party reimbursement, the pharmacy is becoming a hub for routine care because it provides easy access to many types of such care.

Many POC testing (POCTs) can be billed directly to the patient or to third-party insurance provider by the pharmacist. Through the use of tests for which results are available quickly, many simple diseases may be diagnosed earlier. Combining diagnosis and treatment in a single encounter results in better patient compliance. Rather than going to a physician's office for a simple test and then to the pharmacy for a prescription, a single visit to the pharmacy can accomplish both in less time.

Common examples of POCTs include:
- **Influenza:** Rapid testing for types A and B is available. Fast results can allow for antivirals to be given within a 48-hour window

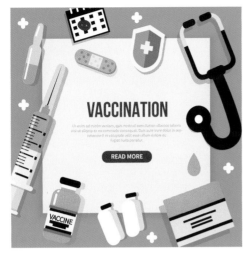

Fig. 19.3 Trained pharmacy technicians can assist in the administration of vaccines through tasks, such as ensure proper documentation and billing, through third-party insurance providers. (Copyright © iStock.com/Irina_Strelnikova.)

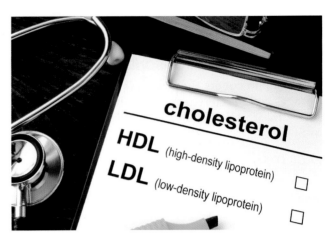

Fig. 19.5 Chronic disease screening includes screening for cholesterol issues. (Copyright © iStock.com/designer491.)

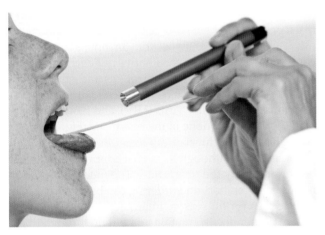

Fig. 19.4 A common example of a point of care testing is a throat culture for group A *Streptococcus*. (Copyright © iStock.com/studio_77-28.)

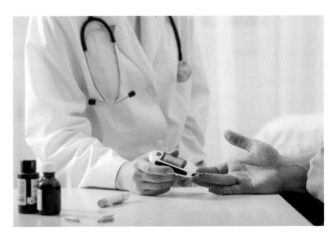

Fig. 19.6 Patients with diabetes should have their A1c levels checked periodically. (Copyright © iStock.com/Maya23K.)

- **Group A *Streptococcus*:** Many patients who experience sore throats do not test positive for group A *Streptococcus* bacteria, but broad spectrum antibiotics are commonly prescribed, leading to antibiotic resistance. The rapid testing involves a simple throat culture (Fig. 19.4).

  POCTs can also include chronic disease screening and chronic disease testing. Examples include:
- Chronic disease screening
  - **HIV:** Patients who engage in high-risk sexual activity are often embarrassed to see a physician in an office for HIV. Several companies offer boxed testing that can be purchased at a community pharmacy and be performed by the patient
  - **Cholesterol (lipid):** Many patients who have elevated cholesterol levels and are unaware until they experience a heart-related event, which could be life-threatening. Early detection with a simple boxed test can allow for possible treatment with a statin drug, such as Lipitor or Tricor (Fig. 19.5)

  - **Hepatitis C:** Screening is recommended for those born between 1945 and 1965, an at-risk group that may be unaware of this condition
  - **Fecal occult blood:** Early detection is important and this test screens for colorectal cancer, which can be performed at home by a patient.
- Chronic disease testing
  - **A1c:** Diabetes is one of the most prevalent diseases today, and those with the disease should have A1c levels checked periodically, to measure long-term glucose control. A pharmacist can test this level, which should be less than 7, in the pharmacy, and may provide counseling to individuals with elevated levels on lifestyle and diet changes to manage the disease (Fig. 19.6).
  - **International normalized ratio (INR)/prothrombin time (PT):** Patients taking anticoagulants, such as warfarin are required to monitor their blood clotting times. This monitoring can be done weekly and require physician's office visit and copay. Monitoring also can be done at a local pharmacy, allowing the pharmacist to work closely with the physician and patient for adjustments, and

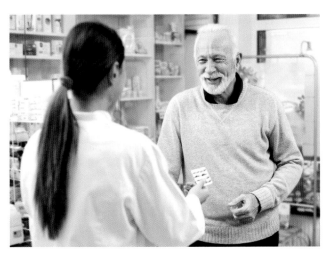

Fig. 19.7 Pharmacy technicians in advanced roles provide support for better medication compliance and disease management. (Copyright © iStock.com/Gligatron.)

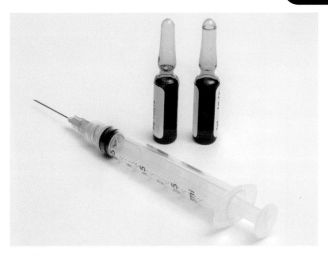

Fig. 19.8 Some larger pharmacy chains offer clinics where patients can go for treatment of minor illnesses. Whereas a physician's office may be required to bill the insurance provider for a full visit when a patient needs an injection (for example, a vaccine or B_{12} injection), the pharmacy clinic can bill for the service provided and save the patient money. (Copyright © iStock.com/trafawma.)

combining the testing and prescription in one location.

Other POCTs include pregnancy, ovulation, drugs of abuse, fecal occult blood, and food pathogens. POCT works well in conjunction with the patient's PPCP, as it is another tool used for diagnosis, monitoring, and follow-up efforts in disease management and improvement. Pharmacy technicians in advanced roles provide support for better medication compliance and disease management. As pharmacists become more involved in the patient's clinical care, the everyday tasks are being performed more and more by the pharmacy technician (Fig. 19.7).

Some larger pharmacy chains are offering clinics where patients can go for treatment of minor illnesses and bill to third-party insurance providers. Whereas a physician's office may be required to bill the insurance provider for a full visit when a patient needs an injection, the pharmacy clinic can bill for the service provided and save the patient money. Common clinic needs include vaccines, injections, such as B_{12} or insulin, or POCT. If provided at the pharmacy, testing is done with pharmacist counseling performed on site and trained pharmacy technicians acting as support staff (Fig. 19.8).

Expanding the roles of trained pharmacy technicians is a key part of a successful interdisciplinary healthcare team according to ASHP. Medication adherence programs are being integrated throughout the country and technicians are often the professional in whom a patient will confide. They may resist taking a medication, not fully understand information received from their practitioner, or just want reassurance of a wellness or disease management program components. The technician who receives this information can relay it to the Pharmacist for counseling or consultation (Fig. 19.9).

As the compounding technician, you could encounter a situation that requires changes in how the patient needs to meet an appointment for their intravenous (IV) treatment. They could be concerned about the

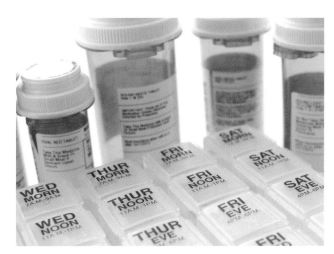

Fig. 19.9 Expanding the role of trained pharmacy technicians has many benefits, including the possibility of improved medication adherence. (Copyright © iStock.com/razmarinka.)

packaging or storage of their sterile compound or need a way to dispose of their sharps. All of these situations can be potential errors if the patient is not confident in the support staff at their pharmacy. If they do not feel comfortable asking questions, they may either not take the medication or may take it the best way they feel is right (Fig. 19.10).

Without national standards for education and training requirements for pharmacy technicians to date, the best way to advance one's career is to participate in any education that expands the knowledge and competency in your field. A better qualified and highly trained pharmacy technician workforce will improve patient safety, bottom-line. Advancing your knowledge in sterile compounding and staying current in the regulations and safety measures will allow the future of pharmacy to be bright.

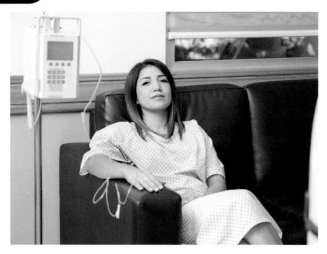

Fig. 19.10 Patient confidence in the support staff at the pharmacy is essential. (Copyright © iStock.com/Antonio_Diaz.)

REVIEW QUESTIONS

1. Which of the following organizations offers an advanced certification known as a CSPT?
   A. NPTA
   B. ASHP
   C. PTCB
   D. PCCA
2. Which of the following organizations publishes the immunization recommendation schedule for adults and children each year?
   A. CDC
   B. USP
   C. US Food and Drug Administration (FDA)
   D. ACA
3. Pharmacy technicians who are properly trained can serve in support roles in all the following EXCEPT?
   A. Immunizations
   B. Medication reconciliation
   C. Preadmission histories
   D. Dosing requirements
4. Which of the following would be considered a common POCT that could be performed at a pharmacy?
   A. EKG
   B. ECG
   C. A1c
   D. Hepatitis A screening
5. Which of the POCTs listed is used to monitor the clotting time for patients taking warfarin?
   A. INR
   B. A1c
   C. Fecal occult blood
   D. Lipid panel
6. Which of the following procedures can a pharmacy clinic bill a third-party insurance company for?
   A. B12 injection
   B. IV push pain medication
   C. IV hydration
   D. IV antibiotic

7. What patient age range is recommended for screening of Hepatitis C?
   A. 1955–1965
   B. 1945–1965
   C. 1935–1965
   D. 1925–1965
8. Which of the following medications is commonly used to treat high cholesterol?
   A. Tricor
   B. Warfarin
   C. B12
   D. Aspirin
9. Which acronym describes the plan that is designed to work with patients to assist them in their overall wellness and disease management?
   A. POC
   B. PPCP
   C. PCCA
   D. NPTA
10. Which of the following CSPT test domains covers the medication safety information found in SDS sheets?
   A. Medications and Components
   B. Facilities and Equipment
   C. Sterile Compounding Procedures
   D. Handling, Packaging, Storage, and Disposal

CRITICAL THINKING

1. As the compounding pharmacy technician in a busy outpatient chemotherapy center, you interact with patients every day. One of the patients receiving Adriamycin IV once a week asks you if it would be alright to dispose of their partially unused IV bags in the regular trash. What would your answer be and why?

BIBLIOGRAPHY

1. Critical Point: For Everything Sterile Compounding. Retrieved April 9, 2019 from https://www.criticalpoint.info/.
2. Davis. *Mosby's pharmacy technician principle and practices instructor addendum*, ed 5, 2019.
3. National Pharmacy Technician Association (NPTA): Sterile Product Certification Course. Retrieved April 7, 2019 from www.pharmacytechnician.org
4. Pharmacy Technician Certification Board (PTCB): NEW! Sterile compounding certification. Retrieved April 10, 2019 from www.ptcb.org.
5. Professional Compounding Centers of America (PCCA): C3. Comprehensive Compounding Course. Retrieved April 10, 2019 from https://pccarx.com.
6. The Society for the Education of Pharmacy Technicians: SEPhT Now Offers ACPE Accredited CEs through Skills Camps and Certifications. Retrieved April 8, 2019 from www.thesepht.org.

Procedure Evaluation Checklists

PROCEDURE 4.1: PROPER HANDWASHING

Student Name: _____ Date: _____

KEY	3: Proficient (can complete task in a timely manner without assistance)
	2: Partially Proficient (can complete most of task but needs some assistance)
	1: Limited (can do the task but requires close assistance and supervision)
	0: Insufficient (cannot perform the task, remediation required)

Task	Student (Self-Evaluation)	Evaluator
Performed handwashing in the ante-room AFTER donning shoe covers, head and facial hair covers, face masks, and NON-sterile gown BEFORE entering the buffer area		
Washed hands and forearms up to the elbows with unscented soap and water for at least 30 seconds.		
Dried hands and forearms to the elbows completely with low-lint disposable towels or wipes.		
Immediately before donning sterile gloves, applied a suitable alcohol-based hand rub.		
Allowed hands to dry thoroughly before donning sterile gloves.		
	Total:	Total:

Evaluator Name _____ **Date** _____
Grade _____

PROCEDURE 4.2: PERSONNEL CLEANSING AND GARBING ORDER

Student Name: _____ Date: _____

KEY	3: Proficient (can complete task in a timely manner without assistance)		
	2: Partially Proficient (can complete most of task but needs some assistance)		
	1: Limited (can do the task but requires close assistance and supervision)		
	0: Insufficient (cannot perform the task, remediation required)		
Task		**Student (Self-Evaluation)**	**Evaluator**
Put on shoe covers.			
Put on head cover.			
Put on head and facial hair covers (i.e., beard cover, if applicable).			
Put on face mask.			
Put on nonsterile gown.			
Performed handwashing (see Procedure 4.1).			
Put on sterile gown.			
Applied hand cleanser and allow to dry.			
Put on sterile gloves.			
		Total:	**Total:**

Evaluator Name _____ **Date** _____

Grade _____

PROCEDURE 7.1: PERFORMING GLOVED FINGERTIP/THUMB SAMPLING PER USP STANDARDS

Student Name: _____   Date: _____

KEY	3: Proficient (can complete task in a timely manner without assistance)		
	2: Partially Proficient (can complete most of task but needs some assistance)		
	1: Limited (can do the task but requires close assistance and supervision)		
	0: Insufficient (cannot perform the task, remediation required)		
Task		**Student (Self-Evaluation)**	**Evaluator**
Performed garbing and handwashing in the ante-room before entering the buffer area (see Procedures 4.1 and 4.2).			
Collected a gloved fingertip and thumb sample from both hands by lightly pressing each fingertip into the agar. Used a separate plate for each hand.			
Covered and recorded date, time, right or left hand, and person identifier on each plate.			
Inverted the plates and incubated the contact sampling devices at 20–35°C for 5 days.			
The results were reviewed with the person and documentation kept to show compliance with USP standards for evaluators and outside agencies.			
		Total:	**Total:**

Evaluator Name _____ **Date** _____
Grade _____

PROCEDURE 7.2: PERFORMING MEDIA FILL

Student Name: _____ Date: _____

KEY	3: Proficient (can complete task in a timely manner without assistance)		
	2: Partially Proficient (can complete most of task but needs some assistance)		
	1: Limited (can do the task but requires close assistance and supervision)		
	0: Insufficient (cannot perform the task, remediation required)		
Task		**Student (Self-Evaluation)**	**Evaluator**
Performed garbing and handwashing in the ante-room before entering the buffer area (see Procedures 4.1 and 4.2).			
Using the commercial kit, followed the instructions in the LAFW using aseptic techniques.			
Incubated the media-filled vials at 20–35°C for a minimum of 14 days. If two temperatures were used for incubation of media-filled samples, incubated the filled containers for at least 7 days at the lower temperature (20–25°C) followed by 7 days at 30–35°C.			
Recorded results in facility documents.			
		Total:	**Total:**

Evaluator Name _____ **Date** _____
Grade _____

PROCEDURE 7.3: PERFORMING SURFACE SAMPLING PER USP STANDARDS

Student Name: _____   Date: _____

KEY	3: Proficient (can complete task in a timely manner without assistance)
	2: Partially Proficient (can complete most of task but needs some assistance)
	1: Limited (can do the task but requires close assistance and supervision)
	0: Insufficient (cannot perform the task, remediation required)

Task	Student (Self-Evaluation)	Evaluator
Performed garbing and handwashing in the ante-room before entering the buffer area (see Procedures 4.1 and 4.2).		
Removed the cover of the contact sampling device aseptically and pressed firmly to the surface being sampled. Covered the contact material back up.		
Inverted the plates and incubated the contact sampling devices at 20–25°C for 5–7 days and then at 30–35°C for 2–3 additional days.		
Examined the sampling devices for growth daily during normal business hours and recorded the observed count at each time point. At the final time point, recorded the total number of discrete colonies of microorganisms (CFU/sample) on the environmental sampling record, based on sample type, sample location, and sample date.		
	Total:	Total:

Evaluator Name _____   Date _____

Grade _____

PROCEDURE 8.1: CLEANING AN LAFW

Student Name: _____   Date: _____

KEY	3: Proficient (can complete task in a timely manner without assistance)
	2: Partially Proficient (can complete most of task but needs some assistance)
	1: Limited (can do the task but requires close assistance and supervision)
	0: Insufficient (cannot perform the task, remediation required)

Task	Student (Self-Evaluation)	Evaluator
Performed nonhazardous garbing and handwashing in the ante-room before entering the buffer area (see Chapter 4).		
Arranged the lint free wipes in a stack, within 6 inches of front of hood edge.		
Poured IPA 70% alcohol on the stack, soaking through to the bottom one.		
Pulled the first wipe off the stack and wiped the ceiling using a side-to-side motion, overlapping strokes starting at the back and moving outward from back to front. Discarded the wipe when done.		
Pulled the second wipe and cleaned the pole and hooks if applicable. Discarded the wipe.		
Pulled the third wipe from the stack and cleaned a side. Started in the back top corner, and used overlapping strokes from top to bottom and working outward (back to front). Discarded the wipe.		
Repeated the same on the other side.		
Used remainder of the stack of wipes to clean the work surface. Started at the back corner, and working in overlapping strokes side to side, cleaned from back to front. Discarded the wipes.		
	Total:	Total:

Evaluator Name _____   **Date** _____
Grade _____

PROCEDURE 10.1: TRANSFERRING LIQUID CONTENTS (VIAL) TO AN IV CONTAINER

Student Name: _____   Date: _____

KEY	3: Proficient (can complete task in a timely manner without assistance)
	2: Partially Proficient (can complete most of task but needs some assistance)
	1: Limited (can do the task but requires close assistance and supervision)
	0: Insufficient (cannot perform the task, remediation required)

Task	Student (Self-Evaluation)	Evaluator
Completed any calculations needed and prepared label before entering the ISO class 8 (ante-area).		
Performed in the ANTE area (ISO class 8)		
Performed handwashing and garbing (see Procedures 4.1 and 4.2).		
Performed the following in Buffer area (ISO class 7). Ensured the LAFW had been cleaned and turned on for at least 30 minutes		
Staged the medication, bag, label, and supplies needed on a (work surface) stainless-steel cart beside the LAFW.		
Placed items in the LAFW one a time, maintaining correct spacing of at least 6 inches, spraying each item with sterile IPA 70% alcohol, and removing outer packaging at the edge of the hood.		
Attached the needle and syringe without touching the critical site areas (needle hub or syringe tip) and laid to the side.		
Removed the plastic cap from the vial and wiped the top (critical site) with an alcohol swab.		
Wiped the port of the IV container.		
Withdrew the appropriate contents from the vial using the see saw method.		
Replaced needle and removed air bubbles.		
Injected the medication into the IV bag and affixed a seal on the port of the bag.		
Inspected the bag for leaks, cloudiness, or particulate matter.		
Removed from PEC and label.		
Removed needle from syringe used and drew back the amount injected into the container.		
Rechecked calculations.		
Allowed the Pharmacist to check with the syringe, medication, and labeled bag staged.		
	Total:	Total:

Evaluator Name _____ **Date** _____
Grade _____

PROCEDURE 10.2: STEPS FOR RECONSTITUTING A POWDER VIAL AND TRANSFERRING LIQUID CONTENTS TO AN IV CONTAINER

Student Name: _____   Date: _____

KEY	3: Proficient (can complete task in a timely manner without assistance)
	2: Partially Proficient (can complete most of task but needs some assistance)
	1: Limited (can do the task but requires close assistance and supervision)
	0: Insufficient (cannot perform the task, remediation required)

Task	Student (Self-Evaluation)	Evaluator
Completed any calculations needed and prepared label before entering the ISO class 8 (ante-area).		
Performed in the ANTE area (ISO class 8)		
Performed handwashing and garbing (see Procedures 4.1 and 4.2).		
Performed the following in Buffer area (ISO class 7). Ensured the LAFW had been cleaned and turned on for at least 30 minutes		
Staged the medication, bag, label, and supplies needed on a (work surface) stainless-steel cart beside the LAFW.		
Placed items in the LAFW one a time, maintaining correct spacing of at least 6 inches, spraying each item with sterile IPA 70% alcohol, and removing outer packaging at the edge of the hood.		
Attached the needle and syringe without touching the critical site areas (needle hub or syringe tip) and laid to the side.		
Removed the plastic cap from the vials (diluent and powder vial) and wiped the tops (critical site) with an alcohol swab.		
Wiped the port of the IV container.		
Withdrew the appropriate contents from the diluent vial using the seesaw method.		
Replaced needle and removed air bubbles.		
Injected the powder vial with the diluent withdrawn to reconstitute, allowing pressure to escape. Did not fight any push-back from the syringe, as liquid was added.		
Swirled the powder vial to mix contents well. Withdrew the calculated amount.		
Injected calculated amount into the container.		
Placed a foil seal over the port and inspected the bag for leaks, cloudiness, or particulate matter.		
Removed from PEC and labeled.		
Removed needle from syringe used and drew back the amount injected into the container.		
Rechecked calculations.		
Allowed the Pharmacist to check with the syringe, medication, and labeled bag staged.		
	Total:	Total:

Evaluator Name _____   Date _____

Grade _____

PROCEDURE 10.3: STEPS FOR WITHDRAWING CONTENTS FROM AN AMPULE AND ADDING CONTENTS TO AN IV CONTAINER

Student Name: _____   Date: _____

KEY	3: Proficient (can complete task in a timely manner without assistance)
	2: Partially Proficient (can complete most of task but needs some assistance)
	1: Limited (can do the task but requires close assistance and supervision)
	0: Insufficient (cannot perform the task, remediation required)

Task	Student (Self-Evaluation)	Evaluator
Completed any calculations needed and prepared label before entering the ISO class 8 (ante-area).		
Performed in the ANTE area (ISO class 8)		
Performed hand washing and garbing (see Procedures 4.1 and 4.2).		
Performed the following in Buffer area (ISO class 7). Ensured the LAFW had been cleaned and turned on for at least 30 minutes		
Staged the medication, bag, label, and supplies needed on a (work surface) stainless-steel cart beside the LAFW.		
Placed items in the LAFW one a time, maintaining correct spacing of at least 6 inches, spraying each item with sterile IPA 70% alcohol, and removing outer packaging at the edge of the hood.		
Attached the filter needle or straw and syringe without touching the critical site areas (needle hub or syringe tip) and laid to the side.		
Cleaned the ampule with an alcohol swab and broke it on the score line. Placed the glass top in the sharps container immediately.		
Withdrew the appropriate contents from the ampule. No need to use seesaw method.		
Replaced filter needle or straw with a regular needle and removed air bubbles.		
Injected the medication into the IV bag and affixed a seal on the port of the bag.		
Inspected the bag for leaks, cloudiness, or particulate matter.		
Removed from PEC and labeled.		
Removed needle from syringe used and drew back the amount injected into the container.		
Rechecked calculations.		
Allowed the Pharmacist to check with the syringe, medication, and labeled bag staged.		
	Total:	Total:

Evaluator Name _____ **Date** _____

Grade _____

PROCEDURE 12.1: PREPARING TPN

Student Name: _____   Date: _____

KEY	3: Proficient (can complete task in a timely manner without assistance)		
	2: Partially Proficient (can complete most of task but needs some assistance)		
	1: Limited (can do the task but requires close assistance and supervision)		
	0: Insufficient (cannot perform the task, remediation required)		
Task	**Student (Self-Evaluation)**		**Evaluator**
Completed any calculations needed and prepared label before entering the ISO class 8 (ante-area).			
Performed in the ANTE area (ISO class 8)			
Performed handwashing and garbing (see Procedures 4.1 and 4.2).			
Performed the following in Buffer area (ISO class 7). Ensured the LAFW had been cleaned and turned on for at least 30 minutes			
Staged the bases and additives, TPN bag, label, and supplies needed on a (work surface) stainless-steel cart beside the LAFW.			
Marked each base with amount needed, and placed base items (Amino acid, Dextrose, and Lipids) and TPN empty container with leads in the LAFW one a time, hanging the bags and maintaining correct spacing of at least 6 inches. Sprayed each port with sterile IPA 70% alcohol, after removing outer packaging at the edge of the hood.			
Attached the leads to each one of the base solutions, without touching the critical site area, port tops, and hang up.			
Undid the roller clamp on the lead to each base hanging up. Stopped by rolling the clamp down when the marked line was reached.			
Laid the base aside for checking by Pharmacist. Once completed, discarded the remaining bags of base fluid and put the TPN base to the side.			
Added each additive vial to the LAFW by spraying or wiping critical sites.			
Added a syringe and needle beside each additive to the amount required to be withdrawn. Allowed this to be checked before proceeding.			
Withdrew each amount from each vial needed and kept the syringe and medication vials separated by laying the syringe/needle with medication in it next to its perspective vial.			
Once verified, added each additive to the port of the base bag. Did not discard syringes, just needles at this point. Affixed a seal to any multiple-dose vials and the port of the finished TPN bag.			
Inspected the bag for leaks, cloudiness, or particulate matter.			
Rechecked calculations.			
Allowed the Pharmacist to check with the syringes, medication, and labeled bag staged.			
	Total:		**Total:**

Evaluator Name_____ **Date** _____

Grade_____

PROCEDURE 13.1: CLEANING A BIOLOGICAL SAFETY CABINET

Student Name: _____   Date: _____

KEY	3: Proficient (can complete task in a timely manner without assistance)
	2: Partially Proficient (can complete most of task but needs some assistance)
	1: Limited (can do the task but requires close assistance and supervision)
	0: Insufficient (cannot perform the task, remediation required)

Task	Student (Self-Evaluation)	Evaluator
Performed hazardous garbing and handwashing in the anteroom before entering the buffer area (see Procedures 4.1 and 4.2).		
Placed the chemo-waste container inside the BSC on the mat.		
Sprayed cleaning agent or alcohol on the front lip (tray area near edge of BSC) and wiped with cloth. Discarded in the container inside the BSC.		
Next, cleaned the IV pole and sides. Wiped with overlapping strokes, from top to bottom, downward toward the work surface. Discarded in the container inside the BSC when finished.		
Cleaned the work surface with from back to front, around the mat, moving outward with overlapping strokes.		
Cleaned the inner view screen (glass front) of the BSC. Discarded the cloth in waste container.		
Pinched the mat and placed in the waste container.		
Removed the outer pair of gloves and discarded them in the waste container.		
Cleaned the outside of the view screen. Discarded cloth in the waste container.		
Removed the container and placed it in the outer trash container marked Hazardous.		
Degowned and placed all PPE in the same trash container.		
	Total:	Total:

Evaluator Name _____ **Date** _____
Grade _____

PROCEDURE 14.1: PREPARING A HAZARDOUS (CHEMOTHERAPY) PREPARATION

Student Name: _____ Date: _____

KEY	3: Proficient (can complete task in a timely manner without assistance)
	2: Partially Proficient (can complete most of task but needs some assistance)
	1: Limited (can do the task but requires close assistance and supervision)
	0: Insufficient (cannot perform the task, remediation required)

Task	Student (Self-Evaluation)	Evaluator
Completed any calculations needed and prepared label before entering the ISO class 8 (ante-area).		
Performed in the ANTE area (ISO class 8)		
Performed handwashing and garbing (see Procedures 4.1 and 4.2).		
Performed the following in Buffer area (ISO class 7) Ensured the BSC had been cleaned and turned on.		
Staged the medication, bag, label, and supplies needed on a (work surface) stainless-steel cart beside the LAFW.		
Laid out the mat in the BSC and items needed for priming the bag.		
Primed the IV bag with clean fluid by attaching the spike end of the tubing to the bag and allowing fluid to reach the end of the tubing and then clamping the line off.		
Placed primed bag with its tubing to the side and added other items in the BSC one a time, maintaining correct spacing of at least 6 inches, spraying each item with sterile IPA 70% alcohol, and removing outer packaging at the edge of the hood.		
Before spiking the vial of HD medication, discarded all trash possible (before exposure to the chemo drug) in regular trash or sharps, if needed.		
Attached the CTSD to the medication vial without touching the critical site areas (spike end).		
Withdrew the contents using just a syringe attached via Luer lock to the CSTD. No need to use the seesaw method or remove air bubbles, as the CSTD is a vented, closed-transfer system.		
Added a needle to the filled syringe and injected the medication into the IV bag and affixed a seal on the port of the bag.		
Inspected the bag for leaks, cloudiness, or particulate matter. Placed the labeled bag in a labeled or marked as HAZARDOUS/CHEMO delivery bag. Wiped the bag with an alcohol wipe.		
Discarded items not needed except vial, mat, and prepared compound. Laid out syringe, drew back to amount added and drug inside the BSC and asked for a Pharmacist check.		
Once the bag was checked, it was removed. While still sitting at the BSC, discarded trash and medication in the appropriate containers (yellow sharps for the syringe, needle, medication) and yellow container for the mat, only the OUTER pair of gloves, supplies, and any other items left in BSC.		
Removed PPE (HD), including the INNER (second) set of gloves outside of BSC and placed in larger hazardous waste container in the ISO class 7 area.		
Washed hands again in the ante-area before leaving the sterile compounding area.		
	Total:	Total:

Evaluator Name _____ Date _____

Grade _____

Practice Exercises

Verifying the CSP label with the Physician's order is a critical part of the compounding technician's job. Each exercise in this appendix includes questions that are followed by items needed to answer the questions, such as orders and labels. See your instructor for the correct answers.

EXERCISE 1

1. What class of medication is vancomycin?
2. What is the diagnosis for this patient?
3. What is the rate of infusion?
4. What is the solution?
5. What is the additive?
6. Is this an SVP or an LVP?

Heartland Memorial Hospital

Date _____ 7/30/19 _____   Physician: Stephen Fineman
Pt. Name: Ahmer, Saleem   Room: CCU-01
Pt. ID#: 1223323   Rx#: 186599
Vancomycin 500 mg
Dextrose 5% 250 mL
Infuse at 125 mL/h
Once daily for 14 days
BUD ___ 8.13.19 ____
Tech _____ KDD _____
RPh _____ KW _____
Refrigerate [x] Yes [ ] No
Special Instructions: _____

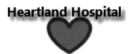

Heartland Hospital

Name	**Ahmer, Saleem**
Birthdate	**3.7.76**
Room	**CCU-01**
ID#	**1223323**
Diagnosis	**COPD, INF UNK**
Allergies	**NKDA**
Diet	**AS TOL WT 125lbs HT 6'2"**

Attending PHYSICIAN   Stephen Fineman

Orders Should be BLOCK PRINTED for Clarity

The following abbreviations are disallowed: u (unit), MS and MSO4 (morphine), MgSO4 (magnesium sulfate), QD (daily), QOD (every other day), IU (International Units)

	Other Orders		Medication Orders
Date/Time:	**ASA 81mg QD**	Date/Time:	**Vancomycin 500mg/D5W 250L @ 125ml/hr QD x 14 days**
	Lasix 40 mg QD		**Phenergan 25mg IVP Q 4-6 HRS PRN N&V**
	Tylenol #3 1 to 2 Tabs PRN q 6 hrs		
	MOM 30cc TID		

Safe Prescribing Practices: Verify all orders by reading the order back to the prescriber. Do not use zeros following a decimal point. Use a zero
before a decimal point. Order IV medications by dose per time (e.g., mg/hr). Order levothyroxine in "mcg" (not "mg") doses.

Order Set Faxed to Pharmacy by:
‒   **(name / time)**   **Unit:**

☐

Form ID: XXX   Last Revision   Date: 07.23.19

EXERCISE 2

Note: To answer these questions, you may need to reference the physician's order for this patient in Exercise 1.
1. What class of medication is Phenergan?
2. If using a stock ampule of Phenergan with a concentration of 25 mg/mL, what would be the procedure to prepare the first dose?
3. How many milliliters will be required for this dose?
4. What is the strength of the medication ordered?
5. What additional documentation is required for this CSP?

Heartland Memorial Hospital

Date _____today_____   Physician: Stephen Fineman
Pt. Name: Ahmer, Saleem   Room: CCU-01
Pt. ID#: 1223323   Rx#: 186599
VPhenergan 50 mg
Intramuscular
Give every 4–6 hours as needed for nausea and vomiting
BUD _____
Tech ____KDD____
RPh ____KW____
Refrigerate ☐ Yes ☐ No
Special Instructions: _____

EXERCISE 3

1. What class of medication is Rocephin?
2. If using a stock powder vial of Rocephin with a concentration of 250 mg/mL, what would be the procedure to dilute the powder contents?
3. How many milliliters will be required for this dose?
4. Is this an SVP or an LVP?
5. Where would you find the "recipe" or instructions for preparing this CSP?
6. What are this patient's diagnoses?
7. What does the abbreviation CXR stand for?
8. What does the abbreviation LTC stand for?
9. What does the abbreviation CBC stand for?
10. What does the abbreviation TID stand for?

Heartland Memorial Hospital

Date _____   Physician: Adams, John
Pt. Name: Harper, Glenn   Room: 224
Pt. ID#: 124463   Rx#: 186570
Rocephin 500 mg IVPB
sodium chloride 0.9% 100 mL
Rate: Give over 30 minutes
BUD _____
Tech ____KDD____
RPh ____KW____
Refrigerate ☒ Yes ☐ No
Special Instructions: _____

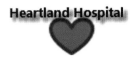

Heartland Hospital

Name	**Harper, Glenn**
Birthdate	**12.1.53**
Room	
ID#	**124463**
Diagnosis	**MRSA, OA**
Allergies	**NKDA**
Diet	**REG WT 221lbs HT 6′2″**

Attending PHYSICIAN   Adams, John

Orders Should be BLOCK PRINTED for Clarity

The following abbreviations are disallowed: u (unit), MS and MSO4 (morphine), MgSO4 (magnesium sulfate), QD (daily), QOD (every other day), IU (International Units)

Other Orders		Medication Orders	
Date/Time:	**Motrin 600mg TID**	Date/Time:	**Rocephin 500mg/NS 100ml IVPB x 3 days**
	CXR in AM		**LR 1L with magnesium sulfate 25mEq @75ml/hr**
	CBC and BUN in AM		
	Schedule transfer for LTC in AM		

Safe Prescribing Practices: Verify all orders by reading the order back to the prescriber. Do not use zeros following a decimal point. Use a zero before a decimal point. Order IV medications by dose per time (e.g., mg/hr). Order levothyroxine in "mcg" (not "mg") doses.

Order Set Faxed to Pharmacy by:
(name / time)   **Unit:**

☐

EXERCISE 4

Note: To answer these questions, you may need to reference the physician's order for this patient in Exercise 3.
1. What class of medication is magnesium sulfate?
2. If using a stock vial of magnesium sulfate with a concentration of 4 mEq/mL, how many milliliters will be required for this dose?
4. What size syringe would be most appropriate for withdrawing the contents from the vial of magnesium sulfate?
5. Is this an SVP or an LVP?

Heartland Memorial Hospital

Date _____   Physician: Adams, John
Pt. Name: Harper, Glenn   Room: 224
Pt. ID#: 124463   Rx#: 186655
Magnesium sulfate 25 mEq
Lactated Ringers 1000 mL
Rate: 75 mL/h
BUD _____
Tech _____KDD_____
RPh _____KW_____
Refrigerate ☒ Yes ☐ No
Special Instructions: _____

EXERCISE 5

1. What class of medication is clindamycin?
2. If using a stock vial of clindamycin with a concentration of 300 mg/mL, how many milliliters will be required for this dose?
4. What size syringe would be most appropriate for withdrawing the contents from the vial of magnesium sulfate?
5. What is the flow rate for this medication?

Heartland Memorial Hospital

Date _____   Physician: Edwards, Linda
Pt. Name: Hernandez, Elza   Room: Med Surg
Pt. ID#: 144331   Rx#: 186657
Clindamycin 600 mg IVPB
D5W 100 mL
Give over 30 minutes
Every 12 hours
BUD _____
Tech _____KDD_____
RPh _____KW_____
Refrigerate ☒ Yes ☐ No
Special Instructions: _____

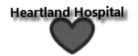

Heartland Hospital

Name	**Hernandez, Elsa**
Birthdate	**8.5.32**
Room	**Med Surg**
ID#	**144331**
Diagnosis	**MVA, broken rt arm**
Allergies	**NKDA**
Diet	**NPO × 24 hrs WT 117lbs HT 5′4″**

Attending PHYSICIAN   Edwards, Linda

Orders Should be BLOCK PRINTED for Clarity

The following abbreviations are disallowed: u (unit), MS and MSO4 (morphine), MgSO4 (magnesium sulfate),
QD (daily), QOD (every other day), IU (International Units)

	Other Orders		Medication Orders
Date/Time:	Schedule consultation with rehab for AM	Date/Time:	Clindamycin 600mg/D5W 100mls IVPB x 7 days
	Vital signs Q2 hrs		D5W 1L w/KCL 25mEq q12 hrs
	Maalox 30ml PO q4hours prn GI complaints		
	Continue routine LTC meds per Dr. Rodriguez orders		

Safe Prescribing Practices: Verify all orders by reading the order back to the prescriber. Do not use zeros following a decimal point. Use a zero
before a decimal point. Order IV medications by dose per time (e.g., mg/hr). Order levothyroxine in "mcg" (not "mg") doses.

Order Set Faxed to Pharmacy by:
– **(name / time)**   **Unit:** _____

☐

Form ID: XXX   Last Revision   Date: 07.23.19

EXERCISE 6

Note: To answer these questions, you may need to reference the physician's order for this patient in Exercise 5.
1. What is the medication to be given on this label?
2. What is the solution the medication is to be mixed in?
3. If using a stock vial of potassium chloride with a concentration of 15 mEq/mL, how many milliliters will be required for this dose?
4. What size syringe would be most appropriate for withdrawing the contents from the vial of magnesium sulfate?
5. If the maximum recommended dose for KCL is 10 mEq/day, is this order appropriate?

Heartland Memorial Hospital

Date _____   Physician: Edwards, Linda
Pt. Name: Hernandez, Elza   Room: Med Surg
Pt. ID#: 144331   Rx#: 186657
Potassium Chloride 25 mEq
Dextrose 1000 mL
Infuse over 12 hours
BUD _____
Tech _____KDD_____
RPh _____KW_____
Refrigerate ☒ Yes ☐ No
Special Instructions: warm to room temperature before administration

---

EXERCISE 7

Preparing a CSP must include completing a CR (compounding record) along with the label. Verifying that the information between the two documents are correct is a critical part of the compounding technician's job and the Pharmacist's verification process.

Check to make sure the CR record matches the CSP label.

Once this is verified, use the CSP label and the CR provided to answer the following questions:
1. What class of medication is Zosyn?
2. What is the manufacturer's lot number for the medication?
3. What is the prescription number assigned?
4. What is the MFR number used?
5. What is the BUD assigned to the medication prepared on the CSP?

Heartland Memorial Hospital

Date ____7/30/19____   Physician: Davis, Karen
Pt. Name: Taynor, Terrance   Room: 332-A
Pt. ID#: 1344563   Rx#: 17740
Zosyn 3.375 g IVPB
NS 100 mL
Infuse over 30 minutes
Every 6 hours
BUD ____8.6.19____
Tech _____KDD_____
RPh _____KW_____
Refrigerate ☒ Yes ☐ No
Special Instructions: Do not freeze

Compounding Record   Drug ___Zosyn 3.375 g/NS 100 mL___   Date _7/30/19_

Prescription Number or ID Assigned	Master FR Record # Used	Name and Strength of Compound	Quantity	Actual Net Measurements	Expiration Date	MFG Lot Number	MFG Expiration Date	BUD Assigned	Date Packaged	Tech Initials	RPh Initials
17740	1330	Zosyn 3.375	4	3.375 g/NS 100	2/2022	BL4001	2/2022	8/6/19	7/30/19	KD	KW

Attach a prescription/patient label if applicable.
ID, Identification; *FR*, formula record; *MFG*, manufacturer; *BUD*, beyond use date; *RPh*, registered pharmacist.

EXERCISE 8

1. What class of medication is Zithromax?
2. What is the diagnosis for this patient?
3. What is the rate of infusion?
4. What is the solution?
5. What is the additive?
6. What is the BUD assigned to this compounded CSP?

Heartland Memorial Hospital

Date _____ 7/30/19 _____   Physician: Stephen Fineman
Pt. Name: Tate, Lucia   Room: 433
Pt. ID#: 1244556   Rx#: 186512
Zithromax 500 mg
NS 250 mL
125 mL/h
Every 6 hours
BUD _____ 8.13.19 _____
Tech _____ KDD _____
RPh _____ KW _____
Refrigerate [X] Yes [ ] No
Special Instructions: _____

Heartland Hospital

Name	**Tate, Lucia**
Birthdate	**3.3.41**
Room	**122**
ID#	**1223323**
Diagnosis	**CHF, diabetes, DVT**
Allergies	**PCN**
Diet	**1500cal_ADA** **WT 303lbs** **HT 5'6"**

Attending PHYSICIAN __Epps, Breanna__

Orders Should be BLOCK PRINTED for Clarity

The following abbreviations are disallowed: u (unit), MS and MSO4 (morphine), MgSO4 (magnesium sulfate), QD (daily), QOD (every other day), IU (International Units)

	Other Orders		Medication Orders
Date/Time:	**Condition: stable**	Date/Time:	**Heparin drip 18units/kg/hr**
	Attending Physician to review home meds in AM		**Morphine 2mg q4h prn anxiety**
	Reg Insulin sliding scale (AC and HS)		**Schedule IV to start 0600 Zithromax (azithromycin) 500mg/NS250ml @125ml/hr q24 hrs**
	Plavix 75mg PO daily		
	Lopressor 5mg PO BID		
	Nystatin 100.ooo units/ml susp Swish and swallow tid		

Safe Prescribing Practices: Verify all orders by reading the order back to the prescriber. Do not use zeros following a decimal point. Use a zero
before a decimal point. Order IV medications by dose per time (e.g., mg/hr). Order levothyroxine in "mcg" (not "mg") doses.

Order Set Faxed to Pharmacy by:
– (name / time)   Unit: _____

☐

EXERCISE 9

Note: To answer these questions, you may need to reference the physician's order for this patient in Exercise 8.
1. How many kilograms does the patient weigh, based on the order provided?
2. If the order is 18 mg for every kilogram the patient weighs per hour, what amount of heparin has been ordered to infuse in ONE hour?
3. Is the CSP being prepared an appropriate compounded bag for the order (18 mg/kg per day)?
4. If you are using a stock bottle of heparin with a concentration of 10,000 units/mL, how many milliliters would be needed for this CSP?
5. What special instructions are included, and why?

Heartland Memorial Hospital

Date _____ 7/30/19 _____ Physician: Stephen Fineman
Pt. Name: Tate, Lucia Room: 433
Pt. ID#: 1244556 Rx#: 186512
Heparin 59,000 units
Dextrose 5% 500 mL
Infuse continuous
BUD _____
Tech _____ KDD _____
RPh _____ KW _____
Refrigerate ☒ Yes ☐ No
Special Instructions: Precaution: "HIGH ALERT" Drug

EXERCISE 10

Note: To answer these questions, you may need to reference the physician's order for this patient in Exercise 8.
1. How will this CSP be packaged?
2. According to the physician's order, how often can the patient receive this medication?
3. What size syringe would be needed for the 2-mg dose?
4. What drug class is morphine?

Heartland Memorial Hospital

Date _____ 7/30/19 _____ Physician: Stephen Fineman
Pt. Name: Tate, Lucia Room: 433
Pt. ID#: 1244556 Rx#: 186513
Morphine 2 mg IVP
BUD _____
Tech _____ KDD _____
RPh _____ KW _____
Refrigerate ☒ Yes ☐ No
Special Instructions: _____

EXERCISE 11

1. What does the abbreviation TPN stand for?
2. When should a new bag of TPN be hung?
3. What is the rate of infusion?
4. What components make the BASE (macronutrients) of the TPN?
5. What are the additives (micronutrients) of the TPN?
6. What is the BUD assigned to this compounded CSP?
7. What type of IV line does this patient have?
8. What is the total volume of the TPN?
9. What is the rate for the TPN ordered?
10. Verify the amount of sodium chloride on the CSP against the order of 40 mEq/L. Check the calculations.
11. Verify the amount of potassium chloride on the CSP against the order of 30 mEq/L. Check the calculations.
12. Verify the amount of Liposyn on the CSP label against the order. Is this correct?
13. If the TPN is interrupted, what is the procedure?
14. For the following, match the descriptions to the component. The components may be used more than once.

DESCRIPTION	COMPONENT
Liposyn: _____	fat
Dextrose: _____	protein
Aminosyn: _____	electrolyte
Sodium chloride: _____	carbohydrate
Potassium chloride: _____	

Heartland Memorial Hospital

Date _____ 7/30/19 _____ Physician: Stephen Fineman
Pt. Name: Campbell, Erma Room: 116
Pt. ID#: 1244599 Rx#: 1865787
TPN (central line)
Aminosyn II 10% 500 mL
Dextrose 70% 400 mL
Liposyn II 10% 100 mL
Sodium Chloride 4 mEq/mL 10 mL
Potassium chloride 2 mEq/mL 15 mL
Infuse at 83 mL/h
BUD _____
Tech _____ KDD _____
RPh _____ KW _____
Refrigerate ☒ Yes ☐ No
Special Instructions: Warm to room temp before administering.
Change bags q 24 hr. Use tubing with in-line filter

Patient Name   Campbell, Erma   HT: 5/5   cm   WT: 64   kg

Adult Total Parenteral Nutrition Order Form TPN (Central Line Only)

Date **7.31.19**	Is central line access in place? [ ]No [x] Yes
Time **0725**	Type: **Groshong** _____ Date placed: 7.30.19 _____

Please note: Prescribers must make selections in section 1-6 of form

1. Base Formula (Check one)	2. Infusion Schedule
[ ] Standard Base: Dextrose 20% 3.4kcal/gm) and Amino acids 10% (50gm/500ml) QS with SWFI for final volume as ordered	Rate:___83_____ mL/hour_____
[x] Individual base: Dextrose_____% and AA____%:	**Cycling Schedule (home TPN only)**
(final concentration)	Cycle _____ mL fluid over _____ hours
OR	
Dextrose___70___%___400___mL	Begin at _____
AA _____10___%___500___mL	

3. Standard Electrolytes/Additives	OR Specify Individualized Electrolytes/Additives	
Check here [ ]	Specify amount of electrolyte	Check all the apply
NaCl 40 mEq / L	NaCl _____4 0____ mEq / L	[ ] Adult MVI 10 mLs / day
NaAc 20 mEq / L	NaAc _____ mEq / L	[ ] MTE – 5 3 mLs / day
KCl 20 mEq / L	NaPhos _____ mEq / L	[ ] Regular Human Insulin
Kphos 22 mEq / L	KCl _____30_____ mEq / L	_____ units / Liter
CaGlu 4.7 mEq / L	KAc _____ mEq / L	[ ] Vitamin C 500 mg / day
MagSO4 8 mEq / L	Kphos _____ mEq / L	[ ] H 2 antagonist _____ mg / day
Adult MVI 10 mLs / day	CaGlu _____ mEq / L	drug _____
MTE-5 3 mLs / day	Mag SO4 _____ mEq / L	[ ] Other additives
DO NOT USE IN RENAL DYSFUNCTION!	Maximum Phosphate (Na phos _____	
	40 mEq / L or K phos 44 mEq / L _____	
	and maximum clearance 10 mEq / L	

4. Lipids (Check one)	5. Blood Glucose monitoring orders
	Blood glucose monitoring every __24_ hours with
[ ] 20% (2kcal/ mL) 500ml daily	sliding scale regular human insulin.
[ ] 20% (2kcal/ml) 500ml every other day	Route **SQ**
[ ] 10% (1.1kcal/ml) 500ml daily	**Sliding Scale** (Check one)
[ ] 10% (1.1kCal/ml) every other day	[x] Sliding scale per T and T protocol
_____	[ ] Individualized sliding scale (write below)
[x] Liposyn 10% 100ml daily	_____
_____	

Additional Orders (All patients)	6. Routine Laboratory Orders (Check all that apply)
1. Consult Nutrition Support Team.	[ ] BMP, Mg, Phos every AM X 3 days then every Monday & Thursday
2. CMP, Mg, Phos, triglyceride, prealbumin in the AM.	[ ] Prealbumin every Monday
3. Weigh patient daily.	[ ] Metabolic study (if required by RT only)
4. Strict I/O & document in chart.	[ ] 24 hour UUN and creatinine clearance
6. If TPN interrupted for any reason, hang D10W @ current TPN rate.	

Physician Signature   *Walter Gantry*

Glossary

absorption: Movement of a drug into the circulatory system

ACPH: Air changes per hour

Active Pharmaceutical ingredient (API): Any substance or mixture of substances used in the compounding process

additives: Drugs commonly added to an intravenous (IV) solution

admixture: The preparation of an IV medication that requires a mixture of medications

adverse effects: Drug effects that are unexpected and unwanted and are usually reported in only a few patients

ALARA: Represents "as low as (is) reasonably achievable". The effort of maintaining exposures to ionizing radiation as low as possible.

anorexia: Extreme loss of appetite

Antagonistic effect: The action of one drug preventing the action of another drug or preventing the action of a messenger on a receptor site in the body

ante area: International Organization for Standardization (ISO) Class 8 area where personal hand hygiene, garbing, and staging of components, order entry, labeling, and high particulate activities are performed before entering the buffer area

antifungal: Medication that destroys or inhibits the growth of fungi

antineoplastic agent: An agent that prevents the development or growth of malignant cells

antiviral: Medication used to treat viral infections

asepsis: Condition free from germs, infection, or any form of life

Batch: more than one unit of a product compounded in a single process

beyond use date (BUD): The date or time when a compounded sterile preparation (CSP) should no longer be stored or transported; it begins at the time of the preparation of the compound

biological safety cabinet (BSC): Special hood where air flows downward through a high-efficiency particulate air (HEPA) filter; used for chemotherapy preparation

bolus: Also known as *direct injection* or *intravenous push (IV push; IVP)*; small amount of medication injected into a port usually in an existing IV line (see also, IV push)

buffer area: International Organization for Standardization (ISO) Class 5 area where laminar airflow workbench (LAFW) or other primary engineering controls (PECs) are physically located and aseptic manipulations occur (see also, cleanroom)

C-PEC: Controlled primary engineering control, such as the class II BSC (biological safety cabinet)

C-SEC containment secondary engineering control: Room with fixed walls with airflow and pressure requirements where the C-PEC is placed

CACI, CAI: Compounding aseptic isolator or compounding aseptic containment isolator

Contamination: Introduction of pathogens or microbes into or on normally clean or sterile objects, surfaces, or spaces

Category 1 CSP: This is a CSP which has been assigned a BUD of 12 hours or less at room temperature or 24 hours or less refrigerated

Category 2 CSP: This is a CSP which has been assigned a BUD of greater than 12 hours at room temperature or greater than 24 hours refrigerated.

Centers for Disease Control and Prevention (CDC): United States Federal Agency under the Department of Health and Human Services concerned with control and prevention of diseases

Certificate of Analysis (COA): A report provided by manufacturer or supplier to indicate specifications and results of testing for the item.

chemotherapy: Treatment of disease with chemicals that destroy disease-causing cells

chronic anemia: Condition in which there is an extreme loss of red blood cells

clarity: Clear and free of visible particulate matter

cleanroom: Term sometimes used for *buffer area*

closed system: Used to describe a vial, which is a sealed container of solution where air is not allowed to move freely in and out of the container

compatibility: Ability to combine drugs or substances without interfering with their action

compounded sterile preparation (CSP): Medications prepared using sterile technique

Compounding record (CR): A document created by the compounder to describe the compounding process for a specific CSP

concentration: Amount of medication per amount of fluid

contamination: Introduction of pathogens or microbes into or on normally clean or sterile objects, surfaces, or spaces

coring: Breaking off small pieces of the rubber closure when withdrawing contents of a vial and allowing them to enter the solution or IV fluid

critical area: International Organization for Standardization (ISO) Class 5 environment where aseptic manipulations take place

critical site: Any location that includes fluid pathway surfaces, such as vial tops, bag ports, injection sites, or necks of ampules; areas to never touch, such as needle tips, tops of vials, and syringe plunger, to avoid cross-contamination during aseptic manipulations

CSPT (Certified Sterile Processing Technician): An advanced certification in sterile compounding offered by Pharmacy Technician Certification Board (PTCB)

Current Procedural Technology (CPT) codes: A set of codes used to identify surgical, diagnostic, and medical procedures used for billing services

cytotoxic agents: Antineoplastic agents that kill dividing cells

Deactivation: Changing an HD to a less hazardous substance on surfaces by use of heat, sterilization, light

Decontamination: Using chemicals to remove or deactivate or neutralize an HD substance

diluent: Solution used to dilute a powder form of an injectable medication

direct compounding area (DCA): Area within the International Organization for Standardization (ISO) Class 5 primary engineering control (PEC) where manipulations are performed (such as the laminar flow workbench [LAFW] and biological safety cabinet [BSC])

disaster: An emergency that requires outside assistance

Disaster Medical Assistance Team (DMAT): Team that sets up temporary treatment medical sites to treat burns and mental health emergencies.

Disaster Mortuary Operations Response Teams (DMORT): Made up of mortuary directors, pathologists, dental assistants, medical examiners, medical record technicians, and mental health staff, who are responsible for identification of victims and support family members in the grieving process in a disaster or emergency event.

disinfectant: Chemical agent used to destroy bacteria, fungi, and viruses

distribution: Movement of a drug through the body into tissues, membranes, and then organs

docking: Procedure used to attach bag and vial used with proprietary bag and vial systems

DUR/DUE (drug use review, drug use evaluation): A review of the drugs within an organization to determine where improvements in the process can occur

dynamic operation condition: Existing conditions in the segregated radiopharmaceuticals compounding processing area (SRPA) or classified area where compounding activity is taking place.

electrolytes: Dissolved mineral salts, usually found in IV fluids, such as total parenteral nutrition (TPN) or lactated Ringer's solution

electronic health record (EHR): Computer-based record that records patients information to include demographic information and overall medical and medication information

emergency: An event which affects public safety, health, or welfare

epidural injection: Injection into the epidural space

excretion: Removal of a drug from the body

FEMA: The Federal Emergency Management System

first air: Direct flow of air exiting the high-efficiency particulate air (HEPA) filter inside the direct compounding area (DCA), which should never be interrupted and is essentially particle-free

flow rate: Amount of medication to be infused over a specific period of time

garbing: donning (putting on) protective personal equipment in a specific method during aseptic preparation

gauge (ga): Size of the needle shaft (thickness); the finer the needle, the higher the gauge number

Hazardous Drugs (HD): antineoplastic and other drugs considered hazardous as identified by the NIOSH organization.

HCPCS: Health Care Financing Administration (HCFA) Common Procedures Coding System Uniform language using codes to describe procedures, services, and diagnoses for billing purposes for Medicare and third-party providers

high-efficiency particulate air (HEPA) filter: Special filter used in the LAFW designed to remove 99.97% of particles that are 0.3 microns or larger. This creates a bacteria free environment to perform aseptic technique manipulations in.

hot-cell: A device made of lead that is used to shield or contain radioactive materials

hot lab: A nonclassified radiopharmaceutical processing area without a PEC

hypermetabolic state: Condition in which an abnormal rate of metabolism occurs, such as in trauma, fever, or severe burns

hypertonic: Any solution containing a higher concentration of dissolved substances than red blood cells

hypoglycemia: Abnormally low level of glucose in the blood

hypotonic: Any solution containing a concentration of dissolved substances less than red blood cells

incompatibility: Drugs and drugs, or drugs and fluids, which cannot be put together because of the incident of unwanted or unexpected effects

infection control: Policies and procedures organizations put in place to prevent the spread of infection

International Medical Surgical Response Team (IMSRT): This team performs as an operating room in the field and manages major traumas

International Organization for Standardization (ISO): Organization whose goal is to make products and services safe, reliable, and of good quality

intraarterial injection: Injection into an artery

intracardiac (IC) injection: Injection into the cardiac muscle or the heart

intradermal (ID) route: Injection into the dermal layer of the skin

intramuscular (IM) injection: Injection into the muscle

intrathecal (IT) route: Injection into the spinal canal

intravenous (IV) injection: Injection into the vein

isolator: Type of PEC that provides isolation from outside areas while maintaining a Class 5 environment required to prepare CSPs.

isotonic: Any solution containing a concentration of dissolved substances, such as salts, that are the same as the concentration found in human red blood cells

IV push (IVP): Also known as *bolus*; small amount of medication injected into a port usually in an existing IV line (see also, bolus)

The Joint Commission: The shortened term for the Joint Commission on Accreditation of Healthcare Organizations; a nonprofit, private organization that evaluates medical facilities to ensure good patient care

kilocalorie (kcal): A unit of measurement in nutrition describing a large calorie

kit: A commercially available kit that contains everything to compound a radiopharmaceutical EXCEPT the radionuclide

kit-splitting (fractionation): Dividing a kit's vial contents to transfer aliquots into other containers

lactated ringer's solution (LR): Sterile isotonic intravenous fluid used for electrolyte or fluid replacement

laminar airflow workbench (LAFW): Also known as the *"hood."* This area is designed to be used to perform aseptic technique in because it uses a HEPA filter to create an environment that produces sterile air

large volume parenteral (LVP): Containers of sterile solution used for intravenous medications; usually 500 mL to 3000 mL in volume

macronutrients: A source of carbohydrates, protein, and fat

malignant: Tending to or threatening to produce death; a neoplasm that is cancerous as opposed to benign

malnutrition: Any disease-promoting condition that results from either inadequate or excessive exposure to nutrients

Master Formulation Record (MFR or FR): Document to record the general processes used in compounding CSPs and can be used as a basis for the CR

media fill test: A process simulating compounding processes or products to ensure that microbial growth is not present

metabolism: Changing of the chemical structure of a drug by the body

metastasize: Spreading of cancer cells to other organs or tissues

micronutrients: Additives in a total parenteral nutrition (TPN), such as vitamins, electrolytes, and trace elements

microorganism: An organism, such as a bacterium, virus, or protozoan, of microscopic size

Natural Disaster Medical System (NDMS): A department of the Federal Government, which is responsible for sending out medical teams, equipment, and supplies to the disaster areas affected

National Incident Management System (NIMS): Established by the Department of Homeland Society to manage the coordination and support of needed facilities and establish guidelines for responders to understand ways to assist before, during, and after an emergency

National Pharmacy Response Team (NPRT): An organization which provides mass immunizations and is made up of pharmacy technicians and Pharmacists

National Veterinary Response team (NVRT): Team responsible for the treatment and care of working and victim animals in affected area

NIOSH: National Institute for Occupational Safety and Health.

normal flora: Bacteria that resides on the skin's outer surface but does not cause disease

normal saline (NS): Sterile intravenous solution, also known as *sodium chloride*, used as a source of water or for fluid replacement

NPTA: National Pharmacy Technician Association

osmolarity: Number of dissolved particles in a solution per liter of solution

osmosis: Movement of a solvent (water) across a cell membrane from a lower osmolality to a higher osmolality

pancreatitis: Inflammation of the pancreas

parenteral: Any medication route other than the alimentary canal (digestive system)

parenteral route: Puncture, injection, or some method to enter the bloodstream directly

pathogen: Any disease-causing agent or microorganism

patient-centered care: Practice model of taking care of patients and their families.

PCCA: Professional Compounding Centers of America

peritonitis: Inflammation of the lining of the abdominal cavity

personal protective equipment (PPE): Equipment including shoe and hair covers, beard covers, gowns, masks, and gloves

pH: Degree of alkalinity or acidity of a solution. Acidity is usually between 0 and 6, whereas alkaline is between 8 and 14. Neutral pH is around 7.

Pharmacy Patient Care Process (PPCP): plan designed to assist patients in their overall wellness and disease management

piggyback (PB): Containers of sterile solution used to administer medications through a secondary set or intermittent infusion; usually 50 to 250 mL in volume

point-of-care (POC) testing: immediate tests performed in pharmacies

PPE: Personal protective equipment to include gown, gloves, hair, foot covers, masks, and eye protection.

precipitation: Solid material or deposits that are separated from a solution often caused from reactions between drugs or drugs and certain fluids

preservative: A substance used to prevent microbial growth

primary engineering control (PEC): Controls, such as laminar airflow workbenches (LAFWs), compounding aseptic isolators, or biological safety cabinets (BSCs) located in the buffer area

process validation: A systematic testing of aseptic technique and processes used in preparing compounded sterile preparations (CSPs) to ensure sterility

pyrogen: Fever-producing substance

pyrogen-free: A substance that lacks fever-inducing toxins

quality assurance (QA): A system of procedures, activities, and management to ensure a set of predetermined standards are met

quality control (QC): The actual sampling, testing, and documentation of quality assurance results or evidence to ensure a quality product.

radioactive materials (RAM) license: Document that is issued by the US or an agreement state that allows for various activities involving radioactive materials, such as compounding, distribution, medical use, and possession.

radio assay: Measurement with a special device for amount of radioactivity present in a container

radiopharmaceutical: A finished dosage form that contains a radioactive substance. Term is interchangeable with "radioactive drug".

reconstitution: The process of adding a sterile solution to a vial of powdered medication in order to make a liquid

release testing: Testing that ensures a product meets required quality characteristics. Process to ensure a CSP meets a predetermined set of requirements or characteristics

responsible person: An individual that is held accountable for an activity

Restricted Access Barrier System (RABS): ISO class 7 or better area that uses glove ports to separate the surrounding areas to allow aseptic manipulations to take place inside

SDS (Safety Data Sheet): Product safety information sheet that records chemical, physical, and health-related hazards

secondary set: When a piggyback infusion is hung higher than the main IV solution, which allows it to run into the vein faster. An example would be an antibiotic that would be ordered to infuse in 30 minutes.

segregated compounding area (SEC): Unclassified area separated from a facility's main workflow areas where category 1 CSPs may be compounded.

segregated radiopharmaceutical processing area (SRPA): The designated area that contains the PEC when radiopharmaceutical compounding takes place

segregated unclassified compounding area (SCA): A designed space, (area or room) that contains a PEC where category 1 compounds can be prepared

SEPhT: The Society for the Education of Pharmacy Technicians

side effects: Drug effects that are predictable, widely reported, and can be found in literature

small volume parenteral (SVP): Containers of sterile solutions used for intravenous medications; usually 50 to 100 mL or less in volume

specific gravity: Weight of a substance measured in grams per milliliters as compared to an equal volume of water

spill kit: A special kit used to clean a spill for HDs

sporicidal: A concentrated agent that destroys bacterial and fungal spores when used in a specific time period

Stability: The time that a CSP retains physical and chemical properties throughout its assigned BUD

stage: Term used to describe how the final preparation is prepared for the pharmacist check of a sterile compound

standard of care: Precautions, such as hand washing, use of PPE, proper disposal of waste, and respiratory hygiene

standard operating procedures (SOPs): Set of procedures, including environmental controls, personnel training, and validation of technique, to ensure sterility of all compounded sterile preparations (CSPs)

Standard Precautions: Centers for Disease Control and Prevention (CDC) guidelines that promote hand hygiene and the use of personal protective equipment (PPE)

sterile: Free of living organisms, especially microorganisms

Strategic National Stockpile (SNS): The United States national repository for medications and supplies needed for disasters or emergencies

subcutaneous route of administration (Sub-Q): Injection just below the skin into the subcutaneous fat layer

supplemental engineering control: an additional control used along with a primary or secondary engineering control, such as a BSC (biological safety cabinet) that is used to enhance protection from an HD

synergistic effect: The action of two drugs working together to produce effects

therapeutic effect: The intended effect of a drug

tonicity: The osmolarity of a solution or the effect of the concentration of dissolved particles in the solution

total parenteral nutrition (TPN): Nutritional support in an intravenous preparation for patients who cannot take in sufficient calories because of trauma or certain diseases

transmission: Interaction between infectious agents and a susceptible host

trypticase soy agar (TSA): General microbiological growth medium that supports bacterial and fungi growth used to perform sampling

United States Pharmacopoeia (USP): Nongovernmental, not-for-profit public health organization that set standards for over-the-counter (OTC) and prescription medicines and other healthcare products in the United States; its main goal is to ensure public health.

universal precautions: Methods to prevent contamination or transference of infection, such as protective barriers

USP<797>: Chapter in the United States Pharmacopoeia (USP) concerning parenteral medications compounding and equipment endorsed by The Joint Commission and American Society of Health-System Pharmacists (ASHP)

U.S. Public Health Service (USPHS): A bank of trained healthcare professionals ready to act once needed in a disaster or emergency

vented needle: A specialty needle used when compounding with vials of powdered medications that require reconstitution

verification: Confirmation of a process, method, or system that occur under normal conditions

Index